Cancer Survival
in Developing Countries

International Agency for Research on Cancer

The International Agency for Research on Cancer (IARC) was established in 1965 by the World Health Assembly, as an independently financed organization within the framework of the World Health Organization. The headquarters of the Agency are at Lyon, France.

The Agency conducts a programme of research concentrating particularly on the epidemiology of cancer and the study of potential carcinogens in the human environment. Its field studies are supplemented by biological and chemical research carried out in the Agency's laboratories in Lyon, and, through collaborative research agreements, in national research institutions in many countries. The Agency also conducts a programme for the education and training of personnel for cancer research.

The publications of the Agency are intended to contribute to the dissemination of authoritative information on different aspects of cancer research. Information about IARC publications and how to order them, is also available via the Internet at: **http://www.iarc.fr/**

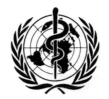

WORLD HEALTH ORGANIZATION

INTERNATIONAL AGENCY FOR RESEARCH ON CANCER

Cancer Survival in Developing Countries

Editors: R. Sankaranarayanan, R.J. Black and D.M. Parkin

IARC Scientific Publications No. 145

International Agency for Research on Cancer
Lyon, France
1998

Published by the International Agency for Research on Cancer,
150 cours Albert Thomas, 69372 Lyon cédex 08, France

Distributed by Oxford University Press, Walton Street, Oxford OX2 6DP, UK
(fax: +44 1865 267782)
and in the USA by Oxford University Press, 2001 Evans Road, Carey,
NC 27513 (fax: +1 919 677 1303). All IARC publications can also be ordered directly from IARCPress
(fax: +33 04 72 73 83 02; E-mail: press@iarc.fr).

IARC Library Cataloguing in Publication Data

Cancer survival in developing countries / editors, R. Sankaranarayanan,
R. J. Black, D. M. Parkin

(IARC scientific publications ; 145)

1. Neoplasms – epidemiology 2. Developing countries I. Sankaranarayanan,
R. II. Black, Roger J. III. Parkin, D. M. IV. Series

ISBN 92 832 2145 1 (NLM Classification: W1)
ISSN 0300–5085

Printed in France

Contents

Foreword

Survival estimates of unselected groups of cancer patients from population-based cancer registries offer an important index for the evaluation of cancer diagnosis and treatment in a community. Like the other comparative measures of cancer control, i.e., incidence of and mortality from cancer, survival data provide a means to assess the effectiveness of overall cancer services. Comparisons of such data from different regions are instrumental for the planning or improvement of national and regional cancer control strategies.

Previously, survival estimates were available only from the United States, Canada, western Europe, and some countries in central and eastern Europe, Japan and Australia. Survival data are strikingly lacking from populations in developing countries where more than half of the global cancer burden occurs (52% of global incidence in 1995). The present volume provides, for the first time, systematic, centrally analysed survival data from 10 population-based cancer registries in developing countries, and this constitutes the outcome of another fruitful international collaboration. It provides not only a context to compare the results obtained in developing countries with those from developed countries but also to investigate deficiencies in cancer registration, clinical follow-up and health services planning, organization and delivery. The differences in cancer survival experienced in populations from developed and developing countries provide important clues to public health authorities in all countries on policies and investments to achieve attainable objectives in cancer control. It is hoped that this effort will further encourage more refined studies to identify technologically and economically viable, i.e. feasible and cost-effective, policies for cancer control.

P. Kleihues
Director, IARC

Acknowledgements

The authors gratefully acknowledge the generous support of the following organizations for the studies on cancer survival reported in this book and for the publication itself:

Association for International Cancer Research (AICR), St. Andrews, UK

Finnish Cancer Society, Helsinki, Finland

Gunnar Nilsson Cancer Research Trust Fund, Stanmore, UK

International Union Against Cancer (UICC), Geneva, Switzerland

Contributors

IARC
R.J. Black[1]
S.A. Bashir
D.M. Parkin
R. Sankaranarayanan

International Agency for Research on Cancer
150 cours Albert Thomas
F-69372 Lyon cedex 08
France

Tel: 33 472 73 84 85
Fax: 33 472 73 85 75
E-mail: parkin@iarc.fr
        sankar@iarc.fr

[1]Present address
Scottish Cancer Intelligence Unit
NHS in Scotland, Information and Statistics Division
Trinity Park House
Edinburgh EH5 3SQ
United Kingdom

Tel: 44 131 551 8903
Fax: : 44 131 551 1392
E-mail: roger.black@isd.csa.scot.nhs.uk

Qidong, People's Republic of China
Jian-Guo Chen
Wen-Guang Li
Zhuo-Cai Shen
Hong-Yu Yao
Bao-Chu Zhang
Yuan-Rong Zhu

Qidong Cancer Registry
Department of Epidemiology
Qidong Liver Cancer Institute
785 Jianghai Zhong Road
Jiangsu 226200
People's Republic of China
Tel: 86 513 331 2557
Fax: 86 513 331 8224

Shanghai, People's Republic of China
Fan Jin
Yong-Bing Xiang
Yu-Tang Gao

Shanghai Cancer Registry
Shanghai Cancer Institute
2200/25 Xie Tu Road
Shanghai 200032
People's Republic of China

Tel: 86 21 640 46 550
Fax: 86 21 640 41 428
E-mail: Fanjin@fudan.ihep.ac.cn

Cuba
Leticia Fernandez Garrote
Margarita Graupera Boschmonar
Yaima Galan Alvarez,
Marta Lezcano Cicilli
Antonio Martin Garcia
Rolando Camacho Rodriguez

National Institute of Oncology and Radiobiology
Calle 29 y F Vedado
Havana
Cuba

Tel: 53 7 552577
Fax: 53 7 552587/662227
E-mail: dinor@infomed.sld.cu

Bangalore, India
A. Nandakumar
N. Anantha
T.C. Venugopal

National Cancer Registry Programme
Kidwai Memorial Institute of Oncology
Hosur Road
Bangalore 560029
India

Tel: 91 80 6632302
Fax: 91 80 6644801
E-mail: ank@blr.vsnl.net.in

Barshi, India
K. Jayant
B.M. Nene
K.A. Dinshaw[1]
A.M. Budukh
P.S. Dale

Rural Cancer Registry
Tata Memorial Centre Rural Cancer Project
Nurgis Dutt Memorial Hospital
Agalgaon Road
Barshi 413401
Solapur District
Maharashtra
India

Tel.: 91 2184 22699, 22784
Fax: 91 2184 23295, 23024

[1]Tata Memorial Hospital
Dr Ernest Borges Road
Parel
Mumbai (Bombay) 400012
India

Mumbai (Bombay), India
B.B. Yeole
D.J. Jussawalla
S.D. Sabnis
Lizzy Sunny
Bombay Cancer Registry
Indian Cancer Society
74 Jerbai Wadia Road, Parel
Mumbai (Bombay) 400 012
India
Tel: 91 22 412 1578
　　91 22 412 2351
Fax: 91 22 416 1447
E-mail: ostomy@bom3.vsnl.net.in

Chennai (Madras), India
V. Shanta
Cancer Institute (WIA)
Adyar
Chennai (Madras) 600020
India

C.K. Gajalakshmi
R. Swaminathan
Cancer Institute (WIA)
18, Sardar Patel Road
Chennai (Madras) 600036
India

Tel: 91 44 2350131
Fax: 91 44 4912085
E-mail: caninst@md2.vsnl.net.in

Rizal, Philippines
D. Esteban
C. Ngelangel
L. Lacaya
E. Robles
M. Monson

Department of Health-Rizal Cancer Registry
Rizal Medical Centre
Pasig Blvd., Pasig City
1600 Metro Manila
Philippines

Tel: 63 2 671 9740 to 9743
Fax: 63 2 671 4216
E-mail: desteban@skyinet.net

Chiang Mai, Thailand
Nimit Martin
Songphol Srisukho
Orathai Kunpradist
Maitree Suttajit

Maharaj Nakorn Chiang Mai Hospital
Faculty of Medicine
Chiang Mai University
Chiang Mai 50200
Thailand

Tel: 66 53 221122, 221788
Fax: 66 53 217144
E-mail: ssrisukh@suandok01.medicine.cmu.ac.th

Khon Kaen, Thailand
Vanchai Vatanasapt
Supannee Sriamporn
Supot Kamsa-ard
Krittika Suwanrungruang
Prasit Pengsaa
D. Jintakanon Charoensiri
Jitjaroen Chaiyakum
Montien Pesee

Cancer Unit, Faculty of Medicine
Khon Kaen University
Khon Kaen
Thailand 40002

Tel: 66 43 24133
Fax: 66 43 243088
E-mail: vanchai@kku1.kku.ac.th

Chapter 1

Introduction

D.M. Parkin

International Agency for Research on Cancer
Lyon,
France

The World Health Organization's guidelines for preparing national cancer control programmes (WHO, 1995) emphasize the different approaches to cancer control — (primary) prevention and early diagnosis and treatment. While primary prevention reduces the incidence of cancer, early detection strategies and treatment regimes aim to improve the outcome of incident cancer cases, by curing the cancer or by improving the quality and/or duration of life after diagnosis. Alongside information on incidence and mortality, survival statistics are a means of quantifying the effectiveness of these two interventions at the population level. Thus, information on survival has long been recognized as an important component in monitoring cancer control activities (WHO/IARC, 1979).

Like all other health indices, survival statistics are useful primarily as comparative measures — showing how survival differs between different populations over time, and between population subgroups (defined by, for example, age, sex, ethnicity or socioeconomic status). It is these comparisons that help us to suggest possible reasons for the variations and provide targets for improvement and a means of monitoring progress towards them.

For all these reasons, there has long been an interest in comparative statistics on survival from different countries. Because, as discussed below, it is essential to ensure that the different datasets really are comparable, the only meaningful comparisons concern outcome (survival) for the entire patient population, as obtained from population-based cancer registries, rather than statistics from single institutions. The factors governing admission to particular hospitals introduce a selection bias which invalidates any comparison of the effectiveness of therapy, which is generally the main concern of such hospital-based analyses, at least implicitly.

Of course, population-based survival cannot normally be used to assess the efficacy of specific anticancer therapies. That is the role of the randomized controlled clinical trial, in which the effect of therapy can be evaluated irrespective of other prognostic factors. Population-based cancer registries also provide very limited information on variations in survival with respect to different prognostic factors (size and spread of the tumour, presence or absence of tumour markers, etc.) compared with data derived from specialized oncology services. Rather, population-based data summarize the experience of the totality of cancer patients — including those who receive no treatment whatsoever — and so permit valid and unbiased comparisons between populations and over time. Their weakness lies in the limited information available about the reasons for the differences observed. This point is discussed further in Chapter 4 'Interpretation of population-based cancer survival data'.

Compilations of population-based survival statistics from several countries have been published over the years (Cutler *et al.*, 1964; Logan, 1978; Berrino *et al.*, 1995). All concern data from cancer registries in Europe and the USA. To date, there have been no comparative analyses of data from other areas of the world, although by 1990 about 55% of new cancer cases annually were occurring in Asia, Africa, Latin America and the Caribbean. This volume aims to fill this important gap by providing such data, which have been analysed using a common methodology, and are presented so as to facilitate comparisons both within the volume, and with data from cancer registries elsewhere. As well as being important for the planning and evaluation of cancer control activities in the countries concerned, the datasets presented in this volume permit comparison with statistics from countries where facilities for diagnosis and treatment are more readily available to cancer patients, as well as being more advanced technologically. This should highlight areas where improvement in outcome is technically feasible. Whether resources should be devoted to securing improvements, and the optimum mix of services to achieve them, will require careful weighing of priorities in the face of limited resources.

References

Berrino, F., Sant, M., Verdecchia, A., Capocaccia, R., Hakulinen, T. & Estève, J., eds. (1995) *Survival of Cancer*

Patients in Europe: the EUROCARE Study (IARC Scientific Publications No. 132). Lyon, International Agency for Research on Cancer

Cutler, S.J. (1964) *International Symposium on End Results of Cancer Therapy.* (National Cancer Institute Monograph No. 15). Washington, DC, National Cancer Instititute

Logan, W.P.D. (1978) Cancer survival statistics: international data. *World Health Statistics Quarterly,* **31**, 62–73

WHO (1995) *National Cancer Control Programmes: Policies Managerial Guidelines.* Geneva, World Health Organization

WHO/IARC (1979) *Cancer Statistics: Report of a WHO/IARC Expert Committee* (WHO Technical Report Series, No. 632). Geneva, World Health Organization

Chapter 2

Statistical methods for the analysis of cancer survival data

R.J. Black[1] and R. Swaminathan[2]

[1]International Agency for Research on Cancer
Lyon,
France

[2]Cancer Institute (WIA)
Chennai (Madras) 600036
India

Introduction

In the context of population-based cancer registry data, the aim of survival analysis is to estimate the probability of survival, expressed as time elapsed since diagnosis, for individuals within groups defined by, say, type of cancer diagnosed, sex, age and place of residence. Even though it is common practice to use the term 'survival rate' to describe this quantity, it is important to realize that we seek to estimate an individual probability rather than a 'rate'. Despite this, the terms 'survival rate', 'survival probability' and simply 'survival' are used interchangeably in this publication, since these will be commonly understood as having the same meaning by many readers. This chapter sets out some basic concepts in survival analysis, and describes how these have been used to estimate the survival of subjects from the developing-country populations included in the study. The methods of analysis used are essentially the same as those of the EUROCARE study (Berrino *et al.*, 1995), the only other recent systematic comparative analysis of survival in a number of cancer registry populations. A comprehensive description of survival analysis methods for cancer registry data is given by Estève *et al.* (1994).

Follow-up of subjects in a survival study

If we were able to obtain *complete* follow-up information for each individual in a group under study, then the probability of survival during a time period t could be estimated simply from the proportion of survivors at the end of the period among all subjects alive at the beginning of t. It would be sufficient to know each individual's survival status at the beginning of the period, t_i and at its end, t_{i+1}. With cancer registry data, we are usually concerned with periods of elapsed time between the date of incidence and some fixed point of follow-up time, such as five years after the date of incidence ('five-year survival'). In practice, follow-up of persons registered with cancer is not complete, either because subjects become 'lost to follow-up' during the period t (say by moving out of the area of surveillance of the cancer registry), or because the end of the period of possible follow-up by the registry occurs before the end of t. This is illustrated in Fig. 1, which shows follow-up of three subjects A, B and C.

Fig. 1 is divided into two parts. The first shows follow-up of the three subjects in terms of calendar time, while the second shows the same information in terms of the duration of follow-up. It will be noted that the period of registration is less than the follow-up period. This is typical of the data analysed in this publication and other cancer registry datasets. Subject A is diagnosed with cancer during the first year of the period of registration, with the date of incidence shown as i, and dies between y_3 and y_4, shown as d, which is within the period of possible follow-up by the registry. In the second part of the figure, this is shown in terms of the duration of follow-up, as three units of time t between incidence and death. Subject B is diagnosed at the beginning of y_1 but is lost to follow-up (lf) between y_2 and y_3, after a duration of follow-up 1.5 units of t. Finally, subject C is diagnosed between y_1 and y_2 and is still alive at the end of the follow-up period of the study y_4: subject C is thus said to be 'withdrawn alive' after 2.5 units of follow-up time t. It will be seen that the characters d, lf and w have been replaced with the values 1, 0 and 0, respectively, in the second part of the figure. This reminds us that, when we come to enumerate the number of deaths during follow-up, only subject A's death is known to us. Subjects B and

3

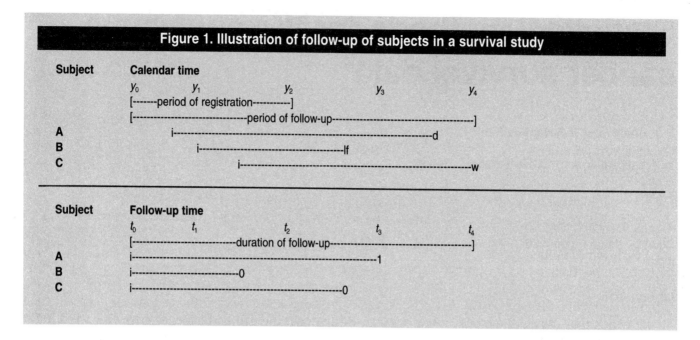

Figure 1. Illustration of follow-up of subjects in a survival study

Subject	Calendar time
	y_0 y_1 y_2 y_3 y_4
	[-------period of registration----------]
	[------------------------------period of follow-up----------------------------------]
A	i---d
B	i--------------------------------------lf
C	i--w

Subject	Follow-up time
	t_0 t_1 t_2 t_3 t_4
	[----------------------------duration of follow-up--------------------------------]
A	i--1
B	i-------------------------0
C	i--0

C have incomplete follow-up and will be *censored* from the analysis at the point in follow-up time at which they were either lost to follow-up or withdrawn. We are not aware of the deaths of subjects B and C, but we can use the information that they did not die during the period in which they were being followed up in estimating the probability of survival for the study group as a whole. This, indeed, is the key to formal survival analysis.

In practical terms, to prepare data for survival analysis, we require the time elapsed between the date of incidence and the date of death *or* date of loss to follow-up *or* date of withdrawal for each individual in the group under study, whichever occurs first. The accuracy of these survival times calculated from cancer registry data depends on the method of follow-up used by the registry. Some registries employ *passive* follow-up, which relies on notifications of deaths of cancer patients to the registry by national statistical organizations. Other registries use *active* follow-up, in which information on the survival status of patients is sought by the registry at fixed points in time after the date of incidence, usually on the anniversaries of this date. Active follow-up by cancer registries can be achieved by using clinical follow-up systems, by contacting patients' physicians, or by contacting the patients or their families directly by means of postal enquiries or even home visits. In the present study, most registries used a mixture of active and passive methods. Typically, registries undertook special follow-up exercises specifically for this study, in order to augment incomplete passive notification systems. The precise methods used by each registry are detailed in their respective chapters. The mixture of active and passive follow-up methods means that the data for analysis were composed of exact survival times for some subjects and less precise data representing cases censored as a result of follow-up enquiries.

Table 1. Calculation of the cumulative probability of survival using the actuarial method

Interval (years)	Alive at beginning of interval	Last known alive during interval (censored)	No. of deaths during interval	Effective no. at risk	Conditional probability of death	Conditional probability of survival	Cumulative prob. of survival (to end of year)
t_i-t_{i+1}	n_i	w_i	d_i	N_i	q_i	s_i	S_{i+1}
0-1	3289	166	365	3206.0	0.114	0.886	0.886
1-2	2758	275	301	2620.5	0.115	0.885	0.784
2-3	2182	37	278	2163.5	0.128	0.872	0.683
3-4	1867	30	191	1852.0	0.103	0.897	0.613
4-5	1646	20	106	1636.0	0.065	0.935	0.573

Estimation of survival

There are two related approaches to the estimation of survival: the Kaplan-Meier and the actuarial, or life table, methods. The former is particularly useful when exact survival times are available, since smooth estimates of survival as a function of time since diagnosis can be obtained. Given the data available, and in order to achieve consistency with other studies, the actuarial method was used in the present study of survival in developing countries. The actuarial method involves the construction of a life table, which permits the calculation of the cumulative probability of survival at time t_{i+1} from the conditional probabilities of survival during consecutive intervals of follow-up time up to and including t_{i+1}. The layout and method of calculation of the elements of a life table are shown in Table 1.

For each time period t_i to t_{i+1}, n_i is the number of subjects at risk of death at the beginning of the interval. The number of cases censored during the interval, because they were lost to follow-up or withdrawn alive at the end of the follow-up period, is shown as w_i. The symbol d_i denotes subjects who died during each interval. Values for n_i, w_i and d_i can be obtained directly from the survival times and outcomes (1=death, 0=censored) from the data set out in Fig. 1. The effective number of subjects at risk during each interval is calculated as

$$N_i = n_i - (w_i/2)$$

In this way, subjects who were alive and at risk of death during the interval t_i to t_{i+1}, but who were censored at some point during the interval, are assumed to have been followed up for, on average, half of the interval. Having estimated the effective number of subjects at risk, it is possible to calculate the probability of death during the interval from

$$q_i = d_i/N_i$$

The probability of survival during the interval beginning t_i is then calculated as

$$s_i = 1 - q_i$$

from which the cumulative probability of survival up to time t_{i+1} is derived from the product of the s_i,

$$S_{i+1} = \prod_{j=0}^{i} s_j$$

The final quantity estimated, S_{i+1}, is often multiplied by 100 to give the 'percentage survival' at

time t_{i+1}. In the context of the present study, use of the actuarial method has the advantage that information from all cases is used in the estimation of survival, including cases which were lost to follow-up at the point of time at which they were last 'known to be alive' by registries using active follow-up methods. However, the estimation of the effective number of subjects at risk in the actuarial method assumes that censored cases are actually followed up for, on average, half the length of a given interval and that such cases are subject to the same probability of death as the cases with complete follow-up during the same interval. In the analysis of registry data, these assumptions may be invalid. For example, at the beginning of follow-up, when cases are under short-term clinical surveillance but are then lost to follow-up by the registry, the average survival times of the censored cases may be less than half of the length of the first interval, as assumed. Furthermore, the true probability of death of the censored cases may be greater than assumed if cases of poor prognosis are more likely to be lost to follow-up.

Relative survival

The above method of calculating observed survival relates to deaths from all causes among the group of cancer patients under follow-up. However, cancer patients are at risk of death both from the cancer with which they have been diagnosed and from other causes of death. The observed survival is therefore influenced by mortality both from the cancer of interest and from other causes. Indeed, the presence of a tumour may increase an individual's risk of death from other causes. If we wish to compare survival in groups which are heterogeneous in terms of their risk of death from causes other than a particular cancer of interest, then observed differences between the groups concerned may be due in part to variations in the risk of death from these other causes, rather than the risk from the cancer under study. Estève et al. (1990) describe 'net survival', which is the survival which would pertain if deaths from other causes did not occur. In other words, net survival is the inverse of cause-specific mortality. One way of estimating the net survival is to censor cases at the point of death from causes other than the cancer of interest. This is called the 'corrected survival'. In the present study, and indeed in many other contexts, information about the cause of death of cancer patients is not available. This may be because of incomplete follow-up of all subjects, or because the death certification system is not sufficiently accurate to discriminate between deaths due to the cancer under study and deaths due to other causes. Recognition of this problem has led to the development of 'relative survival' methodology. The relative survival at the end of an interval beginning at t_i is defined as

$$R_{i+1} = S_{i+1}/S_{i+1}^*$$

where S_{i+1} is the *observed* survival for subjects with a particular cancer and S_{i+1}^* is the *expected* survival of a group of individuals with the same demographic characteristics who are at risk of death only from causes of death other than the cancer under study (Ederer *et al.*, 1961). As long as the cancer of concern does not make a large contribution to overall mortality, we can estimate the probability of survival, in the absence of this cancer, of an individual of a given age from t_0 to t_{i+1} from life tables based on general population mortality. Life tables present age-specific probabilities of surviving intervals of age, usually of one year, given an initial age x. Separate tables for males and females are generally available. The probability of survival at t_{i+1} of each subject h alive at t_0 is calculated as

$$e_h(t_{i+1}) = l_{x+0.5+t}/l_{x+0.5}$$

where $l_{x+0.5}$ is the average of the values of the survival function at ages x and $x+1$ from the life table and t represents the units of time elapsed between t_0 to t_{i+1}. Age $x+0.5$ is used to find the baseline value for the survivor function, since the average of cancer patients who have attained age x will be closer to $x+0.5$ than exactly x. Similar adjustments can be made when using abridged life tables in which values of the survivor function are given at intervals of five years of age. The overall expected survival of the group of subjects under study at t_{i+1} is obtained from expected number of survivors at t_{i+1} divided by the number of subjects alive at t_0,

$$S_{i+1}^* = \left(\sum_{h=1}^{n_0} e_h(t_{i+1})\right) / n_0$$

In the present study, detailed general population mortality life tables were not generally available. Instead, we relied on published life tables which were representative of the period of registration of the subjects under study, or generic life tables for developing countries published by the United Nations (UN, 1982). The life tables used for each population are detailed in the relevant chapters.

The above method of estimating expected survival has some important limitations, particularly in analysing long-term survival. There are three possible end-points for each subject: death from the cancer under study, death from another cause, and withdrawal from the study due to, for example, emigration from the cancer registry area. Normally we are obliged to estimate survival in quite large groups, which may be heterogeneous with respect to the probability of these events occurring. This means that the composition of a group changes over time (since subjects with relatively high probabilities of death or withdrawal would tend to be removed from the study before others), and the expected survival of all subjects alive at the beginning of follow-up becomes less representative of the surviving subjects. In the context of cancer registry data, age is commonly associated with risk of death from the cancer of concern (young patients may be more likely to withstand treatment), risk of death from other causes (young patients may be less likely to die from an unrelated condition such as heart disease), and the probability of becoming a censored case (young patients may be more likely to emigrate from the cancer registry area).

Despite our concern in the present study with survival up to only five years, we have used a computer package which takes account of heterogeneity in expected survival and withdrawal of subjects (Hakulinen *et al.*, 1994). Specifically, the method used was that of Hakulinen (1982), both for overall and for age-specific and sex-specific estimates of relative survival.

Age-standardized survival

It is important to realize that, when comparing survival in different groups, the method of relative survival takes account of variations in the age structure of the groups only to the extent that age is correlated with risk of death from causes other than the cancer under study. For many types of cancer, the risk of dying as a result of the cancer itself is clearly associated with the subject's age at diagnosis. In the present study we were interested in comparing survival in developing and developed country populations, in which the age structures of cancer patient groups are grossly different. For this reason, we used direct standardization of age-specific relative survival estimates to derive an overall summary statistic, *age-standardized relative survival (ASRS)*

$$\text{ASRS}_i = \left(\sum_x r_{ix} w_x\right) / \sum_x w_x$$

where r_{ix} are age-specific relative survival estimates at the end of the follow-up period t_i and w_x are age-specific proportions from the World Standard Cancer Patient Population for the appropriate site of cancer (*see Chapter 3*).

References

Berrino, F., Sant, M., Verdecchia, A., Capocaccia, R., Hakulinen, T. & Estève, J., eds. (1995) *Survival of Cancer Patients in Europe: the EUROCARE Study* (IARC Scientific Publications No. 132). Lyon, International Agency for Research on Cancer

Ederer, F., Axtell, L.M. & Cutler, S.J. (1961) The relative survival rate: a statistical methodology. *Monogr. Natl. Cancer Inst.*, **6**, 101–121

Estève, J., Benhamou, E., Croasdale, M. & Raymond, L. (1990) Relative survival and the estimation of net survival: elements for further discussion. *Stat. Med.*, **9**, 529–538

Estève, J., Benhamou, E. & Raymond, L. (1994) *Statistical Methods in Cancer Research*. Volume IV: *Descriptive Epidemiology*. (IARC Scientific Publications No. 128). Lyon, International Agency for Research on Cancer

Hakulinen, T. (1982) Cancer survival corrected for heterogeneity in patient withdrawal. *Biometrics*, **38**, 933–942

Hakulinen, T., Gibberd, R., Abeywickrama, K.H. & Soderman, B. (1994) *A Computer Program Package for Cancer Survival Studies, Version 2.0*. Tampere, Finnish Cancer Registry/University of Newcastle, Australia

UN (1982) *Model Life Tables For Developing Countries* (Population Studies No. 77). New York, United Nations Department of International Economic and Social Affairs

Chapter 3

World standard cancer patient populations: A resource for comparative analysis of survival data

R.J. Black and S.A. Bashir

International Agency for Research on Cancer
Lyon,
France

Introduction

As noted in Chapter 2 'Statistical methods for the analysis of cancer survival data', cancer patient survival is influenced by age in two ways: the risk of dying as a result of the cancer with which a patient has been diagnosed tends to be greater for elderly persons, and elderly subjects tend to be at greater risk of death from other causes. In comparing two groups of subjects, one of which has a larger proportion of elderly patients than the other, the relatively greater risk of death from causes other than the cancer under study will be reflected in a lower value for expected survival in the older group. However, relative survival is determined by deaths from the cancer under study as well as other causes of death. In these circumstances, comparisons of relative survival within age bands can be recommended. However, it is common for investigators to seek to summarize differences between groups using overall estimates of survival. For this purpose, direct standardization of relative survival estimates has been advocated (Parkin & Hakulinen, 1991). In the EUROCARE study, for example, the data from all registries were combined, within categories of tumour site, in order to establish the standard populations of persons registered with cancer to which individual registry survival estimates were standardized (Berrino et al., 1995). This approach was not possible in the present study, since we wished to make comparisons between the developing country populations and published data for European and US populations. For this reason, we constructed a set of abstract World Standard Cancer Patient Populations for use in the present study and, we hope, other comparative studies of cancer survival.

Data and methods

We obtained global estimates of incidence rates of major cancers in 1985 from Parkin et al. (1993). The data were in the form of rates for the age groups 15–44, 45–54, 55–64 and 65+. In order to provide standard populations for the more detailed five-year age groups (0–4, 5–9, ..., 85+), we used polynomial regression models to estimate incidence rates for intermediate points in the age range 15–64. Worldwide incidence rates for childhood cancer were obtained from Parkin et al. (1988). For age groups from 65–69 to 85+, incidence rates were estimated by linear projection of the trend in incidence between the point estimates of rates at ages 55–59 and 60–64. These incidence rates were then applied to United Nations estimates of the total world population in 1985 (UN, 1991) to obtain estimates of annual numbers of new cases. Finally, for each cancer site, percentages of cases in each age group were calculated.

Results

The standard populations (in percentage terms) are presented in Table 1.

Discussion

As described in Chapter 2, the standard populations are required for direct standardization (i.e. by summing age-specific relative survival estimates weighted by the standard percentages). The standard populations presented are approximations to the true age distributions of new cases of cancer globally. The accuracy of the estimates is not of great concern, since the intention is that they should be used in the intermediate calculations necessary to calculate age-standardized relative survival. Further refinements would not have any material bearing on such results. The regression method used to obtain age-specific estimates of global incidence rates imposes a degree of smoothing on the proportions. Therefore their use is unlikely to produce distorted standardized survival

Table 1. World standard cancer patient populations (percentages): males and females combined

Age	Tumour site (ICD-9 codes)									
	140–208	140–149	150	151	153–154	155	157	161	162	172
0–4	0.5	0.1	0.0	0.0	0.0	0.1	0.0	0.0	0.0	0.0
5–9	0.6	0.2	0.0	0.0	0.0	0.3	0.0	0.0	0.0	0.1
10–14	0.7	0.4	0.0	0.0	0.1	0.4	0.0	0.1	0.0	0.4
15–19	0.9	0.7	0.1	0.1	0.2	0.8	0.0	0.2	0.1	0.9
20–24	1.3	1.2	0.2	0.2	0.4	1.3	0.1	0.4	0.2	1.8
25–29	1.8	1.9	0.5	0.7	0.8	2.1	0.4	0.9	0.5	3.3
30–34	2.5	3.1	1.4	1.7	1.5	3.2	1.3	1.7	1.1	4.9
35–39	3.4	4.6	3.1	3.6	2.3	4.7	3.2	3.0	2.1	6.6
40–44	4.7	6.5	5.3	5.7	3.4	6.5	5.3	5.1	3.6	7.8
45–49	6.3	8.6	7.5	7.3	4.7	8.3	6.6	7.7	5.6	8.7
50–54	8.0	10.5	9.1	8.2	6.1	10.0	7.1	10.7	8.0	9.0
55–59	9.7	11.9	10.3	8.6	7.5	11.1	7.5	13.2	10.4	8.9
60–64	10.5	11.2	12.4	10.8	9.5	11.6	9.9	12.9	12.6	9.1
65–69	10.5	10.0	11.8	11.0	10.6	10.2	10.6	11.5	12.3	8.7
70–74	10.3	8.9	11.0	10.9	11.7	9.0	11.2	10.1	11.9	8.3
75–79	9.9	7.8	10.1	10.7	12.8	7.8	11.8	8.7	11.3	7.8
80–84	9.5	6.8	9.1	10.5	13.8	6.8	12.2	7.4	10.5	7.2
85+	8.9	5.6	8.2	10.0	14.6	5.8	12.8	6.4	9.8	6.5
Total	100.0	100.0	100.0	100.0	100.0	100.0	100.0	100.0	100.0	100.0

Age	Tumour site (ICD-9 codes)									
	174	180	182	183	185	186	188	189	200-203	204-208
0-4	0.0	0.0	0.0	0.2	0.0	0.6	0.0	4.5	2.8	8.1
5-9	0.0	0.0	0.0	0.4	0.0	0.1	0.0	2.1	2.7	6.3
10-14	0.1	0.1	0.1	0.7	0.0	0.1	0.1	1.3	2.7	5.3
15-19	0.3	0.3	0.2	1.1	0.0	3.8	0.2	1.0	2.8	4.6
20-24	0.9	1.1	0.4	1.9	0.0	12.5	0.4	1.0	3.1	4.3
25-29	2.1	2.7	0.8	2.9	0.0	18.6	0.6	1.3	3.5	4.1
30-34	4.0	5.2	1.6	4.2	0.1	19.0	1.1	1.6	4.0	4.2
35-39	6.4	8.2	3.0	5.8	0.2	16.1	1.8	2.3	4.6	4.3
40-44	8.5	10.8	5.1	7.5	0.3	9.8	2.8	3.5	5.4	4.5
45-49	10.0	12.1	7.9	9.0	0.8	6.3	4.2	5.3	6.2	4.8
50-54	10.5	12.0	11.0	10.2	1.6	3.9	6.0	7.7	7.0	5.2
55-59	10.2	10.9	13.6	10.9	3.3	2.9	7.9	10.6	7.7	5.6
60-64	9.7	9.8	13.6	10.4	6.2	1.8	10.0	10.9	8.5	6.2
65-69	9.0	8.0	11.7	9.2	8.7	1.3	11.1	10.6	8.4	6.4
70-74	8.2	6.5	9.9	8.0	12.1	1.1	12.2	10.1	8.2	6.6
75-79	7.5	5.2	8.3	6.9	16.4	0.9	13.1	9.4	7.9	6.6
80-84	6.7	4.1	6.9	5.9	21.8	0.7	13.9	8.8	7.5	6.6
85+	5.9	3.0	5.9	4.8	28.5	0.5	14.6	8.0	7.0	6.3
Total	100.0	100.0	100.0	100.0	100.0	100.0	100.0	100.0	100.0	100.0

values, as long as there is reasonable precision in the original estimates of age-specific relative survival. If the original survival data are very sparse, it may be wise to combine them in larger age groups, for which the standard proportions can be combined additively. A further recommendation would be to show a truncated standardized relative survival, say to age 74, as we have done in the present report. If an investigator wishes to standardize data for a cancer which has not been included in the tables, then it would be a reasonable approach to choose a set of proportions for a similar type of cancer, or for all cancer combined. It should be noted that the site-specific cancer patient populations are not suitable for comparisons of survival of patients in a single population with different types of cancer. If this is an aim of a particular study, then, again, the standard populations given in Table 1 for all cancers combined should be used.

The effect of standardizing using a worldwide standard is that greater weight is given to younger patients than would be the case if an age distribution based on developed countries only had been used. For developed countries in which elderly cancer patients predominate, use of the World Standard Cancer Patient Populations tends to raise the age-standardized relative survival above the unstandardized value. The interpretation of results of this kind is that they indicate the overall relative survival which would pertain if the developed country's age-specific survival values applied in a 'worldwide average' group of patients. This may seem artificial but, in the spirit of the World Standard Population (Segi, 1960), which has now gained universal acceptance, use of the World Standard Cancer Patient Populations will enhance the comparability of survival results published by individual cancer registries.

References

Berrino, F., Sant, M., Verdecchia, A., Capocaccia, R., Hakulinen, T. & Estève, J., eds. (1995) *Survival of Cancer Patients in Europe: the EUROCARE Study* (IARC Scientific Publications No. 132). Lyon, International Agency for Research on Cancer

Parkin, D.M. & Hakulinen, T. (1991) Analysis of survival. In: Jensen, O.M., Parkin, D.M., MacLennan, R., Muir, C.S. & Skeet, R.G. *Cancer Registration: Principles and Methods* (IARC Scientific Publications No. 95). Lyon, International Agency for Research on Cancer

Parkin, D.M., Stiller, C.A., Bieber, C.A., Draper, G.J., Terracini, B. & Young, J. (1988) *International Incidence of Childhood Cancer* (IARC Scientific Publications No. 87). Lyon, International Agency for Research on Cancer

Parkin, D.M., Pisani, P. & Ferlay, J. (1993) Estimates of the world-wide incidence of eighteen major cancers in 1985. *Int. J. Cancer*, **54**, 594–606

Segi, M. (1960) *Cancer Mortality for Selected Sites in 24 Countries (1950-1957)*. Sendai, Japan, Tohoku University School of Medicine, Department of Public Health

UN (1991) *World Population Prospects 1990* (Population Studies No. 120). New York, United Nations Department of International Economic and Social Affairs

Chapter 4

Interpretation of population-based cancer survival data

R. J. Black, R. Sankaranarayanan and D.M. Parkin

International Agency for Research on Cancer
Lyon,
France

Introduction

In order to describe completely the experience of cancer in a population, it is necessary to know not only its incidence and mortality, but also the survival of cancer patients. There are three main sources of information about survival: the randomized controlled clinical trial, which represents the 'gold standard' for the evaluation of forms of treatment; the hospital-based study, which aims to provide information about the outcome of treatment in particular settings; and population-based survival from cancer registries, which reflects a broader range of cancer control activities, including screening and the organization of treatment services. Each of these has its limitations: survival information from trials and published hospital series is often biased by patient selection, whereas population-based survival data may lack the details of stage and treatment which are of particular interest to the clinician.

The rationale of a randomized clinical trial is to eliminate the confounding effects of factors such as age and comorbidity in order to isolate the effects of treatment. This is achieved in two ways: by adopting selection criteria which exclude some subjects (such as those with comorbid conditions) and random allocation of the remainder into groups in which the only systematic differences are the treatments to be received. This approach is essential in order to determine the *efficacy* of particular treatments. However, the *effectiveness* of cancer services in general depends not only on the efficacy of particular treatments but also on the context in which they are applied.

Evaluating effectiveness requires estimation of survival in unselected groups of cancer patients, which is a key aim of most cancer registries. Estimates of survival in such groups may be influenced by a range of prognostic and other factors (see Table 1). In accounting for these, the methodology of clinical trials cannot be deployed, since selection would invalidate the generality of results and it is impossible, of course, to randomize cancer patients to different health care systems. Therefore another approach is required when evaluating survival at the population level and making comparisons between population groups which are heterogeneous in respect of prognostic factors. Some factors such as age and sex can be accounted for in the statistical methodology used to estimate survival. Information on other factors such as comorbidity may not even be present in cancer registry data. For these, the best we can do is to be aware of their possible influences or, as has been attempted in the EUROCARE study (Berrino *et al.*, 1995), augment the basic cancer registry information with 'high resolution' data. The remainder of this chapter provides a review of comparability issues: that is, data quality factors (e.g. methods of ascertainment and follow-up), host factors (e.g. age, sex, risk of death from other diseases), tumour-related factors (e.g. extent of disease) and health care factors (e.g. availability and quality of diagnosis and treatment services) which influence population-based estimates of survival.

Data quality factors

Inevitably, the quality of cancer registration data will vary according to the availability of source data, the experience of registry staff and other factors. This variation complicates the interpretation of survival data based on routine cancer registry data (Hanai & Fujimoto, 1985). Of particular concern is the completeness of ascertainment. If cases of cancer which are not registered represent a random sample from the total, then there should be no systematic bias in survival results. However, this is unlikely to be the case, since the probability of being registered tends to be correlated with prognosis: for example, elderly patients not seen in hospital are less likely to be registered than younger patients, for whom curative treatment may have been attempted. Estimates of survival may therefore be artificially

Table 1. Factors influencing population-based survival data

Data quality factors
- Completeness of ascertainment
- Accuracy of registration
- Completeness of follow-up
- 'Death certificate only' (DCO) registrations

Host factors
- Age
- Sex
- Race/Ethnicity
- Comorbidity
- Socioeconomic status
- Behaviour (including awareness of cancer symptoms and compliance with treatment)

Tumour-related factors
- Extent of disease
- Site (including subsite) of tumour
- Morphology of tumour
- Tumour biology

Health care-related factors
- Screening
- Diagnostic facilities
- Treatment facilities
- Quality of treatment
- Follow-up care

raised for a particular registry area if ascertainment is not complete. Similarly, the accuracy of diagnostic information for cancer patients tends to be correlated with prognosis. For example, a registry relying exclusively on a particular pathology laboratory for diagnostic information might tend to classify cases from other sources in nonspecific categories for primary site. Such cases would be excluded from tumour-site-specific survival analyses, whereas data for another registry might include cases with clinical diagnoses. Again, the effect of this aspect of data quality would be to increase the survival estimate for a registry which allocated a large proportion of cases to nonspecific diagnostic categories.

In cancer registry data, there are usually some subjects for whom the registration of cancer was based on information from the death certificate only (DCO). By convention, such cases are excluded from survival analyses since — by definition — their survival time is zero. This convention was adopted in the present study. If the proportion of DCO cases is relatively low, say less than 10%, then excluding them from the analysis does not greatly influence survival estimates. However, larger proportions of DCO cases are problematic, since they may mean that cases of poor prognosis (which would have been registered by other means if the registry had had better ascertainment procedures) are excluded, thus artificially increasing estimates of survival. Some of the registries in the present study have quite large proportions of DCO cases.

Under either active or passive follow-up systems, individuals can be lost due to migration, breaking off contacts with local authorities or other changes in living conditions. Normally, registries assume that a subject is alive until a notification of death is received, or active follow-up results in a confirmation of death. Many of the individuals who are lost to follow-up will, in fact, have died, so that a registry with a large proportion of individuals with whom they have lost contact will report artificially high survival. However, the direction of the bias is unpredictable, and will depend on local circumstances. For example, loss to follow-up may occur when subjects with a relatively good prognosis are obliged to move away from their original cancer registry area to receive treatment.

A common feature of most of the aspects of data quality discussed above is that poor data quality tends to increase estimates of survival. A key aim of the international network of cancer registries is to standardize data collection methods and indicators of data quality. We believe that the differences in survival between the registries reported in the present study are mainly due to factors other than data quality (see the discussion in Chapter 16). However, it is important to be aware that apparently high survival rates for some registries may have been influenced by data quality factors. Detailed information on data quality, including data quality indicators such as the proportion of DCO registrations and the proportion of cases with histological verification, can be seen in the individual registry chapters.

Host factors

Age at diagnosis is an independent prognostic factor for many types of cancer. This operates in two ways: age may be correlated both with the risk of dying from a particular type of cancer and with the risk of dying from some other cause. In the present study, we adjusted for age using age-standardized relative survival (to take account of variations in age-specific background mortality and differences in the age distributions of the populations being compared).

Sex is less commonly associated with variations in survival and, for this reason, many registries combined data for males and females in the interests of increasing the precision of survival estimates. However, survival from some cancers, such as malignant melanoma, has been seen to be greater for women in some developed countries, which is probably due to a greater recognition of early symptoms and a willingness to seek medical attention.

Comorbid conditions experienced by cancer patients may vary substantially between registry populations. Comorbidity affects survival by presenting an additional source of risk of death, making it less likely that a patient will be offered curative treatment and, if it is offered, less likely that the patient will be able to withstand the effects of the treatment itself.

Socioeconomic differences in survival have been reported for many sites of cancer within populations in Europe (Kogevinas, 1991) and the USA (Berg et al., 1977). Socioeconomic status tends to be correlated with strong prognostic factors such as extent of disease at diagnosis, but it has been shown to have a residual effect which may be due to inequalities in access to medical care facilities, compliance with treatment regimens, coping strategies or social support. Within developed countries, race is also associated with survival, although the extent to which this operates independently of socioeconomic status is unclear (Howard et al., 1991). Berg et al. (1977) propose a host vulnerability hypothesis in which the poor nutritional status, general health and immunological status (related to alcoholism) of some social and racial groups leads to lower survival from cancer. Clearly, socioeconomic conditions in developed and developing countries are grossly different, to the extent that inequalities in access to medical care are likely to be of particular significance in the present study.

Tumour-related factors

By convention, cancer registry data are aggregated within categories defined by the anatomical site of the tumour. When comparing international survival data, caution must be exercised when the distributions of tumour subsites vary. The same point applies to variations in the frequency of morphological types of tumour within categories of site, and variations in tumour biology, as expressed by differences in natural history and aggressiveness of clinical course (e.g. breast cancers with variations in the frequencies of tumour markers such as hormonal receptor status; variations in the grade of non-Hodgkin lymphomas).

The stage of disease at diagnosis is generally the most important factor determining the survival of cancer patients. This is because certain treatments may be available only for early-stage tumours, and any treatment is more likely to be successful if initiated before metastasis has occurred. Therefore variations in the stage distributions of tumours in populations being compared are of particular concern. Some of the registries involved in the present study were able to supply data on extent of disease, which we have used in interpreting results for these regions. However, even when such data are available, variations in diagnostic technology such as those between developed and developing countries are likely to lead to measurement error. Stage of disease at diagnosis is influenced both by the general level of health awareness in the population, and by the presence or absence of programmes of early detection for cancer. The effect of the former is seen clearly with respect to cervical cancer statistics recorded in patients admitted to the Radiumhemmet Hospital, Stockholm, Sweden since 1920. Even before the introduction of screening programmes, there was a dramatic change in the proportion of cases diagnosed at early stages (I and II), from less than 20% in 1920 to some 80% in 1965. (Pontén et al., 1995).

Health care-related factors

Factors relating to the health care of cancer patients in developed and developing countries are of particular concern in the present study. There are a number of ways in which the availability of, and access to, screening services and diagnostic and treatment facilities can influence survival. Screening programmes aim to detect early-stage cancers or premalignant tumours so that the disease can be treated at an early stage, which is generally more effective. However, interpreting survival statistics in terms of the benefit to patients resulting from screening is problematic, since one consequence of early detection is to bring forward the date of diagnosis of a condition, whether or not this has the desired effect of reducing risk of death from the disease. This is called 'lead-time bias'. In addition, screening programmes may result in the detection of disease that would not otherwise have been diagnosed at all during the life of the patient — so-called 'overdiagnosis bias' (Morrison, 1985). This latter will necessarily result in a marked improvement in survival, and one that is independent of any 'downstaging' effect of screening which, theoretically at least, could be monitored in cancer registry data. Overdiagnosis almost certainly accounts for the huge increases recently observed in the reported incidence of prostate carcinoma in the USA, and the corresponding changes in survival (Kosary et al., 1995). As far as the results in this volume are concerned, however, they are likely to be little influenced by screening programmes. With certain exceptions (described in the relevant chapters), screening programmes are not extensive or systematically implemented in developing countries and, where information on extent of disease is available, it will be observed that, for many cancers, more patients are presenting late in the course of their disease than would be expected from experience in Europe or North America.

Diagnostic facilities may also influence survival by ensuring that a specific and correct diagnosis can be made. Improvements in the sensitivity of diagnosis may have the effect of inducing 'stage migration' in which, for example, tumours of limited metastatic activity which at one time would have been inaccurately described as simply invasive, may be reallocated to the metastatic category, thus increasing estimates of survival of individuals in both metastatic and the nonmetastatic groups (Feinstein et al., 1985). This phenomenon can operate on a geographical as well as a temporal basis (Farrow et al., 1995). Therefore, comparisons of stage-specific survival data from settings with very different diagnostic facilities cannot be made with confidence. It should be noted that comparisons of survival of groups comprising patients with tumours of all stages combined are not subject to this problem, as long as there is no selection bias due to greater diagnostic specificity in one population compared with another.

The availability of treatment facilities for cancer patients affects the survival of those for whom curative treatment would have the potential to succeed. Therefore the issue of availability of treatment facilities is bound up with the availability of other facilities, such as screening programmes and diagnostic facilities. Survival data from cancer registries cannot be used to make direct comparisons of populations in terms of the quality of care available, although some studies have shown that the survival of some cancer patients is prolonged after treatment at specialized cancer centres (Stiller,

1994). However, results of this kind are difficult to interpret because of selection criteria for specialized care, which may determine the apparently better results rather than the quality of care received per se.

Conclusions

The previous discussion indicates the difficulty of making meaningful comparisons of survival among groups of cancer patients with varying demographic and socioeconomic characteristics, and served by very different health care infrastructures, using retrospectively collected data from cancer registries. It is certainly important to realize that variations are not simply due to the availability and quality of medical services. However, as will be seen from the discussion in Chapter 16 'An overview of cancer survival in developing countries', a comparison of the magnitude of differences between countries provides at least an indirect indication of the relative importance of early detection and treatment for certain major cancers.

References

Berg, J.W., Ross, R. & Latourette, H.B. (1977) Economic status and survival of cancer patients. *Cancer*, **39**, 467–477

Berrino, F., Sant, M., Verdecchia, A., Capocaccia, R., Hakulinen, T. & Estève, J., eds. (1995) *Survival of Cancer Patients in Europe: the EUROCARE Study* (IARC Scientific Publications No. 132). Lyon, International Agency for Research on Cancer

Farrow, D.C., Hunt, W.C. & Somet, J.M. (1995) Biased comparisons of lung cancer survival across geographic areas: effects of stage bias. *Epidemiology*, **6**, 558–560

Feinstein, A.R., Sosin, D.M. & Wells, C.K. (1985) The Will Rogers phenomenon: stage migration and new diagnostic techniques as a source of misleading statistics for survival in cancer. *New Engl. J. Med.*, **312**, 1604–1608

Hanai, A. & Fujimoto, I. (1985) Survival as an index in evaluating cancer control. In: Parkin, D.M., Wagner, G. & Muir, C.S., eds., *The Role of the Registry in Cancer Control* (IARC Scientific Publications No. 66). Lyon, International Agency for Research on Cancer

Howard, J., Hankey, B.F., Greenberg, R.S., Austin, D.F., Correa, P., Chen, V.W. & Duraho, S. (1992) A collaborative study of differences in the survival rates of black patients and white patients with cancer. *Cancer*, **69**, 2349–2360

Kogevinas, M. (1991) *Longitudinal Study: Socio-demographic Differences in Cancer Survival* (OPCS Series LS No. 5). London, HMSO

Kosary, C.L., Ries, L.A.G., Miller, B.A., Hankey, B.F., Harras, A. & Edwards, B.K., eds. (1995) *SEER Cancer Statistics Review, 1973-1992: Tables and Graphs* (NIH Publication No. 96-2789). Bethesda, MD, National Cancer Institute

Morrison, A.S. (1985) *Screening in Chronic Disease.* New York, Oxford University Press

Pontén, J., Adami, H.O., Bergström, R., Dillner, J., Friberg, J., Gustafsson, L., Miller, A.B., Parkin, D.M., Sparén, P. & Trichopoulos, D. (1995) Strategies for global control of cervical cancer. *Int. J. Cancer,* **60**, 1–26

Stiller, C.A. (1994) Centralised treatment, entry to trials and survival. *Br. J. Cancer,* **70**, 352–362

Chapter 5

Database on cancer survival from developing countries

R. Swaminathan

Cancer Institute (WIA)
Chennai (Madras) 600036
India

R.J. Black and R. Sankaranarayanan

International Agency for Research on Cancer
Lyon,
France

Introduction

Ten population-based cancer registries from five countries in Asia and South America have contributed data on survival for this study. The registries are as follows (Fig. 1):

Qidong, China
Shanghai, China
National Cancer Registry, Cuba
Bangalore, India
Barshi, India
Bombay, India
Madras, India
Rizal, Philippines
Chiang Mai, Thailand
Khon Kaen, Thailand

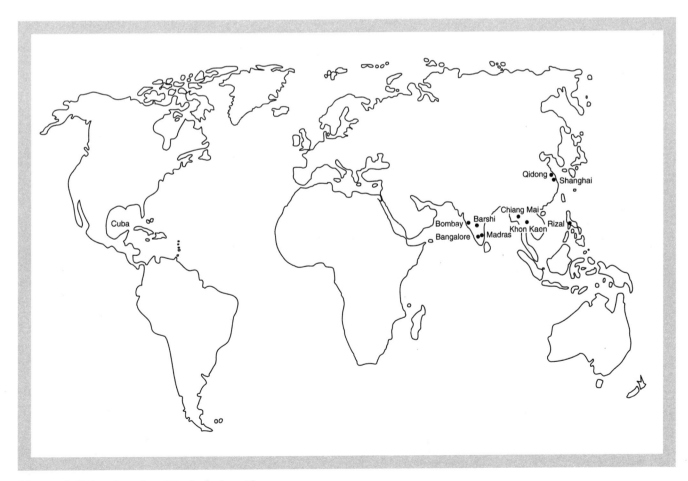

Figure 1. Map showing 10 study locations

Table 1. Cancer registration, coding and follow-up practices in participating registries

| Registry, Country | Cancer registration | | | Coding practices | | Details of follow-up | |
	Period included	Method and population	Year started	Topography	Morphology	Closing date	Methods
Qidong, China	1982–91	Active and passive methods, predominantly rural	1972	ICD-9 (4 digits)	Local codes	31-Dec-94	Predominantly passive - matching with death certificates - scrutiny of medical records - house visits
Shanghai,China	1988–91	Passive notification, rural and urban	1963	ICD-9 (4 digits)	Local codes	31-Dec-94	Predominantly passive - matching with death certificates - scrutiny of medical records - house visits
Cuba	1988–89	Passive notification–voluntary till 1986, compulsory thereafter; entire country covered	1964	ICD-O I ed. (4 digits)	ICD-O I ed. (5 digits)	31-Dec-94	Predominantly passive - matching with death certificates - matching with national identity register - scrutiny of medical records - postal enquiries
Bangalore, India	1982–89	Active data collection by registry staff, totally urban	1982	ICD-9 (3 digits)	ICD-O I ed. (6 digits)	31-Dec-93	Predominantly active - matching with death certificates - repeated scrutiny of case records - postal/telephone enquiries/house visits
Barshi, India	1988–92	Active data collection by registry staff, totally rural	1987	ICD-9 (4 digits)	ICD-O I ed. (6 digits)	31-Dec-95	Predominantly active - matching with death certificates - repeated scrutiny of case records - postal/telephone enquiries/house visits
Bombay, India	1982–86	Active data collection by registry staff, totally urban	1963	ICD-O I ed. ICD-9 (4 digits)	ICD-O I ed. (6 digits)	31-Dec-93	Predominantly active - matching with death certificates - repeated scrutiny of case records - postal/telephone enquiries/house visits
Madras, India	1984–89	Active data collection by registry staff, totally urban	1982	ICD-O I ed. ICD-9 (4 digits)	ICD-O I ed. (6 digits)	31-Dec-93	Predominantly active - matching with death certificates both cancer and not cancer as cause - repeated scrutiny of case records - perusal of area health registers - postal/telephone enquiries/house visits
Rizal, Philippines	1987	Passive notification till 1978 - active since then, mainly urban	1974	ICD-O I ed. ICD-9 (4 digits)	ICD-O I ed. (5 digits)	31-Dec-93	Predominantly passive - matching with death certificates - matching with case finding lists - scrutiny of medical/health records - enquiries with attending physician
Chiang Mai, Thailand	1983–92	Active data collection by registry staff, rural and urban	1963 Hospital-based till 1986. Population-based since then - retrospective data collected from 1983	ICD-O I ed. (4 digits)	ICD-O I ed. (4 digits)	30-Jun-94	Predominantly active - matching with death certificates - repeated scrutiny of medical records - postal enquiries/house visits
Khon Kaen, Thailand	1985–92	Active and passive methods, rural and urban	1984 Hospital-based till 1988. Population-based since then - retrospective data collected from 1984	ICD-O I ed. (4 digits)	ICD-O I ed. (5 digits)	31-Dec-95	Predominantly active - matching with death certificates - scrutiny of hospital records - postal enquiries/house visits

Table 2. Cancers included and variables provided for analysis		
Registry, Country	**Cancer sites included : ICD-9**	**Variables provided by the registry**
Qidong, China	147, 150–5, 157, 162, 174, 180, 188, 191–2*, 203–8	Identification number, age at incidence date, sex, date of birth, most valid basis of diagnosis, incidence date, primary site of cancer, dates of death/last follow-up, vital status, survival time
Shanghai, China	140–208	Identification number, age at incidence date, sex, most valid basis of diagnosis, incidence date, primary site of cancer, dates of death/last follow-up, vital status, survival time
Cuba	140–1, 143–6, 153–4, 162, 174,180, 182–3, 185, 200–8	Identification number, age at incidence date, sex, date of birth, most valid basis of diagnosis, incidence date, primary site of cancer, clinical extent of disease, morphology, dates of death/last follow-up, vital status, survival time
Bangalore, India	174, 180, 200–8	Identification number, age at incidence date, sex, most valid basis of diagnosis, incidence date, primary site of cancer, tumour stage/clinical extent of disease, histology, dates of death/last follow-up, vital status
Barshi, India	180	Identification number, age, sex, religion, most valid basis of diagnosis, incidence date, primary site of cancer, tumour stage,morphology,treatment, dates of death/last follow-up, vital status, survival time
Bombay, India	174, 180	Identification number, age at incidence date, sex, marital status, mother tongue, religion, literacy, most valid basis of diagnosis, incidence date, primary site of cancer, morphology, dates of death/last follow-up, vital status
Madras, India	140–1, 143–6,148,150–1, 157, 161–2, 174, 180, 188, 200–2, 204–8	Identification number, age at incidence date, sex, marital status, mother tongue, religion, literacy, most valid basis of diagnosis, incidence date, primary site of cancer, morphology, dates of death/last follow-up, vital status, survival time
Rizal, Philippines	143–5, 151, 153–5, 162, 174, 180, 185, 204–8	Identification number, age at incidence date, sex, date of birth, most valid basis of diagnosis, incidence date, primary site of cancer, clinical extent of disease, morphology, dates of death/last follow-up, vital status
Chiang Mai, Thailand	140–208	Identification number, age at incidence date, sex, most valid basis of diagnosis, incidence date, primary site of cancer, clinical extent of disease, morphology, treatment, dates of death/last follow-up, vital status
Khon Kaen, Thailand	140–208	Identification number, age at incidence date, sex, marital status, ethnicity, religion, most valid basis of diagnosis, incidence date, primary site of cancer, clinical extent of disease, morphology, dates of death/last follow-up, vital status, survival time

* Includes benign and unspecified neoplasms, number not known

Data on the following variables were requested from each participating registry:
• identification number
• sex
• date of birth
• socioeconomic factors (marital status, mother tongue, religion, ethnicity, education, socioeconomic status, etc.)
• incidence date
• age at incidence date
• most valid basis of diagnosis of cancer
• clinical extent of disease before treatment/tumour stage
• primary site of cancer (ICD-O, ICD-9)
• morphology
• date of death/last follow-up
• vital status at this date (alive/dead/lost to follow-up).

Tables 1 and 2 give the details of the study period, cancers studied, variables provided, cancer registration and follow-up methods, and coding practices followed for each of the registries. Since all these registries were population-based, they were asked to send data on *all* incident cases for the period under study, not merely for the subset of cases for which follow-up information was available. This was done mainly to evaluate the usual indicators of data quality (proportion of cases with a histological verification of cancer diagnosis, proportion of cases registered on the basis of death certificate only) and to permit the entire dataset to be subjected to standard validation checks.

Study period

The participating registries had been in operation for varying periods of time. The years for which follow-up information was available were even more varied. For this reason, it was decided to use the maximum period of data available from each registry, rather than imposing a single time period on all. The periods of registration under study were all between 1 January 1982 and 31 December 1992.

Study material

Not all the participating registries could provide follow-up information on all the cancer sites registered during the study period. Chiang Mai and Khon Kaen from Thailand and Shanghai from China had follow-up information for all cancer sites. Data were available only for selected cancer sites in the other registries: for the most part, these were the most common cancers in their respective regions. Follow-up of breast and cervical cancers in females and lung cancer and other tobacco-related cancers in both sexes had been carried out in most registries (Table 2).

All the incident cancer cases (in the sites chosen for analysis) were included in the study. Only invasive cancers were included. No distinction was made between first and subsequent primary cancers in the same individual. However, in most developing countries, second and subsequent primaries constituted a negligible proportion of the total.

Primary site of cancer

Data on the tumour site had been coded in accordance with the *International Classification of Diseases for Oncology*, First Edition (ICD-O) (WHO, 1976) by all the registries, and some had simultaneously coded the site in accordance with the *International Classification of Diseases, Ninth Revision* (ICD-9) (WHO, 1978). Conversion to ICD-9 codes was done wherever necessary. Details of the diagnostic categories used are shown in Table 3. Only categories with at least 25 cases were considered for analysis.

Morphology

Morphology (and behaviour), coded in accordance with the *International Classification of Diseases for Oncology*, First Edition (WHO, 1976), were available for all the datasets except the two from China, which had used local codes (Chinese characters) for morphology.

Tumour stage/clinical extent of disease

Data on tumour stage, classified by TNM (tumour-node-metastasis) stage categories, were not routinely available in the population-based cancer registries participating in this study. However, data on the clinical extent of disease before treatment were available in all the registries (at least for selected sites) except the two from China. The criteria followed by the participating registries are shown in Table 4. There is bound to be variation in the accuracy of this information between registries, as it depends on the extent of investigative procedures and on registration practices. Because of this variability, comparison of survival estimates by clinical extent of disease was confined to selected sites within individual registries.

Index date

There are several possible starting dates for calculating survival. The one most widely available in population-based cancer registries is the incidence date. This date, as provided by the registries, was taken as the index date for this study. A review of the definitions used by the registries for coding the incidence date did not reveal any substantial variation. Such a variation might lead to minimal differences in short-term survival (<2 years) and will be less evident in long-term survival (Berrino *et al.*, 1995). The index dates in this study ranged from 1 January 1982 and 31 December 1992.

Closing date

The closing date, or date of last follow-up, varied between registries and ranged between 31 December 1993 and 31 December 1995. Each patient's vital status was classified as dead, alive or lost to follow-up as on the closing date.

Survival time

This was calculated as the time (in months) between the index date and the date of death from any cause *or* date of loss to follow-up *or* the closing date, whichever was earliest. The date of loss to follow-up was assumed to be the middle of the year/month if only the year/month was known; it was taken to be 31 December of the calendar year if it occurred in the same calendar year as diagnosis and the precise date of loss to follow-up was not known.

Data quality indicators

Two indices of data quality were calculated: (1) the percentage of cases with histological verification of cancer diagnosis and (2) the percentage of cases registered on a death certificate only (DCO) basis. Other aspects of data quality, especially those concerned with the completeness of ascertainment and follow-up, are discussed in the chapters dealing with individual registries.

Exclusions

Two categories of cases were excluded from the analysis.

(1) Cases based on DCO registrations (i.e. ones for which no information prior to death certificate could be traced) and cases first identified at autopsy. The percentage of cases so excluded ranged from 0% to 42.7%, as specified in the registry results chapters.

(2) Cases for which no follow-up information was available after the incidence date. The percentage excluded for this reason ranged from 0% to 11.9% in different registries.

Study database

The following variables were included in the database created for analysis.

1. Registry identification number (two-digit code for each registry).
2. Sex (1: male; 2: female).
3. Age at incidence date.
4. Primary site of cancer (ICD-9: 140-208).
5. Morphology (ICD-O, first edition, where available).
6. Clinical extent of disease (1: localized; 2: regional; 3: distant metastasis; 4: unknown; where available).
7. Incidence date (mm/dd/yy).
8. Date of death/closing date/date of loss to follow-up (mm/dd/yy).
9. Vital status of patients at this date (0: dead, 1: alive, 2: lost to follow-up).
10. Survival time (in months).

Validation checks

A set of validation checks was performed prior to survival analysis. A list of the checks undertaken, with the range of errors encountered among the registries, is given in Table 5. The CHECK program (Parkin *et al.*, 1994) was used to detect inconsistencies in age, site and histology combinations. The CONVERT program (Ferlay, 1994) was used to convert primary site codes in ICD-O, first edition (WHO, 1976) and ICD-O, second edition (WHO, 1990) to ICD-9 (WHO, 1978) wherever necessary. Age at diagnosis was recalculated whenever the date of birth was available.

A list of any potential errors was returned to the registry for clarification and correction. The validation checks were then repeated on the revised data. Tables showing the proportion of cases finally excluded from the study by site are given separately in the chapters dealing with the individual registries.

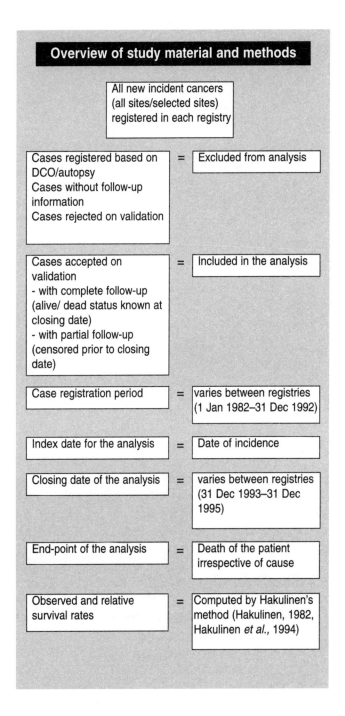

Overview of study material and methods

All new incident cancers (all sites/selected sites) registered in each registry

Cases registered based on DCO/autopsy Cases without follow-up information Cases rejected on validation	= Excluded from analysis
Cases accepted on validation - with complete follow-up (alive/ dead status known at closing date) - with partial follow-up (censored prior to closing date)	= Included in the analysis
Case registration period	= varies between registries (1 Jan 1982–31 Dec 1992)
Index date for the analysis	= Date of incidence
Closing date of the analysis	= varies between registries (31 Dec 1993–31 Dec 1995)
End-point of the analysis	= Death of the patient irrespective of cause
Observed and relative survival rates	= Computed by Hakulinen's method (Hakulinen, 1982, Hakulinen *et al.*, 1994)

Table 3. Description of sites chosen for survival analysis

ICD-9 code	Title	ICD-9 description
140	Lip	Lip
141	Tongue	Tongue
142	Salivary gland	Major salivary glands
143–5	Oral cavity	Gum, floor of mouth, unspecified parts of mouth
146	Oropharynx	Oropharynx
147	Nasopharynx	Nasopharynx
148	Hypopharynx	Hypopharynx
150	Oesophagus	Oesophagus
151	Stomach	Stomach
152	Small intestine	Small intestine
153	Colon	Colon
154	Rectum	Rectum, rectosigmoid junction, anal canal and anus
153–4	Colorectal	Colon and rectum
155	Liver	Liver
156	Gallbladder	Gallbladder
157	Pancreas	Pancreas
161	Larynx	Larynx
162	Lung	Bronchus, trachea and lung
170	Bone	Bone
171	Connective tissue	Soft and connective tissues of all regions
172	Skin melanoma	Melanoma of the skin of any part
173	Skin non-melanoma	Non-melanomatous skin of any part
174	Breast	Female breast
180	Cervix	Cervix uteri
182	Corpus uteri	Corpus uteri
183	Ovary	Ovary and other uterine adnexa
184	Vagina	Vagina, vulva and unspecified female genital organs
185	Prostate	Prostate
186	Testis	Testis
187	Penis	Penis, scrotum and unspecified male genital organ
188	Bladder	Urinary bladder
189	Kidney	Kidney, urethra and other urinary organs
191–2	Brain, nervous system	Brain and other central nervous system
193	Thyroid	Thyroid
201	Hodgkin's disease	Hodgkin's disease
200,202	Non-Hodgkin lymphoma	Lymphosarcoma and non-Hodgkin lymphoma
203	Multiple myeloma	Multiple myeloma
204	Lymphatic leukaemia	Acute, chronic and other lymphatic leukaemia
205	Myeloid leukaemia	Acute, chronic and other myeloid leukaemia
204–8	All leukaemia	All types of leukaemia
195–9	Primary site uncertain	Ill-defined sites, primary site unknown

Table 4. Criteria used for classification of clinical extent of disease

Category	Description
Localized	Tumour confined to the organ of origin, without invasion into the surrounding tissue/organ and without involvement of any regional or distant lymph nodes or organs
Regional	Tumour not confined to the organ of origin, with invasion into the surrounding tissue/organ, with or without the involvement of the regional lymph nodes and not involving the nonregional lymph nodes or organs
Distant metastasis	Tumour involving the nonregional lymph nodes or distant organs
Unknown	The above information is unknown

Table 5. Validation checks and range of errors detected among registries

Validation check	Range (%) of errors
Age or sex unknown	0.0–1.40
Date of diagnosis — out of range	0.0–0.02
Date of death/last follow-up — out of range	0.0–0.02
Cases with negative duration of survival time	0.0–0.10
Primary site code — out of range	0.0–0.03
Unlikely age and site combination	0.0–0.04
Unlikely sex and site combination	0.0–0.10
Conversion error of site code from ICD-O to ICD-9	0.0–0.01
Histology codes — out of range	0.0–0.60
Unlikely site and histology combination	0.0–0.70
In situ cancers	0.0–0.30
Invalid vital-status codes	0.0–0.30

References

Berrino, F., Sant, M., Verdecchia, A., Capocaccia, R., Hakulinen, T. & Estève, J., eds. (1995) *Survival of Cancer Patients in Europe: the EUROCARE Study* (IARC Scientific Publications No. 132). Lyon, International Agency for Research on Cancer

Ferlay, J. (1994) *ICD Conversion Programs for Cancer* (IARC Technical Report No. 21). Lyon, International Agency for Research on Cancer

Hakulinen, T. (1982) Cancer survival corrected for heterogeneity in patient withdrawal. *Biometrics*, **38**, 933–942

Hakulinen, T., Gibberd, R., Abeywickrama, K.H. & Soderman, B. (1994) *A Computer Program Package for Cancer Survival Studies, Version 2.0.* Tampere, Finnish Cancer Registry/University of Newcastle, Australia

Parkin, D.M., Chen, V.W., Ferlay, J., Galceran, J., Storm, H.H. & Whelan, S.L. (1994) *Comparability and Quality Control in Cancer Registration* (IARC Technical Report No. 19). Lyon, International Agency for Research on Cancer, pp. 61–65

WHO (1976) *International Classification of Diseases for Oncology, First Edition.* Geneva, World Health Organization

WHO (1978) *International Classification of Diseases, Ninth Revision.* Geneva, World Health Organization

WHO (1990) *International Classification of Diseases for Oncology, Second Edition.* Geneva, World Health Organization

Chapter 6

Population-based cancer survival in Qidong, People's Republic of China

Jian-Guo Chen, Wen-Guang Li, Zhuo-Cai Shen, Hong-Yu Yao, Bao-Chu Zhang, Yuan-Rong Zhu

Qidong Cancer Registry
Qidong Liver Cancer Institute,
Jiangsu 226200, People's Republic of China

Introduction

Qidong, in Jiangsu province on the east coast of China, is located at the mouth of the Yangtze river (*Chang Jiang*), to the north of Shanghai (Fig. 1). It is situated in Shanghai Economic Zone, at latitude 31°40′–32°06′ N and longitude 121°22′–121°55′ E. It is surrounded by water on three sides like a peninsula, covering an area of about 1600 km², and had a population of 1.16 million around 1994 (population density: 750/km²). The climate is generally warm and moist in spring and summer, pleasantly cool in autumn and slightly cold in winter. The annual temperature is around 14°C, the humidity is >80%, and the annual rainfall is 100–110 cm.

Administratively, there are two towns and six districts directly subordinate to the municipality. Each district is further subdivided into six townships (*Xiang*), each with about fifteen villages (*Cun*). Farming is still the major occupation,

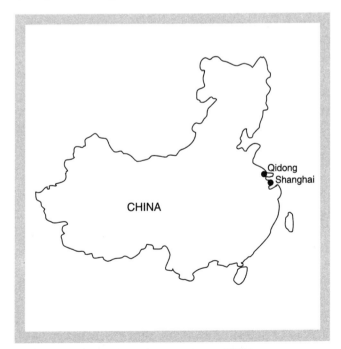

Figure 1. Map showing location of Qidong

although industrialization has been increasing in recent years.

This report describes survival from selected cancers registered in Qidong Cancer Registry during the period 1982–91.

The Qidong cancer registry

A population-based cancer registry covering the whole region and all its residents has been in existence since 1972, when the Qidong Liver Cancer Institute was established. The main aim of cancer registration in the beginning was to promote epidemiological and etiological research into liver cancer and to monitor treatment outcomes. The data from the cancer registry and the mortality registration system (which was established in 1974 as one of the seven national rural sites for disease monitoring under the supervision of the Ministry of Health of the People's Republic of China) are now widely used not only for epidemiological research into liver cancer, but also for monitoring cancer incidence and mortality for all cancer sites and evaluating cancer control programmes (Chen *et al.*, 1991a).

The registry covers a population of 1.16 million people (1994). The age structure of the population (Fig. 2) is quite different from that generally seen in developing countries, and is more like that of a developed country. The sex ratio is 1018 females to 1000 males. The proportion of subjects aged under 15 years is 18.8%, and the proportion of those aged over 65 years is 8.8%.

The cancer incidence data for the periods 1983–87 and 1988–92 from this registry were published in Volumes VI and VII of *Cancer Incidence in Five Continents* (Parkin *et al.*, 1992, 1997).

Case-finding in the Qidong cancer registry involves both active and passive methods. At district and township hospitals, there are small registries with one full-time physician or health worker from

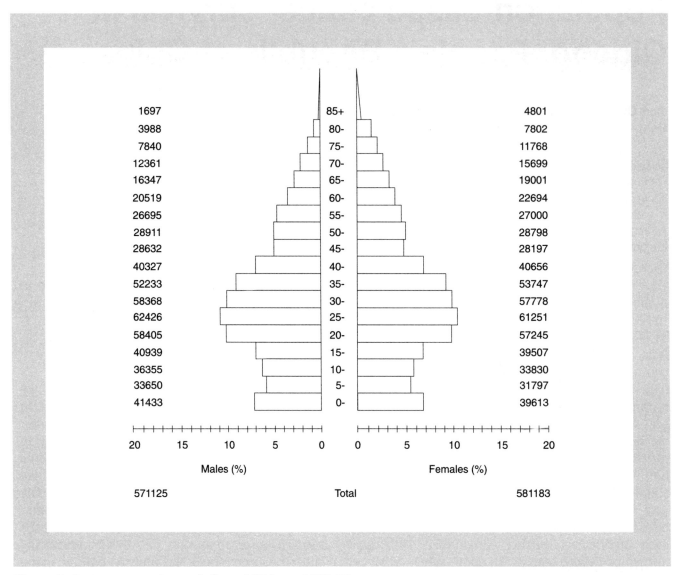

1697	85+	4801
3988	80-	7802
7840	75-	11768
12361	70-	15699
16347	65-	19001
20519	60-	22694
26695	55-	27000
28911	50-	28798
28632	45-	28197
40327	40-	40656
52233	35-	53747
58368	30-	57778
62426	25-	61251
58405	20-	57245
40939	15-	39507
36355	10-	33830
33650	5-	31797
41433	0-	39613

20 15 10 5 0   0 5 10 15 20

Males (%)   Females (%)

| 571125 | Total | 581183 |

Figure 2. Average annual population of Qidong, 1988–92

the Qidong Anti-Cancer Network acting as one of the registration personnel. The units providing primary care are also responsible for reporting incident cancer cases and cancer deaths in their region. Upon discovering any new patient with cancer in their area, the registration official will first check whether the case is an incident cancer. For confirmed incident cases, details such as name, sex, age at diagnosis, marital status, address and occupation, and basic information on date and basis of diagnosis, treatment, hospital name and outcome are collected using a special form provided by the Qidong registry. When the person eventually dies, at home or in hospital, the registration official adds the date of death to the record. Sometimes the registration official may receive information after the person's death, as a death certificate notification (DCN), rather than at the time of diagnosis, and in this case the person's medical records are reviewed or a home visit is carried out to obtain information.

Because of these efforts to trace cases back, the proportion of cases registered on a death-certificate-only (DCO) basis is very low.

The data collected by the village and district registries are reported each month to the central registry, located in the epidemiology unit of the Qidong Liver Cancer Institute. All data files received from lower-level registries and other hospitals are checked with cancer report lists and DCN cards in order to track down missing cases and exclude duplicate registrations. Until 1985, registry operations and indexing were performed manually. Computers were installed at the cancer registry in 1985, and a computerized database is now available.

Cancer incidence in Qidong

Table 1 gives the crude and age-standardized incidence rates (ASR) of all cancers in males and females in Qidong during the period 1988–92

	MALES			FEMALES		
Site	Number	Crude rate	ASR	Number	Crude rate	ASR
Lip	4	0.1	0.1	2	0.1	0.1
Tongue	4	0.1	0.1	6	0.2	0.2
Salivary gland	11	0.4	0.4	3	0.1	0.1
Mouth	8	0.3	0.3	8	0.3	0.2
Oropharynx	1	0.0	0.0	5	0.2	0.1
Nasopharynx	58	2.0	1.9	40	1.4	1.1
Hypopharynx	3	0.1	0.1	0	0.0	0.0
Oesophagus	347	12.2	11.5	181	6.2	4.6
Stomach	1292	45.2	42.7	780	26.8	20.7
Small intestine	15	0.5	0.5	17	0.6	0.4
Colon	64	2.2	2.1	79	2.7	2.0
Rectum	224	7.8	7.4	262	9.0	7.0
Liver	2336	81.8	72.1	648	22.3	19.1
Gallbladder	41	1.4	1.4	37	1.3	1.1
Pancreas	212	7.4	7.0	180	6.2	4.8
Larynx	19	0.7	0.7	2	0.1	0.1
Lung	1053	36.9	35.0	405	13.9	11.0
Bone	46	1.6	1.6	37	1.3	1.1
Connective tissue	9	0.3	0.3	6	0.2	0.2
Melanoma of skin	12	0.4	0.4	11	0.4	0.3
Other skin	40	1.4	1.4	48	1.7	1.1
Breast	3			371	12.8	11.2
Cervix uteri				97	3.3	2.6
Corpus uteri				19	0.7	0.6
Ovary				37	1.3	1.2
Prostate	15	0.5	0.5			
Testis	8	0.3	0.2			
Penis	17	0.6	0.5			
Bladder	118	4.1	4.0	30	1.0	0.7
Kidney	15	0.5	0.5	15	0.5	0.5
Brain, nervous system	97	3.4	3.2	62	2.1	2.0
Thyroid	5	0.2	0.1	17	0.6	0.5
Hodgkin's disease	2	0.1	0.1	1	0.0	0.0
Non-Hodgkin lymphoma	104	3.6	3.7	64	2.2	1.8
Multiple myeloma	37	1.3	1.3	20	0.7	0.5
Lymphoid leukaemia	31	1.1	1.1	20	0.7	0.7
Myeloid leukaemia	53	1.9	1.8	57	2.0	1.8
All sites	6400	224.1	207.1	3691	127.0	102.9
All sites without skin	6360	222.7	205.7	3643	125.4	101.9

Table 1. Annual average cancer incidence per 100 000 person-years in Qidong, People's Republic of China, 1988–92

ASR: Age-standardized incidence rate (world population).

(Parkin *et al.*, 1997). The overall ASR is twice as high in males (207.1) as in females (102.9). Liver cancer is the most common cancer in both sexes, accounting for 36.5% of male and 17.6% of female cancers. More than two-thirds of the cases occurred in those aged 30–59 years. Qidong has the highest reported incidence rate for hepatocellular carcinoma in the world, in both males and females. Hepatitis B infection has been identified as a major cause of liver cancer in Qidong (Zhu *et al.*, 1989).

The prevalence of hepatitis B surface antigen (HBsAg) in the general population is around 15% (Lu *et al.*, 1987). Aflatoxin exposure is another major risk factor (Fujimoto *et al.*, 1994; Groopman *et al.*, 1995).

The stomach is the second most common cancer site among both sexes and accounts for 20.2% of male and 21.1% of female cancers. This is followed by lung cancer, which constitutes 16.5% of male and 11.0% of female cancers. Liver, stomach and lung cancers together account for almost three-quarters of all male cancers and half of female cancers in Qidong. Breast cancer (10.1%) is the fourth most common cancer in females. Cervical cancer incidence (ASR: 2.6) is rather low in this population.

Health care services

Health care and social welfare schemes have developed rapidly in Qidong since the 1970s. There is a special office in charge of primary health care activities, as part of the work of the local health bureau. Health care services in Qidong have two systems. One is free of charge for professional persons (teachers, medical staff, scientific researchers, government staff, etc.); the other is the cooperative medical service for all inhabitants. In the near future, the two systems are likely to be merged into a health-insurance-based system.

At the basic level, there are village clinics staffed by one to three health workers with responsibilities in extended primary health care. In each township, there is a hospital with 20–50 beds, with responsibility for primary medical care. At the district level, there is a district hospital with 100–150 beds, where more specialized diagnostic and therapeutic care for various diseases is available. The tertiary care institutions include five city hospitals with 200–500 beds and the Qidong Liver Cancer Institute with 100 beds. All the city hospitals and six district hospitals are State-run; the township hospitals and village clinics are supported by local governments. Public health authorities implement health care projects mainly through hospitals at the four levels of the city, district, township and village — the so-called 'health care network'. In the past, there were almost no private clinics or practitioners in this region. Of late, a few have been established: this is a recent phenomenon accompanying the development of the market-based economy.

Pathology, cytology and haematology diagnostic services are available at all district hospitals, city hospitals and the Qidong Liver Cancer Institute. City hospitals and the Qidong Liver Cancer Institute provide radiological diagnostic facilities for cancer as well as cancer surgery and chemotherapy. Radiotherapy facilities are not available in Qidong, and patients who require this treatment are referred to Shanghai, Nanjing or Nantong.

Early detection and prevention activities

Liver cancer screening has been carried out since 1970, for early detection of liver cancer using the health care network (Zhu et al., 1989). Between 1972 and 1979, mass screening was carried out in the population using alpha-fetoprotein (AFP) assay. More than two million residents aged 15 years and over participated in this programme. Since the 1980s, a screening programme with AFP assay and testing for HBsAg has been conducted for people aged 30–69 years (Chen et al., 1991b). Several thousand subjects have been subjected to this testing, which has yielded a cohort of HBsAg carriers and non-carriers, who are currently being followed up. A randomized controlled screening trial with serial AFP estimation and ultrasonography was carried out among 5581 male HBsAg carriers, who were identified by screening the high-risk population during the period 1989–95 (Chen et al., unpublished). They were randomly assigned to a screening group (N=3712) and a control group (N=1869). Although screening resulted in early detection of liver cancer, there was little difference in mortality from liver cancer in the two groups (mortality rate 1138.1 per 100 000 person-years in the intervention group vs. 1113.9 per 100 000 in the control group).

In 1983, a hepatitis B vaccination pilot project started after the hepatitis B virus had been identified as a major cause of liver cancer in this area (Sun et al., 1991; Zhu & Sun, 1996). The target population for the vaccination study was neonates from eight townships in the pilot study, and it was later extended to 26 townships in the area. Vaccinations were given at birth, one month and six months after delivery. This programme was initially supported by the World Health Organization, the Imperial Cancer Research Fund and the Chinese Academy of Medical Sciences, and has now become a part of the extended immunization programme in the area.

Survival analysis

Subjects

A total of 17 331 incident cases in selected cancer sites, registered during the period 1982–91 in Qidong, formed the basis for the survival analysis. The distribution of these cases, the proportion of cases registered on the basis of death certificates only (DCO), the proportion of histologically verified cases and the number of cases ultimately included in the survival analysis for individual cancer sites are shown in Table 2. The percentage of DCO cases is less than 1% for all sites. The proportion of histologically verified cases ranged

Table 2. Cases of cancer registered and data quality indices, Qidong, People's Republic of China, 1982–91

Site	ICD 9	No. of cases registered	Data quality indices		Cases excluded from analysis		Cases included in survival analysis	
			% DCO	% HV	DCO	Others	No.	%
Nasopharynx	147	171	0.0	84.2	0	3	168	98.2
Oesophagus	150	979	0.1	22.0	1	12	966	98.7
Stomach	151	3861	0.2	44.8	9	98	3754	97.2
Small intestine	152	95	0.0	66.3	0	2	93	97.9
Colon	153	256	0.0	67.2	0	17	239	93.4
Rectum	154	831	0.1	75.8	1	21	809	97.4
Colorectum	153–4	1087	0.1	73.8	1	38	1048	96.4
Liver	155	5950	0.7	6.5	40	35	5875	98.7
Pancreas	157	689	0.0	28.6	0	18	671	97.4
Lung	162	2539	0.2	7.0	5	48	2486	97.9
Breast	174	644	0.0	86.7	0	48	596	92.5
Cervix	180	206	0.5	79.1	1	5	200	97.1
Bladder	188	257	0.0	68.9	0	17	240	93.4
Brain, nervous system*	191–2	277	0.4	31.8	1	4	272	98.2
Multiple myeloma	203	134	0.0	51.5	0	3	131	97.8
Myeloid leukaemia	205	134	0.0	71.6	0	6	128	95.5
All leukaemias	204–8	442	0.2	69.9	1	19	422	95.5
Total	-	17331	0.3	29.3	59	350	16922	97.6

DCO: Death certificate only; HV: Histological verification.

* Includes benign and unspecified neoplasms, number not known.

from 6.5% in liver cancer to 86.7% in breast cancer. DCO cases and 350 cases with either no follow-up information or incomplete information on date of diagnosis or death were excluded, leaving 16 922 cases (97.6% of all incident cases) for survival analysis. The proportion of cases excluded varied from 1.3% in oesophageal and liver cancer to 7.5% in breast cancer.

Follow-up methods

A mixture of passive and active methods was employed to collect information on the vital status of subjects. Certificates of death from all causes were matched with the registry database annually as a routine procedure. For cancer patients presumed to be still alive, active follow-up was conducted, which involved house visits by health workers from the village clinics. In a few cases, case records were scrutinized at the data sources to ascertain the subject's vital status.

Analytical methodology (see Chapters 2, 3 and 5)

The index date for calculating the duration of survival was the incidence date. The survival time for each case was the time between the index date and the date of death, or the cut-off date, 31 December

1994. Cumulative observed and relative survival rates were calculated using Hakulinen's method (Hakulinen, 1982; Hakulinen et al., 1994). The expected survival rate for a group of people in the general population similar to the patient group with respect to age, sex and calendar period of observation was calculated using the Qidong life tables for the years 1982–91 (Chen et al., 1996). Age-standardized relative survival (ASRS) was calculated for all ages and for the age group 0–74 years by directly standardizing the site-specific and age-specific relative survival to the site-specific age distributions of the estimated global incidence of major cancers in 1985, to facilitate comparison with other reported survival experiences from other countries.

Results

The cumulative observed and relative survival rates by site and sex are given in Table 3. The survival outcomes for sites such as oesophagus, liver, pancreas, lung, multiple myeloma and leukaemia were poor, with five-year relative survival rates less than 6%. Liver cancer had the lowest survival for both sexes combined: a five-year relative survival of 2%. One-year relative survival was greater than 80%

in the case of breast cancer, and ranged between 50% and 60% for nasopharyngeal, rectal, cervical and urinary-bladder cancers. Five-year relative survival for female breast cancer was 55.7%; it was 28.2% for nasopharyngeal cancer, 24.8% for rectal cancer, 33.6% for cervical cancer and 37.7% for cancer of the urinary bladder.

Survival rates among females were higher than among males for cancers of the nasopharynx and small intestine and lower for bladder cancer and leukaemias. There were minimal differences between the sexes in five-year relative survival for other sites.

Table 4 shows the number of cases and five-year relative survival by age group, as well as the ASRS for all ages and 0–74 years of age. Liver cancer had the lowest survival, with no differences between the age groups. There were no evident trends of survival according to age.

Discussion

Population-based survival data are useful for the evaluation of certain aspects of cancer control programmes, such as early detection, effectiveness of therapy and accessibility to diagnostic and treatment facilities across the region. But they are not easy to obtain, especially in developing countries, owing to the lack of population-based information systems and difficulties in obtaining follow-up information on vital status. In mainland China, cancer incidence data are available from population-based cancer registries in Shanghai (since 1963), Qidong (since 1972) and Tianjin (since 1978). Cancer incidence data from these sources have been published (Parkin et al., 1992). They reveal interesting differences in cancer patterns. This is the first concerted effort to obtain survival estimates in our region.

The Chinese health services, which currently rely heavily on primary health care delivery, not only improve the health of the population, but can also contribute to the establishment of information systems which will help to evaluate the impact of available health care services. Cancer registration and follow-up of cancer patients in Qidong have benefited greatly from this extensive network and from the on-going liver cancer control programmes. The very low proportion of DCO cases and cases lost to follow-up, even for cancers in sites with a poor prognosis, is a reflection of input by this integrated primary health care system.

The survival rates observed in various cancers should be interpreted against the background of satisfactory case-finding to ensure registration of all diagnosed cases, adequate follow-up and the availability of a dedicated institution for the control of liver cancer. Though our efforts resulted in the detection of an increasing proportion of early liver cancers, the proportion of early-stage liver cancers or those which underwent effective resection was too limited to influence population-based survival.

Mass screening in the general population during the 1970s (Zhu et al., 1989) and selected screening in a high-risk population since 1989 (Chen et al., 1991b) did result in detection of a higher percentage of early-stage cases. In a more recent report from the area, liver cancer screening resulted in early detection (29.6% of 257 liver cancers at stage I in the intervention group vs. 6.0% of 117 liver cancers in the control group of the randomized screening trial), but the five-year survival rates were similar in both groups (Chen et al., unpublished). This may be because there was no effective treatment for the cases detected and/or because the early-stage cases were not sufficiently numerous to influence survival over the cohort as a whole. It may also reflect the fact that patients with liver cancer need other effective therapy besides resection, as the latter offers very little chance for most patients.

Hepatitis B infection has now been established as a major cause of liver cancer in several regions of the world, including China (IARC, 1994). Vaccination against hepatitis B infection to prevent liver cancer seems to have considerable potential. There is some observational evidence of decreasing incidence of liver cancer among children following a hepatitis B vaccination programme in Taiwan (Chang et al., 1997). Future reductions in the liver cancer burden should result from this practical preventive option, now increasingly used by national governments in their extended immunization programmes.

The exceedingly low survival in cases of oesophageal, pancreatic and lung cancer is not surprising in view of the comparable results seen in developed countries with more sophisticated and technologically advanced health care. The poor survival in the case of colorectal cancers is probably due to late presentation. In cancers such as multiple myeloma and leukaemia, intensive chemotherapy-based treatment is important in improving outcome. This is not consistently available in our health services, whose emphasis is more on primary health care for common diseases. The poor survival from these cancers is therefore not surprising.

Table 3. Observed and relative survival by site and sex, Qidong, People's Republic of China, 1982–91

| Site | ICD 9 | Number included | All ages and both sexes combined | | | | | | % survival by sex at 5 years of follow-up | | | | | |
| | | | Observed survival (OS) | | | Relative survival (RS) | | | Male | | | Female | | |
			1 yr	3 yr	5 yr	1 yr	3 yr	5 yr	Number	OS	RS	Number	OS	RS
Nasopharynx	147	168	56.0	33.3	25.4	57.0	35.4	28.2	113	22.7	24.9	55	30.9	34.8
Oesophagus	150	966	16.4	5.1	3.3	17.1	5.8	4.2	653	3.3	4.2	313	3.2	4.0
Stomach	151	3754	31.6	15.7	11.8	32.7	17.5	14.3	2423	12.3	15.1	1331	11.0	13.0
Small intestine	152	93	31.2	19.4	11.0	32.2	21.4	13.1	41	5.7	6.7	52	14.8	17.9
Colon	153	239	44.4	31.4	26.2	45.8	34.8	31.4	104	25.5	29.8	135	26.9	32.8
Rectum	154	809	48.7	27.1	20.8	50.2	29.9	24.8	355	22.2	26.9	454	19.6	23.1
Colorectum	153–4	1048	47.7	28.1	22.0	49.2	31.0	26.3	459	23.0	27.6	589	21.3	25.3
Liver	155	5875	10.6	3.0	1.9	10.7	3.1	2.0	4574	1.7	1.8	1301	2.6	2.7
Pancreas	157	671	10.1	5.1	4.6	10.5	5.7	5.5	374	4.8	5.8	297	4.3	5.1
Lung	162	2486	13.5	4.1	3.0	14.0	4.6	3.6	1784	2.8	3.4	702	3.5	4.1
Breast	174	596	83.9	63.9	52.3	84.8	66.2	55.7				596	52.3	55.7
Cervix	180	200	57.5	36.5	28.9	59.2	39.9	33.6				200	28.9	33.6
Bladder	188	240	52.5	36.7	30.4	54.6	41.5	37.7	177	35.3	43.7	63	17.1	21.3
Brain, nervous system*	191–2	272	19.5	10.3	7.8	19.7	10.7	8.3	156	7.9	8.5	116	7.5	7.9
Multiple myeloma	203	131	12.2	4.6	2.0	12.6	5.0	2.3	81	1.2	1.4	50	2.9	3.3
Myeloid leukaemia	205	128	21.9	10.9	9.7	22.2	11.4	10.5	72	14.6	15.8	56	3.6	3.8
All leukaemia	204–8	422	16.6	5.9	4.4	16.8	6.2	4.7	234	5.6	6.1	188	3.0	3.2

* Includes benign and unspecified neoplasms, number not known

Five-year relative survival for breast cancer (56%) was the highest among all the sites in our study. The preliminary results of a population-based randomized intervention trial of screening for female breast cancer using breast self-examination in Shanghai, China, indicated no difference between the intervention and the control groups in the proportion of cancer cases diagnosed at an early stage (Thomas *et al.*, 1997). The comparatively higher survival observed in Shanghai is probably due to a high proportion of breast cancers being diagnosed at an early stage, as seen in the above study, possibly because of improved awareness and the extensive network of diagnostic and therapeutic facilities (*see* Chapter 7). A number of advances in understanding the natural history of breast cancer, awareness among women and physicians, early detection and local and systemic adjuvant therapies have led to varying degrees of improvement in prognosis from this cancer in several European countries (Berrino *et al.*, 1995). These advances have not yet reached all community settings in developing countries. However a focus on early detection by increasing awareness further is likely to improve the results even within the scope of existing treatment facilities.

For cervical cancer, the five-year relative survival was rather low in our setting. Early

diagnosis and treatment should be emphasized to improve outcomes for this cancer.

Though the lack of detail about several clinical factors, particularly information on clinical extent, is a severe limiting factor in our study, the results prompt certain realistic interpretations concerning outcomes from major cancers in our region. We are planning future studies with more information about clinical details in order to establish the outcome of patterns of care in our city.

To summarize, the most common cancers in Qidong occur in the digestive system: liver, stomach, oesophagus, rectum, colon and pancreas. Cancer of the lung, ranking third, shows an increasing trend and may emerge as the second major cancer, overtaking stomach cancer, in the near future (Chen *et al.*, 1991a). The above-mentioned cancer sites accounted for some 85% of all cancers in the population of this region. Unfortunately, survival from these kinds of cancers (except colorectal) is generally very poor everywhere. The low likelihood of further improvements in survival in the range of common cancers in Qidong makes it essential to maintain a strong preventive focus in our cancer control programme in order to reduce the burden from these cancers.

Table 4. Site-specific and age-specific number of cases, five-year relative survival and ASRS, Qidong, People's Republic of China, 1982–91

Site	ICD 9	Number of cases						% Relative survival (RS) at 5 years						RS	ASRS	
															All	
		≤34	35–44	45–54	55–64	65–74	75+	≤34	35–44	45–54	55–64	65–74	75+	ages	0–74
Nasopharynx	147	18	26	46	36	28	14	56.1	25.2	36.0	14.0	15.4	24.0	28.2	25.0	25.2
Oesophagus	150	7	19	86	238	351	265	0.0	0.0	9.7	3.6	3.9	3.1	4.2	4.2	4.6
Stomach	151	103	216	442	979	1226	788	16.9	22.2	22.2	17.7	11.0	3.8	14.3	13.0	17.2
Small intestine	152	4	9	9	20	27	24	25.2	22.7	11.6	21.6	6.7	0.0	13.1	8.5	14.4
Colon	153	16	17	38	49	59	60	44.1	48.0	29.2	35.7	30.3	16.0	31.4	26.7	34.1
Rectum	154	42	66	100	178	242	181	19.3	34.8	35.5	29.8	23.8	6.4	24.8	19.4	28.5
Colorectum	153–4	58	83	138	227	301	241	26.1	37.6	33.7	31.1	25.0	8.6	26.3	21.0	29.6
Liver	155	985	1626	1451	1096	540	177	2.3	2.2	1.5	2.2	2.3	0.0	2.0	1.6	2.1
Pancreas	157	17	45	74	158	239	138	11.9	6.8	4.2	4.8	7.2	1.8	5.5	4.4	6.0
Lung	162	32	98	281	710	884	481	9.5	1.0	4.8	4.3	3.3	2.0	3.6	3.3	3.9
Breast	174	50	163	160	110	73	40	59.8	60.8	62.1	47.0	51.8	23.2	55.7	49.7	55.7
Cervix	180	6	12	32	57	45	48	50.3	42.2	47.4	41.6	28.0	6.9	33.6	37.7	42.0
Bladder	188	4	6	21	71	79	59	50.5	68.3	39.3	43.0	38.3	19.2	37.7	33.0	42.8
Brain, nervous system	191–2	66	38	68	59	29	12	8.8	18.2	7.6	3.7	8.2	0.0	8.3	6.6	8.2
Multiple myeloma	203	14	8	23	28	36	22	7.2	0.0	0.0	0.0	3.4	6.4	2.3	3.5	2.7
Myeloid leukaemia	205	49	20	16	13	18	12	10.8	5.1	19.5	0.0	6.5	25.8	10.5	12.3	9.0
All leukaemia	204–8	163	59	52	52	67	29	5.9	1.7	5.0	4.2	3.6	11.2	4.7	6.0	4.7

ASRS: Age-standardized relative survival

Acknowledgements

The authors acknowledge the contribution of the staff of the Qidong Health Care Network to this important work. They thank the International Union Against Cancer (UICC) for the award of an International Cancer Research Technology Transfer (ICRETT) fellowship which enabled the first-named author to study cancer survival analysis and carry out the analysis of the data at the Unit of Descriptive Epidemiology, International Agency for Research on Cancer (IARC), Lyon, France.

References

Berrino, F., Sant, M., Verdecchia, A., Capocaccia, R., Hakulinen, T. & Estève, J., eds. (1995) *Survival of Cancer Patients in Europe: the EUROCARE Study* (IARC Scientific Publications No. 132). Lyon, International Agency for Research on Cancer

Chang, M.H., Chen, C.J., Lai, M.S., Hsu, H.M., Wu, T.C., Kong, M.S., Liang, D.C., Shau, W.Y. & Chen, D.S. (1997) Universal hepatitis B vaccination in Taiwan and the incidence of hepatocellular carcinoma in children. Taiwan Childhood Hepatoma Study Group. *N. Engl. J. Med.*, 336, 1855–1859

Chen, J.G., Peto, R., Sun, Z.T. & Zhu, Y.R. (1991a) Feasibility of a prospective study of smoking and mortality in Qidong, China. In: O'Neill, I., Chen, J. & Bartsch, H., eds., *Relevance to Human Cancer of N-Nitroso Compounds, Tobacco Smoke and Mycotoxins* (IARC Scientific Publications No. 105). Lyon, International Agency for Research on Cancer, pp. 502–506

Chen, J.G., Zhang, B.C., Jiang, Y.H., Lu, J.H., Chen, Q.G., Yun, Z.X. & Shen, Q.J. (1991b) Study on screening for primary liver cancer in high risk population of an endemic area. *Chin. J. Prev. Med.*, 25, 325–328

Chen, J.G., Li, W.G., Shen, Z.C., Yao, H.Y. & Zhu, J. (1996) Analysis of life expectancy of inhabitants in Qidong, 1974-1994. *Chin. J. Health Stat.*, 13, 37–39

Fujimoto, Y., Hampton, L.L., Wirth, P.J., Wang, N.J., Xie, J.P. & Thorgeirsson, S.S. (1994) Alterations of tumor suppressor genes and allelic losses in hepatocellular carcinomas in China. *Cancer Res.*, 54, 281–285

Groopman, J.D., Sheng, J., Scholl, P. & Kensler, T.W. (1995) Induction of aflatoxin carcinogenesis and mutational spectra. *Proc. Am. Assoc. Cancer Res.*, 36, A657–A658

Hakulinen, T. (1982) Cancer survival corrected for heterogeneity in patient withdrawal. *Biometrics*, 38, 933–942

Hakulinen, T., Gibberd, R., Abeywickrama, K.H. & Soderman, B. (1994) *A Computer Program Package for Cancer Survival Studies, Version 2.0*. Tampere, Finnish Cancer Registry/University of Newcastle, Australia

IARC (1994) *IARC Monographs on the Evaluation of Carcinogenic Risk to Humans,* Vol. 59, *Hepatitis Viruses.* Lyon, International Agency for Research on Cancer

Lu, J.H., Chen, J.G., Ni, J.P., Huang, F. & Zhu, Y.R. (1987) HBsAg carriers and hepatocellular carcinoma: a ten-year prospective study. *Chin. J. Prev. Med.*, **22**, 259–262

Parkin, D.M., Muir, C.S., Whelan, S.L., Gao, Y.-T., Ferlay, J. & Powell, J., eds. (1992) *Cancer Incidence in Five Continents,* Volume VI (IARC Scientific Publications No. 120). Lyon, International Agency for Research on Cancer

Parkin, D.M., Whelan, S.L., Ferlay, J., Raymond L. & Young J., eds. (1997) *Cancer Incidence in Five Continents,* Volume VII (IARC Scientific Publications No. 143). Lyon, International Agency for Research on Cancer

Sun, Z.T., Zhu, Y.R., Stjernsward, J., Hilleman, M., Collins, R., Zhen, Y., Hsia, C.C., Lu, J.H., Huang, F., Ni, Z., Ni, T.,

Liu, G.T., Yu, Z., Liu, Y., Chen, M. & Peto, R. (1991) Design and compliance of HBV vaccination trial on newborns to prevent hepatocellular carcinoma and 5-year results of its pilot study. *Cancer Detect. Prev.*, **15**, 313–318

Thomas, D.B., Gao, D.L., Self, S.G., Allison, C.J., Tao, Y., Mahloch, J., Ray, R., Qin, Q., Presley, R. & Porter, P. (1997) Randomized trial for breast self-examination in Shanghai: methodology and preliminary results. *J. Natl. Cancer Inst.*, **89**, 355–365

Zhu, Y.R. & Sun, Z.T. (1996) Long-term protective efficacy of HB vaccination in Qidong. *Bulletin Chin. Cancer*, **5**, 16–17

Zhu, Y.R., Chen, J.G. & Huang, X.Y. (1989) Hepatocellular carcinoma in Qidong County. In: Tang, Z.Y., Wu, M.C. & Xia, S.S., eds., *Primary Liver Cancer.* Beijing, China Academic Publishers/Springer-Verlag, pp. 202–221

Chapter 7

Cancer survival in Shanghai, People's Republic of China

Fan Jin, Yong-Bing Xiang, Yu-Tang Gao

Shanghai Cancer Registry
Shanghai Cancer Institute
Shanghai 200032
People's Republic of China

Introduction

Shanghai is the largest and the most industrialized city on the Chinese mainland and the commercial capital of the People's Republic of China. It is located on the coast of the East China Sea near the mouth of the Yangtze river, at an altitude of 4 m above sea level and at latitude 31°14′N and longitude 121°29′E (Fig. 1). The annual average temperature is approximately 15°C. The Shanghai urban area covers 748 km² and had a population of 7.1 million in 1990.

The Shanghai population-based cancer registry, covering the entire urban population of Shanghai, was established in 1963 at the Department of Epidemiology of the Shanghai Cancer Institute. Cancer incidence data from this registry were included in Volumes IV-VII of *Cancer Incidence in Five Continents* (Waterhouse *et al.*, 1982; Muir *et al.*, 1987; Parkin *et al.*, 1992, 1997). In this chapter, we present the survival experience of cancer patients in Shanghai, with background information on the cancer registration process, the pattern of cancer incidence and the organization of cancer-related health services in the region.

Cancer registration in Shanghai

The population age structure of urban Shanghai in 1990 is shown in Fig. 2. It is distinctly different from the general pattern in most developing countries. It shows comparable proportions of subjects at both ends of the age range (<15 years: 16.5%; ≥60 years: 15.7%), resembling the pattern observed in developed countries. The impact of family planning measures in this region is evident, as well as the excess of young adults commonly observed in urban areas in developing countries.

The registry relies mainly on passive case-finding. In accordance with a law promulgated by the Shanghai Municipal Bureau of Public Health, all new cases of cancer diagnosed and treated in medical facilities in Shanghai (about 160 units) must be reported to the cancer registry using a standardized notification card completed by a physician or medical clerk. The information collected includes name, age, sex, date of birth, address, occupation, primary site of cancer, incidence date, most valid basis of diagnosis, histology and reporting hospital. The notification cards received by the registry are filed by name and district of residence.

From time to time, staff members of the registry visit the medical facilities responsible for case-reporting to facilitate discussion and resolution of problems encountered in the registration process and to assess the completion of reporting. Notification cards received by the registry are checked by means of home visits by health workers from the district offices of cancer control facilities and 'street hospitals' to ascertain the residential status of the patients.

Mortality data are obtained from the Vital Statistics Section of the Shanghai Hygiene and Anti-Epidemic Centre in a standard format every month.

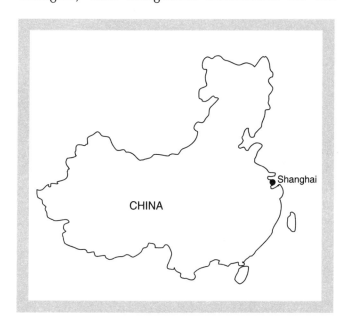

Figure 1. Map showing location of Shanghai, People's Republic of China

CHINA

Shanghai

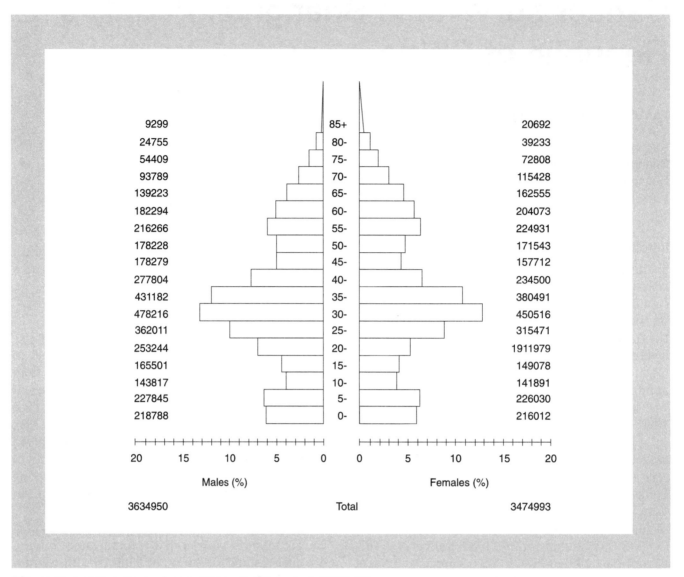

Males	Age	Females
9299	85+	20692
24755	80-	39233
54409	75-	72808
93789	70-	115428
139223	65-	162555
182294	60-	204073
216266	55-	224931
178228	50-	171543
178279	45-	157712
277804	40-	234500
431182	35-	380491
478216	30-	450516
362011	25-	315471
253244	20-	1911979
165501	15-	149078
143817	10-	141891
227845	5-	226030
218788	0-	216012

Males (%) — 20 15 10 5 0   Females (%) — 0 5 10 15 20

| 3634950 | Total | 3474993 |

Figure 2. Average annual population in Shanghai, 1988–92

These are matched with the incidence database of the registry on a routine basis. If a deceased cancer patient was not registered prior to death (a death certificate notification — DCN), his/her relatives are interviewed in a home visit to obtain information about hospital attendance and the care the person received. A misunderstanding of the DCN and death certificate only (DCO) procedures in our registration practice and a failure to search actively for evidence of prior diagnosis of cancer in cases registered from DCNs meant that a relatively high proportion of DCO cases was recorded until 1987. Since 1988, house and hospital visits by registration staff have been pursued more vigorously for all DCN cases. This has reduced the proportion of cases registered as DCO to very low levels and has improved coverage. During the period 1972-87, DCO cases ranged from 21.5% to 34.8% of all registrations; in 1988-91, they fell to 2.1% owing to improved tracing of case information for DCNs.

Records containing similar names, sex, date of birth, address, and cancer site are printed out and examined manually to try to eliminate duplicate records. The data are then coded and entered into the computer using customized computer software in dBASE III in which Chinese characters are read directly. Software written in BASIC and FORTRAN is used for analysis, with outputs produced in both Chinese and English. Initially, *International Classification of Diseases, Ninth Revision* (ICD-9) codes (WHO, 1978) were used to code the cancers registered, and Chinese characters were used to code morphology until 1996. From 1997, *International Classification of Diseases for Oncology, Second Edition* codes (WHO, 1990) have been used to code both the primary site and morphology.

The registry staff consist of a director, deputy director, six nurses, one computer technician, one statistician, two data-entry operators and 150 hospital clerks who spend part of their working time reporting cancer cases to the registry and establishing the residential status of patients.

Cancer incidence in Shanghai

Table 1 shows numbers of new cases and crude and age-standardized incidence rates of cancers in Shanghai in the period 1988-92 (Parkin *et al.*, 1997). In males, the lung (24.8%), stomach (20.5%) and liver (12.3%) are the leading cancer sites, accounting for more than half of all cancers, followed by colorectal (9.4%) and oesophageal (5.4%) cancers. These together account for three-quarters of all male cancers. In females, cancers of the breast (15.8%), stomach (14.5%), lung (12.7%), colorectum (12.1%) and liver (6.7%) predominate; these together represent more than three-fifths of all female cancers. Chinese women have relatively high rates of lung cancer compared with those in many other countries; most cases are adenocarcinomas. The incidence of invasive carcinoma of the cervix is very low.

Shanghai is one of the few cancer registries in the developing world which can provide incidence data for continuous periods of 15 years or more. The availability of incidence data since 1972 has allowed trends in cancer incidence to be studied (Coleman *et al.*, 1993; Jin *et al.*, 1993; Parkin, 1994; Boffetta & Parkin, 1994). Nasopharyngeal, oesophageal, stomach, liver, laryngeal and uterine cervical cancers have shown a declining trend in incidence. The decreasing intake of salt-preserved foods and increasing consumption of fresh fruits and vegetables may have contributed to the decline of these upper-respiratory and upper-digestive tract cancers (Gao *et al.*, 1988). The decline in stomach cancer is less obvious among women. Cervical cancer has rapidly decreased among women; the availability of cytology screening and the general improvements in living standards seem to be responsible for the decline.

Though the initial trends in lung cancer incidence indicated an increase, more recently rates have stabilized in males and even showed a decline in females, although women in Shanghai are still at high risk for lung cancer compared with women in many other countries. Examination of age-specific trends in incidence indicate rising rates only in the very old generations born before 1910 (Parkin *et al.*, 1993). Most men in Shanghai smoke, but the smoking rate among women is low (6-18%). Indoor air pollution from cooking and coal-fired heating stoves, prior history of pulmonary disease and perhaps genetic factors contribute to the high risk of lung cancer in women (Gao *et al.*, 1987; Zheng *et al.*, 1987).

There is a distinct trend of increasing incidence of colon cancer in both sexes. Rectal cancer rates have increased only slightly. Until the early 1980s, rectal cancer was more common than colon cancer in both sexes. Increasing consumption of food of animal origin and less physical activity have been identified as risk factors for colon cancer in Shanghai (Chow *et al.*, 1993; Whittemore *et al.*, 1990) and an increasing prevalence of these risk factors (Lu & Xiu, 1987) has possibly contributed to the rising incidence of colon cancer.

Breast cancer incidence has rapidly increased in Shanghai over the last two decades. A population-based case-control study in Shanghai identified early age at menarche, late age at menopause, late age at first pregnancy, lack of lactation and obesity as major risk factors for breast cancer (Yuan *et al.*, 1987). Changes among successive birth cohorts with respect to these factors, particularly in the context of the family planning programme, which stipulates one child per family, may partly explain the increased risk of breast cancer in Shanghai.

The rates for cancers of the pancreas, gallbladder, corpus uteri, ovary, prostate and brain and that for non-Hodgkin's lymphoma are relatively low. An upward trend is emerging for cancers of the pancreas, gallbladder, corpus uteri and brain, and non-Hodgkin's lymphoma. These changes in the cancer spectrum indicate the dynamics of the underlying risk factors in the community, as well as improvements in health services and reporting.

Health care services in Shanghai

With the country's improving socioeconomic profile, there has been a rapid improvement in the organization and provision of health care in China. The Chinese model of primary health care delivery has already brought improvements in the health indices of the Chinese people and has been a forerunner for development of primary health and medical care services in the developing world (WHO, 1987; Braveman & Tarimo, 1994). There have been impressive improvements in the availability of trained human resources, health services and technology. Medical schools have trained thousands of 'barefoot doctors' with the medical skills to provide basic care. China is the first developing country to manufacture its own linear accelerators at low cost for use in cancer therapy.

Health care services are entirely State-funded, and there are no private hospitals in Shanghai. The city's health facilities include thousands of small clinics associated with factories, schools, retail establishments, government offices and research organizations. There is a well developed network of cancer care services in Shanghai, with more than 100 hospitals in the city providing cancer diagnostic facilities, surgical and chemohormonal therapy for

Table 1. Annual cancer incidence per 100 000 person-years Shanghai, People's Republic of China, 1988–92

Site	MALES			FEMALES		
	Number	Crude rate	ASR	Number	Crude rate	ASR
Lip	26	0.1	0.1	12	0.1	0.0
Tongue	152	0.8	0.7	128	0.7	0.5
Salivary gland	111	0.6	0.5	98	0.6	0.4
Mouth	223	1.2	1.0	200	0.5	0.8
Oropharynx	61	0.3	0.3	35	0.1	0.1
Nasopharynx	999	5.5	4.5	389	2.2	1.8
Hypopharynx	30	0.2	0.1	11	0.1	0.0
Oesophagus	2855	15.7	12.5	1338	7.7	4.8
Stomach	10761	59.2	46.5	5584	32.1	21.0
Colon	2797	15.4	12.2	2762	15.9	10.8
Rectum	2129	11.7	9.3	1890	10.9	7.3
Liver	6459	35.5	28.2	2579	14.8	9.8
Gallbladder	577	3.2	2.5	971	5.6	3.6
Pancreas	1445	8.0	6.3	1118	6.4	4.1
Larynx	767	4.2	3.3	98	0.6	0.4
Lung	13000	71.5	56.1	4898	28.2	18.2
Bone	353	1.9	1.6	286	1.6	1.3
Connective tissue	354	1.9	1.7	273	1.6	1.3
Melanoma of skin	77	0.1	0.3	68	0.4	0.3
Other skin	362	2.0	1.7	276	1.6	1.1
Breast	86	0.5	0.4	6084	35.0	26.5
Cervix uteri				860	4.9	3.3
Corpus uteri				856	4.9	3.7
Ovary				1321	7.6	5.8
Prostate	530	2.9	2.3			
Testis	172	0.9	0.7			
Penis	66	0.4	0.3			
Bladder	1562	8.6	6.9	486	2.8	1.8
Kidney	631	3.5	2.9	371	2.1	1.6
Brain	1180	6.5	5.6	1019	5.9	4.7
Thyroid	241	1.3	1.0	670	3.9	3.0
Hodgkin's disease	88	0.5	0.4	60	0.3	0.3
Non-Hodgkin lymphoma	926	5.1	4.3	579	3.3	2.5
Multiple myeloma	162	0.9	0.7	117	0.7	0.5
Lymphoid leukaemia	235	1.3	1.5	180	1.0	1.1
Myeloid leukaemia	374	2.1	1.7	273	1.6	1.3
All sites	52466	288.7	230.5	38524	221.7	154.3
All sites except skin	52104	286.7	228.8	38248	220.1	153.2

ASR: Age-standardized incidence rate (world population).

cancer management. Forty hospitals in urban Shanghai have radiotherapy facilities. The indigenous manufacture of diagnostic and therapeutic X-ray machines at low cost has enabled the health service to provide adequate radiological imaging and radiotherapy facilities.

Palliative care services for people with advanced cancer are widely available in a number of medical facilities in urban Shanghai, and these are coordinated by the Shanghai cancer control network.

Early detection activities

There is an extensive cancer control network in Shanghai, consisting of city and district cancer control offices. These are responsible for health education, early detection of common cancers and coordination of treatment services.

In the early 1950s, a cervical cytology programme was planned for the prevention of female cervical cancer in Shanghai. This programme was formally implemented in the late 1950s. Cytology screening services have been provided since 1958 through all municipal, district and maternal and child health hospitals with the aim of taking Pap smears every 1–2 years from all sexually active women in Shanghai (Wu, 1997). Socioeconomic improvements and the wide availability of cytology and treatment facilities for cervical precursors in the various medical facilities of Shanghai are responsible for a reduction in incidence of more than 80% over the last two decades. The age-adjusted incidence rate of cervical cancer was 23.3 per 100 000 females in 1975 (Waterhouse et al., 1982) and 3.3 per 100 000 females in the period 1988-92 (Parkin et al., 1997). The experience of cervical cancer screening in Shanghai contrasts favourably with the lack of impact on incidence of and mortality from cervical cancer in other developing countries where cytology-based screening programmes have been in operation for several years (Sankaranarayanan & Pisani, 1997).

A mass screening programme for stomach cancer with miniature barium meal investigations and gastroscopy/biopsy (three-step method) or gastroscopy/biopsy (two-step method) in high-risk groups was initiated by the Shanghai Cancer Institute and the Shanghai Second Medical University in 1986. The subjects were 95 640 male workers aged 45–64 years, employed in 342 factories in urban Shanghai, who were randomized into three groups: a control group (N=26 253), a second group receiving two-step screening (N=35 713) and the third group (N=33 674) receiving three-step screening. Among the screened groups, 28 stomach cancers and 1350 precancerous lesions were diagnosed by two-step screening; 31 cancers and 423 precancerous lesions in the three-step group; 52 cancers were diagnosed in the control group. More than 50% of the cancers diagnosed in the screened groups had stage I or stage II disease, as compared with 10% in the control group. Three-year survival rates were 80% in the two-step group, 56% in the three-step group and 26% in the control group (Qui et al., 1994).

A population-based randomized intervention trial of screening for female breast cancer with breast self-examination is currently under way in Shanghai. This is a collaborative study between the Fred Hutchinson Cancer Research Centre, Seattle, USA and the Shanghai Textile Industry Bureau. The study population comprised 267 040 women aged 30–64 years and born between 1925 and 1958, employed in 520 factory units of the Shanghai Textile Industry Bureau. There are 133 375 women in the intervention group and 133 665 women in the control group. During the period 1990–94, 331 breast cancers were detected in the intervention group, giving an incidence rate of 49.6 per 100 000 person-years; the corresponding figures in the control group were 332 cancers and 49.7 per 100 000 person-years. Interim results indicate that there is no difference in the proportion of cases diagnosed at an early stage in the intervention group (57.5%) and the control group (55%), for all ages (Thomas et al., 1997)

Survival analysis

Subjects

A total of 290 696 new cancer cases were registered between 1972 and 1991 among the residents of urban Shanghai. The proportion of DCOs ranged between 21.5% and 34.8% in 1972–87: it fell sharply in 1988–91 to 2.1%, presumably owing to improved coverage and increased active registration practices. However, the figure for histological verification ranged between 35.8% and 52.1% in 1972–87 and was 47.7% in 1988–91, indicating no change. It was decided not to include incident cases from the period 1972–87 in the survival analysis in view of the high proportion of DCO cases and the likelihood of these representing an entirely different subset of cancer cases. Thus this survival study was based on 72 102 cases registered in Shanghai during the period 1988–91.

Table 2. Cases of cancer registered and data quality indices, Shanghai, People's Republic of China, 1988–91

Site	ICD 9	No. of cases registered	Data quality indices		Cases excluded from analysis		Cases included for survival analysis	
			% DCO	% HV	DCO	Others	No.	%
Lip	140	30	0.0	63.3	0	4	26	86.7
Tongue	141	226	0.9	74.3	2	20	204	90.3
Salivary gland	142	153	0.7	68.7	1	16	136	88.9
Oral cavity	143–5	336	0.3	71.4	1	37	298	88.7
Oropharynx	146	78	0.0	76.9	0	9	69	88.5
Nasopharynx	147	1121	0.6	67.4	7	127	987	88.0
Hypopharynx	148	32	0.0	68.8	0	5	27	84.4
Oesophagus	150	3371	3.3	42.1	110	117	3144	93.3
Stomach	151	13051	2.3	49.4	303	691	12057	92.4
Small intestine	152	199	1.5	64.3	3	13	183	92.0
Colon	153	4365	0.9	61.3	39	323	4003	91.7
Rectum	154	3154	1.4	64.4	44	255	2855	90.5
Colorectum	153–4	7519	1.1	62.6	83	578	6858	91.2
Liver	155	7231	3.4	13.2	245	129	6857	94.8
Gallbladder	156	1220	2.6	35.4	32	34	1154	94.6
Pancreas	157	2019	2.9	17.8	58	36	1925	95.3
Larynx	161	685	0.4	69.2	3	61	621	90.7
Lung	162	14157	2.3	39.0	319	465	13373	94.5
Bone	170	508	7.7	32.3	39	23	446	87.8
Connective tissue	171	504	1.2	70.6	6	46	452	89.7
Skin melanoma	172	125	2.4	72.0	3	10	112	89.6
Other skin	173	507	1.0	74.8	5	62	440	86.8
Breast	174	4811	0.4	71.0	21	555	4235	88.0
Cervix	180	684	0.7	66.9	5	60	619	90.5
Corpus uteri	182	676	0.3	78.2	2	84	590	87.3
Ovary	183	1038	1.3	63.8	13	84	941	90.7
Vagina	184	98	0.0	69.4	0	9	89	90.8
Prostate	185	403	2.2	45.9	9	21	373	92.6
Testis	186	144	1.4	59.0	2	21	121	84.0
Penis	187	83	0.0	73.5	0	13	70	84.3
Bladder	188	1595	1.9	59.5	30	133	1432	89.8
Kidney	189	771	1.7	49.4	13	67	691	89.6
Brain & nervous system*	191–2	1732	3.1	43.7	53	116	1563	90.2
Thyroid	193	677	0.6	70.1	4	99	574	84.8
Hodgkin's disease	201	124	0.0	80.6	0	18	106	85.5
Non-Hodgkin lymphoma	200,202	1217	1.9	69.0	23	81	1113	81.5
Multiple myeloma	203	219	2.3	63.7	5	11	203	92.7
Lymphatic leukaemia	204	329	1.2	72.9	4	28	297	90.3
Myeloid leukaemia	205	525	0.8	77.9	4	29	492	93.7
All leukaemia	204–8	1328	1.4	72.9	19	73	1236	93.1
Primary site uncertain	195–9	1531	1.3	37.8	20	63	1448	94.6
All sites	140–208	72102	2.1	47.7	1498	4155	66449	92.2

DCO : Death certificate only; HV : Histological verification

* Includes benign and unspecified neoplasms, number not known

Table 2 shows the number of cases of cancer of various sites registered in 1988–91, the proportion of histologically verified cases and DCOs, and the number of cases included in the final survival analysis. The percentage of histologically diagnosed cases ranged from 13.2% to 80.6% . The proportion of DCO cases varied from 0% to 7.7% in different sites. The major exclusions were DCO cases (2.1%) and cases without any follow-up information or with incomplete details about the exact date of diagnosis or date of death, or other incompatible follow-up information (5.8%). Thus a total of 66 449 cases (92.2% of the incident cases) were included in the final survival analysis. For each site, at least 80% of all incident cases were included.

Follow-up methods

A mixture of passive and active follow-up procedures was used. The registry receives monthly notifications of deaths from the Vital Statistics division of the Shanghai Hygiene and Anti-Epidemic Centre, which are routinely matched with the incidence database. The vital status (alive/dead) of unmatched cases was established by home visits in early 1995 by the medical workers of various street hospitals. In a few cases, information was also obtained by scrutinizing hospital case-records. The vital status was known in almost all the cases included in the study (99.8%) excepting a very few (0.2%) whose status up to the closing date could not be traced.

Analytical methodology (see Chapters 2, 3 and 5)

The index date for calculating survival time was the incidence date. The closing date for follow-up was 31 December 1994. The survival time for each case was the time between the index date and the date of death *or* date of loss to follow-up *or* 31 December 1994. Cumulative observed and relative survival probabilities were calculated using Hakulinen's method (Hakulinen, 1982; Hakulinen *et al.*, 1994). The expected survival rate for a group of people in the general population similar to the patient population with respect to age, sex, and calendar period of observation was calculated using the Shanghai life tables for 1988–91. Age-standardized relative survival (ASRS) was calculated for all age groups and for the age group 0–74 years by directly standardizing the site-specific and age-specific relative survival rates to the site-specific age distributions of the estimated global incidence of major cancers in 1985 to facilitate comparison with other reported survival experiences from other countries.

Results

The site-specific cumulative observed and relative survival for both sexes is shown in Table 3. The highest five-year relative survival was observed in the case of lip cancer (86%) and the lowest in liver cancer (4.4%). The five-year relative survival was between 70% and 80% for non-melanoma skin cancers and cancers of the breast, corpus uteri and thyroid; it was between 50% and 70% for cancers of the oral cavity, oropharynx, nasopharynx, larynx, connective tissue, cervix, testis, penis and bladder. It was less than 10% for cancers of the liver, gallbladder and pancreas. It ranged between 10% and 20% for cancers of the oesophagus, lung and bone and leukaemias. Survival at one year was already very low for cancers with a poor long-term outcome. For most cancer sites, particularly the major sites, the five-year relative survival was not greatly different between the two sexes.

Table 4 shows the site-specific and age-specific number of cases and their five-year relative survival, ASRS for all ages and ASRS for the age group 0–74 years. Declining survival with advancing age, with minor fluctuations, was observed in most cancer sites, including head and neck, stomach, pancreas, lung, connective tissue, cervix, corpus uteri, ovary, bladder, brain and thyroid, as well as lymphomas.

Discussion

The cancer survival information from Shanghai during the period 1988–91 should be interpreted against a background of changing cancer patterns and risk factors and the developments in cancer care and preventive services in this region over the last three decades. Obviously, the improvements in cancer registration achieved during this period is another factor which must be taken into account in interpreting the survival experience. For some cancers, such as cervix, breast, stomach, oesophagus, liver and lung, the impact of early detection, prevention efforts (health education, dietary advice, vaccination) and socioeconomic changes deserves particular consideration.

The cancer registration process in Shanghai has improved over the years, particularly since 1987, as a result of more active case-finding, using record clerks in the hospitals and the staff of the cancer control offices and intensified home and hospital visits by the registration staff, especially to trace the details of DCN cases. This is demonstrated by the rapid reduction in DCO cases after 1987. The coverage of multiple sources by a large number of

Table 3. Observed and relative survival by site and sex, Shanghai, People's Republic of China, 1988–91

Site	ICD 9	Number included	All ages and both sexes combined Observed survival (OS)			Relative survival (RS)			% Survival rate at 5 years of follow-up Male			Female		
			1 yr	3 yr	5 yr	1 yr	3 yr	5 yr	Number	OS	RS	Number	OS	RS
Lip	140	26	88.5	73.1	73.1	91.2	80.5	86.0	16	68.8	83.4	10	80.0	89.7
Tongue	141	204	59.8	45.6	41.8	61.2	49.1	47.5	105	39.0	44.7	99	44.8	50.5
Salivary gland	142	136	79.4	63.8	56.3	81.3	68.7	64.1	74	49.5	56.8	62	63.7	71.9
Oral cavity	143-5	298	73.5	50.7	45.0	75.6	55.2	52.1	156	45.1	53.2	142	45.0	50.9
Oropharynx	146	69	66.7	50.7	46.8	68.7	55.8	55.3	44	38.7	47.1	25	60.0	67.9
Nasopharynx	147	987	81.1	58.1	50.0	82.1	60.3	53.3	705	46.3	49.7	282	59.1	62.2
Hypopharynx	148	27	40.7	22.2	18.5	42.2	24.8	22.3	19	21.1	25.7	8	12.5	14.2
Oesophagus	150	3144	32.6	11.7	9.0	33.9	13.2	11.2	2131	8.3	10.5	1013	10.5	12.7
Stomach	151	12057	43.5	24.1	20.1	45.0	26.6	23.9	7937	20.5	24.8	4120	19.3	22.3
Small intestine	152	183	51.9	31.1	27.7	53.1	33.5	31.4	103	23.1	26.2	80	33.7	38.1
Colon	153	4003	64.4	43.7	37.7	66.2	47.5	43.5	2007	36.1	43.1	1996	39.3	44.0
Rectum	154	2855	71.1	45.5	37.1	73.0	49.3	42.8	1487	34.9	41.3	1368	39.6	44.3
Colorectum	153-4	6858	67.2	44.5	37.5	69.0	48.3	43.2	3494	35.6	42.3	3364	39.4	44.1
Liver	155	6857	14.2	5.2	3.9	14.6	5.6	4.4	4899	3.8	4.3	1958	4.1	4.8
Gallbladder	156	1154	22.7	10.5	8.0	23.5	11.6	9.5	436	8.8	10.8	718	7.6	8.7
Pancreas	157	1925	14.4	5.7	5.2	14.9	6.3	6.1	1087	5.8	6.9	838	4.4	5.1
Larynx	161	621	72.9	51.5	43.7	75.4	57.0	52.1	547	44.8	53.3	74	35.5	42.7
Lung	162	13373	32.9	12.5	9.9	34.0	13.8	11.9	9717	10.0	12.1	3656	9.7	11.3
Bone	170	446	36.8	19.3	17.0	37.6	20.8	19.4	258	16.7	19.3	188	17.4	19.6
Connective tissue	171	452	74.1	59.7	56.3	75.3	62.7	61.0	261	56.6	61.4	191	55.8	60.1
Skin melanoma	172	112	72.3	49.1	39.1	74.3	53.3	45.3	62	35.9	42.5	50	43.3	48.9
Other skin	173	440	79.5	67.0	59.4	82.9	75.8	72.7	238	61.7	74.6	202	57.0	70.7
Breast	174	4235	89.4	74.7	67.5	90.5	77.6	72.0				4235	67.5	72.0
Cervix	180	619	74.3	53.6	45.0	76.2	58.0	51.9				619	45.0	51.9
Corpus uteri	182	590	90.2	77.6	72.3	91.2	80.3	76.8				590	72.3	76.8
Ovary	183	941	65.9	47.2	41.5	66.6	48.9	44.2				941	41.5	44.2
Vagina	184	89	65.2	42.7	41.6	66.7	46.0	47.1				89	41.6	47.1
Prostate	185	373	62.5	36.2	29.6	66.0	43.0	40.1	373	29.6	40.1			
Testis	186	121	76.0	63.6	62.4	76.9	65.8	65.8	121	62.4	65.8			
Penis	187	70	78.6	64.3	55.8	81.5	71.8	67.9	70	55.8	67.9			
Bladder	188	1432	74.1	55.8	49.2	77.2	63.2	60.9	1089	51.3	64.1	343	42.3	51.2
Kidney	189	691	62.8	46.6	42.2	64.3	50.0	47.7	424	40.5	46.5	267	44.8	49.4
Brain & nervous system*	191-2	1563	48.6	35.7	32.3	49.2	37.3	34.8	860	27.2	29.8	703	38.5	40.8
Thyroid	193	574	85.9	79.6	75.8	86.7	82.0	79.7	164	66.7	71.7	410	79.4	82.8
Hodgkin's disease	201	106	64.2	51.9	45.6	64.9	53.9	48.8	69	48.3	51.0	37	40.5	44.4
Non-Hodgkin lymphoma	200,202	1113	52.2	34.2	29.8	53.4	36.5	33.4	701	28.3	31.8	412	32.3	35.9
Multiple myeloma	203	203	49.8	26.6	20.7	50.8	28.4	23.3	120	23.3	26.4	83	16.7	18.6
Lymphatic leukaemia	204	297	42.4	22.9	17.9	43.0	23.9	19.2	166	17.0	18.3	131	19.3	20.3
Myeloid leukaemia	205	492	42.9	22.4	16.0	43.4	23.2	17.1	281	15.8	16.9	211	16.7	17.8
All leukaemia	204-8	1236	36.9	18.6	14.1	37.5	19.6	15.4	689	13.9	15.1	547	14.6	15.8
Primary site uncertain	195-9	1448	25.9	12.5	9.6	26.7	13.7	11.2	800	10.0	11.8	648	9.0	10.4

* Includes benign and unspecified neoplasms, number not known.

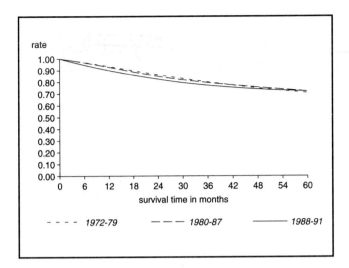

Figure 3. Trend in relative survival from breast cancer in Shanghai, 1972–91

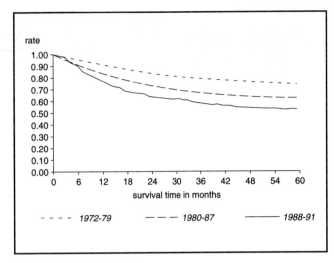

Figure 4. Trend in relative survival from cervical cancer in Shanghai, 1972–91

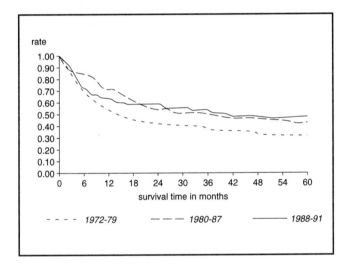

Figure 5. Trend in relative survival from Hodgkin's disease in Shanghai, 1972–91

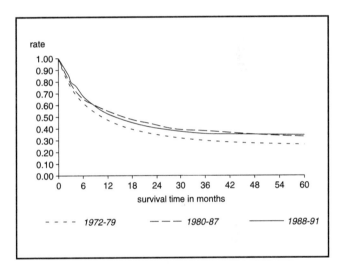

Figure 6. Trend in relative survival from non-Hodgkin lymphoma in Shanghai, 1972–91

staff, thanks to the extensive public health infrastructure of Shanghai and the experience gained over the years, indicates that cancer registration has become stable and is now fairly complete. The possibility of selection bias resulting from the exclusions must be considered. However, it is difficult to guess the direction of bias this might have caused, given the absence of details about known prognostic factors.

In Shanghai, the survival estimates obtained for several major sites (stomach, colorectum, lung, breast) are superior to the range of values generally observed in developing countries (Sankaranarayanan et al., 1996). The fact that the availability of an extensive network of diagnostic and therapeutic facilities in Shanghai ensures equitable access to services also needs to be highlighted when

interpreting the results. We believe that the particularly satisfactory results obtained in respect of some cancer sites in our population is partly due to the possibility of prompt diagnosis and treatment in the highly accessible health care services in our region. Early diagnosis of cancers in sites such as head and neck, stomach, breast, cervix, ovary, corpus uteri and testis is made possible by health education, public awareness and early detection programmes.

A major limitation of our study is the lack of information on factors such as clinical extent of disease at presentation, and treatment. In fact, this is generally a major problem of population-based survival studies, as opposed to hospital-based studies. Since data are collected from a variety of sources, predominantly by passive methods, it is a

Table 4. Site-specific and age-specific number of cases, five-year relative survival and ASRS, Shanghai, People's Republic of China, 1988–91

Site	ICD 9	Number of cases by age group						% Relative survival (RS) at 5 years						RS	ASRS%	
		≤34	35–44	45–54	55–64	65–74	75+	≤34	35–44	45–54	55–64	65–74	75+	All ages	0–74	
Lip	140	0	2	3	5	11	5	-	100.7	101.6	84.3	75.0	101.5	86.0	84.7	80.4
Tongue	141	11	18	30	61	48	36	63.9	61.5	50.8	45.8	46.0	27.7	47.5	46.3	51.0
Salivary gland	142	11	26	10	40	27	22	91.2	72.9	46.6	64.1	52.1	55.3	64.1	59.8	60.9
Oral cavity	143–5	17	17	24	88	108	44	88.1	70.6	80.8	62.1	35.7	13.6	52.1	53.8	64.0
Oropharynx	146	1	3	3	20	30	12	100.3	100.5	68.1	47.4	60.4	38.8	55.3	62.1	67.9
Nasopharynx	147	109	187	216	254	178	43	68.0	60.6	58.7	50.0	34.4	41.9	53.3	49.6	51.6
Hypopharynx	148	1	0	0	8	12	6	0.0	-	-	26.4	29.5	0.0	22.3	11.6	14.6
Oesophagus	150	9	44	146	828	1307	810	11.2	18.0	20.7	15.0	9.6	5.0	11.2	12.1	14.8
Stomach	151	420	705	920	3224	4318	2470	40.2	39.0	33.2	26.6	20.0	10.5	23.9	22.7	28.2
Small intestine	152	4	11	21	62	59	26	25.1	45.8	38.9	35.6	25.2	18.1	31.4	26.7	32.7
Colon	153	150	298	401	1167	1316	671	39.3	45.9	53.7	45.4	42.0	32.9	43.5	40.2	45.4
Rectum	154	139	262	311	807	851	485	37.9	45.4	55.7	47.4	40.7	21.3	42.8	35.7	45.7
Colorectum	153–4	289	560	712	1974	2167	1156	38.7	45.7	54.5	46.2	41.5	28.2	43.2	38.4	45.5
Liver	155	283	554	934	2180	1936	970	6.0	7.3	6.9	4.3	2.7	2.9	4.4	4.7	5.1
Gallbladder	156	11	26	79	347	447	244	27.4	5.8	17.2	9.3	9.4	5.5	9.5	10.6	12.6
Pancreas	157	23	61	154	550	733	404	13.1	9.9	8.6	6.6	5.3	4.2	6.1	6.1	7.2
Larynx	161	4	10	49	213	229	116	75.4	80.6	71.0	54.6	50.2	31.6	52.1	54.3	60.9
Lung	162	120	335	795	3929	5626	2568	24.0	17.0	17.0	14.0	10.1	7.8	11.9	11.9	13.8
Bone	170	67	27	37	106	150	59	38.4	52.2	28.7	12.5	7.8	11.4	19.4	18.9	21.9
Connective tissue	171	122	58	61	86	89	36	57.6	76.7	70.2	61.2	54.5	37.3	61.0	55.3	62.4
Skin melanoma	172	7	8	9	34	37	17	28.6	50.4	56.6	54.1	38.4	37.2	45.3	44.8	46.8
Other skin	173	10	23	47	113	129	118	100.3	87.5	84.1	71.4	61.5	75.2	72.7	74.9	74.8
Breast	174	292	931	891	1059	739	323	70.5	74.9	76.9	69.9	70.0	58.0	72.0	69.7	72.7
Cervix	180	9	21	47	189	232	121	66.9	76.6	59.5	59.8	46.1	36.9	51.9	58.8	61.9
Corpus uteri	182	21	41	143	247	105	33	85.1	88.2	76.8	79.5	67.7	55.1	76.8	72.2	76.7
Ovary	183	115	145	179	267	170	65	66.5	57.4	42.7	38.0	32.4	25.3	44.2	41.5	45.0
Vagina	184	1	4	8	26	34	16	100.3	50.2	25.5	72.1	43.0	8.7	47.1	40.8	48.9
Prostate	185	2	3	10	65	147	146	0.0	0.0	49.2	43.6	42.2	36.1	40.1	38.2	42.3
Testis	186	48	39	6	15	6	7	68.5	80.0	85.3	42.6	18.5	0.0	65.8	69.3	70.8
Penis	187	2	5	6	17	26	14	100.4	100.8	85.1	75.1	51.0	54.4	67.9	67.3	72.4
Bladder	188	27	55	76	339	567	368	86.1	81.6	67.7	72.0	55.7	44.8	60.9	57.3	66.1
Kidney	189	52	51	92	220	188	88	52.1	73.1	57.3	47.0	38.1	33.1	47.7	45.0	49.2
Brain & nervous system*	191–2	315	233	183	410	324	98	43.8	54.8	41.8	29.3	17.7	5.0	34.8	28.5	34.5
Thyroid	193	121	136	96	112	79	30	91.8	94.3	86.4	80.7	35.7	20.3	79.7	63.4	74.3
Hodgkin's disease	201	42	9	10	20	20	5	71.4	55.9	30.5	31.7	29.7	0.0	48.8	51.2	55.2
Non-Hodgkin lymphoma	200,202	180	116	116	290	271	140	41.1	36.5	38.3	35.4	25.3	23.8	33.4	32.8	35.5
Multiple myeloma	203	5	8	21	72	79	18	60.2	37.8	48.5	22.5	12.7	17.4	23.3	32.8	37.3
Lymphatic leukaemia	204	143	26	20	46	41	21	23.4	7.7	30.6	16.0	15.5	0.0	19.2	16.3	20.2
Myeloid leukaemia	205	156	77	62	84	81	32	18.7	26.0	23.8	13.9	6.3	4.4	17.1	14.9	17.4
All leukaemia	204–8	392	149	116	230	234	115	19.1	20.9	24.1	12.3	6.7	3.1	15.4	14.2	16.9
Primary site uncertain	195–9	71	100	130	397	474	276	16.7	21.5	14.9	9.6	8.7	9.4	11.2	12.3	13.0

ASRS: Age-standardized relative survival

* Includes benign and unspecified neoplasms, number not known.

Table 5. Trend of relative survival from breast cancer, Shanghai, People's Republic of China, 1972–91

Period	Total cases registered	% DCO	Cases included for analysis (%)	Relative survival (%)		
				1 year	3 years	5 years
1972–79	4715	11.8	4157 (88.2)	93.2	79.8	70.5
1980–87	6504	6.6	5469 (84.1)	92.8	79.4	71.8
1988–91	4811	0.4	4235 (88.0)	90.5	77.6	72.0

DCO: Death certificate only

Table 6. Trend of relative survival from cervical cancer Shanghai, People's Republic of China, 1972–91

Period	Total cases registered	% DCO	Cases included for analysis (%)	Relative survival (%)		
				1 year	3 years	5 years
1972–79	4644	7.3	4304 (92.7)	91.1	78.4	73.9
1980–87	1798	12.7	1457 (81.0)	83.0	67.3	61.6
1988–91	684	0.7	619 (90.5)	76.2	58.0	51.9

DCO:Death certificate only

challenge to obtain information about a number of potential prognostic factors in our setting.

The low survival rate observed in cancer sites such as lung, oesophagus, stomach, liver and pancreas indicates the need to emphasize preventive measures to reduce the future burden of these diseases. In the case of liver cancer, a reduction in exposure to aflatoxins and protection against hepatitis B infection by vaccination of infants are the possible preventive measures. For lung and pancreatic cancers, continuing education of the public on the health risks of the tobacco habit and advocacy measures should be continued in a sustained fashion to achieve reductions in exposure to tobacco smoke. Improved nutrition is the only possible preventive action for oesophageal and stomach cancers.

The five-year survival rates observed in breast cancer are impressive. No particular effect of age was evident in breast cancer survival rates across the age groups, except that survival was lower in those aged 75 years and above. Early detection and adequate treatment seem partly to explain these good results. The fact that there was apparently little difference in the proportion of cases diagnosed at an early stage between an intervention group (57.5%) and a control group (55%), for all ages, in a population-based randomized intervention trial of screening for breast cancer in 1990–94 (Thomas et al., 1997) implies that a high proportion of breast cancers in the population are already diagnosed at an early stage.

We wished to examine the survival of breast cancer patients registered in the periods 1972–79 and 1980–87 and compare it with survival in the period 1988–91. There was no appreciable difference observed in the survival rates in the three periods (Table 5; Fig. 3). The reasons could be natural history (i.e. a good proportion of breast cancers in Chinese women are less aggressive) and the advantages of longstanding, well developed and accessible health services leading to early detection of breast cancers. The interim results of the breast self-examination study (Thomas et al., 1997) also suggest that cancers were already being detected early when the study was initiated.

The five-year relative survival in cervical cancer was 52%. Survival rates decreased with advancing age. Examination of survival rates in the three time periods (1972–79, 1980–87 and 1988–91) provides interesting information about the efficacy of the cytology screening programme in Shanghai (Table 6; Fig. 4). The reductions in the annual average number of cases in the three periods indicate that many

Table 7. Trend of relative survival from Hodgkin's disease, Shanghai, People's Republic of China, 1972–91

Period	Total cases registered	% DCO	Cases included for analysis (%)	Relative survival (%)		
				1 year	3 years	5 years
1972–79	290	16.6	242 (83.4)	53.7	37.2	32.7
1980–87	175	8.6	148 (84.6)	72.4	50.2	44.2
1988–91	124	0.0	106 (85.5)	64.9	53.9	48.8

DCO: Death certificate only

Table 8. Trend of relative survival from non-Hodgkin lymphoma, Shanghai, People's Republic of China, 1972–91

Period	Total cases registered	% DCO	Cases included for analysis (%)	Relative survival (%)		
				1 year	3 years	5 years
1972-79	1273	20.6	1011 (79.4)	48.0	30.5	26.2
1980-87	1800	18.9	1383 (76.8)	53.6	37.6	33.2
1988-91	1217	1.9	1113 (91.5)	53.4	36.5	33.4

DCO: Death certificate only

invasive cervical cancers were prevented in successive years owing to the detection and treatment of cervical pre-invasive lesions. The decreasing trend in survival over time is likely to be an indication of an increasing proportion of clinically diagnosed invasive cervical cancers which escaped detection by screening, probably because they were fast-developing or occurred in individuals who had never undergone screening.

We are aware of the concern in some circles that the dramatic reduction in invasive cervical cancer incidence observed in Shanghai may reflect a misclassification of pre-invasive lesions as invasive cancer in the early years of cancer registration. While this may have happened in the initial years to some extent, the reduction in incidence does seem to reflect a reduced risk due to socioeconomic development as well as a genuine screening effect.

The poor survival rate of people with cancers of the colorectum and laryngeal and other head and neck cancers is likely to be due to late diagnosis of cases. Survival rates decreased with old age in head/neck and rectal cancers; the age effect was less evident in colon cancer. The good prognosis associated with cancers of the corpus uteri and thyroid is well known.

The poor survival in lymphomas and leukaemias indicates that therapeutic services for these malignancies must improve considerably in order to increase the survival rate and reduce mortality. It seems that results in the case of lymphomas have improved somewhat over the last 20 years. Tables 7 and 8 show survival in Hodgkin's disease and non-Hodgkin lymphoma respectively in three consecutive time periods (1972–79, 1980–87 and 1988–91). The same information is shown in Figs. 5 and 6. In the first period, the exclusions were mostly DCO cases. In the last two periods, in addition to DCO cases, those without follow-up have been excluded. Even with all the possible data limitations, the improvement in survival is most likely due to some improvement in the availability of treatment over time.

Implications

Despite the difficulties of population-based cancer registration, there should be an attempt to collect information on a number of potential prognostic factors, such as clinical extent of disease (stage of disease) and details of treatment at least for important cancer sites, if cancer registries wish to improve their contribution to the evaluation of cancer control. The cancer survival rates presented here evoke some valid arguments for effective directions in cancer control in Shanghai and in other regions of China. Prevention of tobacco-related cancers by means of tobacco control measures (education and advocacy) is important for the control of these cancers. Among the tobacco-related cancers, there is a role for early diagnosis and treatment as a control measure only in the case of some head and neck cancers. Vaccination against hepatitis B infection is important for the control of liver cancer. Promoting healthy nutrition through education about culinary practices as part of sociocultural measures should receive further attention for the control of digestive-tract cancers. Introduction of treatment protocols agreed by consensus and ensuring the availability of adequate chemotherapeutic drugs and supportive care are important in improving survival and reducing mortality from testicular tumours, ovarian cancers, lymphomas and leukaemias.

Acknowledgements

The authors gratefully acknowledge the contribution of hundreds of health care workers in Shanghai, the outcome of whose work is reflected in this chapter. We also thank the International Union Against Cancer (UICC), Geneva, Switzerland, for awarding an International Cancer Research Technology Transfer (ICRETT) fellowship to Dr Xiang, which enabled him to learn analytical methods in cancer survival and to analyse our data in the Unit of Descriptive Epidemiology, International Agency for Research on Cancer (IARC), Lyon, France.

References

Boffetta, P. & Parkin, D.M. (1994) Cancer in developing countries. *Ca, Cancer J. Clin.*, **44**, 81–90

Braveman, P.A. & Tarimo, E. (1994) *Screening in Health Care. Setting Priorities with Limited Resources*. Geneva, World Health Organization

Coleman, M.P., Estève, J., Damiecki, P., Arslan, A. & Renard, H. (1993) *Trends in Cancer Incidence and Mortality* (IARC Scientific Publications No. 121). Lyon, International Agency for Research on Cancer

Chow, W.H., Dosemeci, M., Zheng, W., Vetter, R., McLaughlin, J.K., Gao, Y.-T. & Blot, W.J. (1993) Physical activity and occupational risk of colon cancer in Shanghai, China. *Int. J. Epidemiol.*, **22**, 23–29

Gao, Y.-T., Blot, W.J., Zheng, W., Ershow, A.G., Levin, L.I., Zhang, R. & Fraumeni, J.F., Jr (1987) Lung cancer among Chinese women. *Int. J. Cancer*, **40**, 604–609

Gao, Y.T., Gao, R.N. & Jin, F. (1988) A changing cancer pattern in Shanghai urban area. *Tumor (Shanghai)*, **8**, 3–6

Hakulinen, T. (1982) Cancer survival corrected for heterogeneity in patient withdrawal. *Biometrics*, **38**, 933–942

Hakulinen, T., Gibberd, R., Abeywickrama, K.H. & Soderman, B. (1994) *A Computer Program Package for Cancer Survival Studies, Version 2.0*. Tampere, Finnish Cancer Registry/University of Newcastle, Australia

Jin, F., Devesa, S.S., Zheng, W., Blot, W.J., Fraumeni, J.F., Jr & Gao, Y.-T. (1993) Cancer incidence, trends in urban Shanghai, 1972–1989. *Int. J. Cancer*, **53**, 764–770

Lu, R.F. & Xiu, D.D. (1987) A study of association between cancer incidence and diet in Shanghai. *Tumor (Shanghai)*, **7**, 68–70

Muir, C., Waterhouse, J., Mack, T., Powell, J. & Whelan, S., eds. (1987) *Cancer Incidence in Five Continents*, Volume V (IARC Scientific Publications No. 88). Lyon, International Agency for Research on Cancer

Parkin, D.M. (1994) Cancer in developing countries. In: Doll, R., Fraumeni, J.F. & Muir, C.S. eds., Trends in cancer incidence and mortality. *Cancer Surveys*, **19/20**, 519–561Parkin, D.M., Muir, C.S., Whelan, S.L., Gao, Y.-T., Ferlay, J. & Powell, J., eds. (1992) *Cancer Incidence in Five Continents*, Volume VI (IARC Scientific Publications No. 120). Lyon, International Agency for Research on Cancer

Parkin, D.M., Pisani, P. & Ferlay, J. (1993) Estimates of the world-wide incidence of eighteen major cancers in 1985. *Int. J. Cancer*, **54**, 594–606

Parkin, D.M., Whelan, S.L., Ferlay, J., Raymond L. & Young J., eds. (1997) *Cancer Incidence in Five Continents*, Volume VII (IARC Scientific Publications No. 143). Lyon, International Agency for Research on Cancer

Qui, X.Y., Shi, K.X. & Shi, R. (1994) Mass screening for gastric cancer-establishment of pattern recognition method and its application. *Chinese J. Hlth. Stat.*, **11**, 47–50

Sankaranarayanan, R. & Pisani, P. (1997) Prevention measures in the third world: are they practical? In: Franco, E. & Monsonego, J., eds., *New Developments in Cervical Cancer Screening and Prevention*. Oxford, Blackwell Science Publishers, pp. 70–83

Sankaranarayanan, R., Swaminathan, R. & Black, R.J. (for Study Group on Cancer Survival in Developing Countries) (1996) Global variations in cancer survival. *Cancer*, **78**, 2461–2464

Thomas, D.B., Gao, D.L., Self, S.G., Allison, C.J., Tao, Y., Mahloch, J., Ray, R., Qin, Q., Presley, R. & Porter, P. (1997) Randomized trial for breast self-examination in Shanghai: methodology and preliminary results. *J. Natl. Cancer Inst.*, **89**, 355–365

Waterhouse, J., Muir, C., Shanmugaratnam, K. & Powell, J., eds. (1982) *Cancer Incidence in Five Continents*,

Volume IV (IARC Scientific Publications No. 42). Lyon, International Agency for Research on Cancer

Whittemore, A.S., Wu-Williams, A.H., Lee, M., Zheng, S., Gallagher, R.P., Jiao, D.A., Zhou, L., Wang, X.H., Chen, K., Jung, D., The, C.Z., Ling, C.D., Xu, J.Y., Paffenbarger, R.S., Jr & Henderson, B.E. (1990) Diet, physical activity, and colorectal cancer among Chinese in North America and China. *J. Natl. Cancer Inst.*, **82**, 915–926

WHO (1978) *International Classification of Diseases, Ninth Revision.* Geneva, World Health Organization

WHO (1987) *The Community Health Worker.* Geneva, World Health Organization

WHO (1990) *International Classification of Diseases for Oncology,* Second Edition. Geneva, World Health Organization

Wu, A.R. (1997) Secondary prevention of cervical cancer. *Bull. Chinese Cancer*, **6**, 8–11

Yuan, J.M., Gao, Y.-T., Yu, M.C. & Henderson, B.E. (1987) The risk factors of female breast cancer in Shanghai. *Tumor (Shanghai)*, **7**, 244–248

Zheng, W., Blot, W.J., Liao, M.L., Levin, L.I., Zhao, J.J., Fraumeni, J.F., Jr & Gao, Y.-T. (1987) Lung cancer and prior tuberculosis infection in Shanghai. *Br. J. Cancer*, **56**, 501–504

Chapter 8

Cancer survival in Cuba

Leticia Fernandez Garrote,
Margarita Graupera Boschmonar
Yaima Galan Alvarez, Marta Lezcano Cicilli
Antonio Martin Garcia, Rolando Camacho Rodriguez

National Institute of Oncology and Radiobiology
Havana, Cuba

Introduction

Cuba is the biggest island of the Caribbean archipelago with an area of 114 524 km^2 (Fig. 1) and 11 million inhabitants in 1995, with a sex ratio of 988 females to 1000 males. The structure of the population is shown in Fig. 2. Less than one-quarter of the population is under 15 years of age and those aged 65 and over constitute just over 8%. The country is divided into 14 provinces. It has a unique national health care system emphasizing primary health and medical care, which is readily accessible to the population throughout the country. Cuba is one of the very few developing countries to have a reliable nationwide death registration system. In this chapter, we discuss survival from selected cancers in Cuba in the context of background information on cancer registration and health services in the country.

Cancer registration in Cuba

The National Registry of Cuba was established in 1964 within the framework of the national health system of Cuba. Its objectives are to describe the

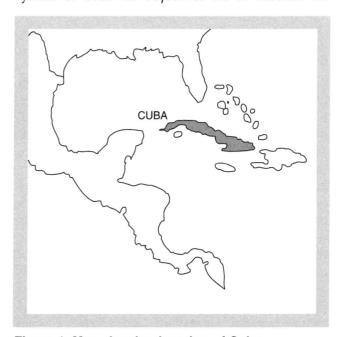

Figure 1. Map showing location of Cuba

annual cancer burden in terms of incidence and mortality, to conduct epidemiological cancer studies and to monitor and evaluate cancer control activities. Until 1986, the registry relied on voluntary reporting of cases and notifications from the death registration system. The Ministry of Public Health of the Cuban Government then made it compulsory for all secondary health facilities and physicians to report cases to the registry.

As already indicated, data collection is passive. The National Registry of Cuba receives information from two major sources: (1) hospitals and (2) death certificates through the National Statistics Directorate. The difficulty of tracing back a large number of death certificate notifications (DCN) has been a persistent problem in the registry, and hence many DCNs ended up as 'death certificate only' (DCO) registrations. Since 1995, efforts have been made to trace the relevant information.

The central office of the National Registry of Cuba is located at the National Institute of Oncology and Radiobiology, Havana, which is the coordinating body for cancer control in Cuba. Until 1991, hospital reports were collected by the provincial health offices and then sent to the registry's central office for processing. Since 1992, provincial cancer registries have been introduced, in which the information reported from the hospitals of the province is entered into the computer and checked for consistency, and duplicates are eliminated. The data are then sent to the central office, where they undergo consistency checking, duplicate checking and coding. The primary site and morphology of the cancers are coded using the *International Classification of Diseases for Oncology,* First Edition (ICD-O) (WHO, 1976). The topography is converted to *International Classification of Diseases, Ninth Revision* (ICD-9) codes for reporting purposes (WHO, 1978).

For several years, the National Registry of Cuba has published annual reports containing a detailed analysis of incident cases. Data on cancer incidence from the registry for the periods 1968-72 and 1973-77 and the year 1986 were included in Volumes III and

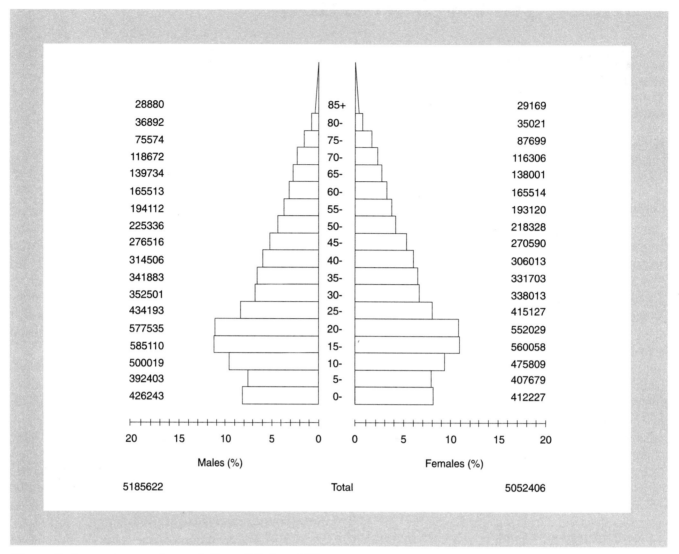

28880	85+	29169
36892	80-	35021
75574	75-	87699
118672	70-	116306
139734	65-	138001
165513	60-	165514
194112	55-	193120
225336	50-	218328
276516	45-	270590
314506	40-	306013
341883	35-	331703
352501	30-	338013
434193	25-	415127
577535	20-	552029
585110	15-	560058
500019	10-	475809
392403	5-	407679
426243	0-	412227

Males (%) — 20 15 10 5 0 — Females (%) — 0 5 10 15 20

| 5185622 | Total | 5052406 |

Figure 2. Average annual population of Cuba, 1986

IV (Waterhouse *et al.*, 1976, 1982) and VI (Parkin *et al.* 1992) of *Cancer Incidence in Five Continents*. Mortality data from Cuba have been used to study cancer trends (Coleman *et al.*, 1993). A survival study has also been reported using an earlier series of cases registered by the National Registry of Cuba (Graupera *et al.*, 1994).

Cancer incidence in Cuba

The number of cancer cases, crude and age-standardized incidence rates for males and females in 1986 are given in Table 1 (Parkin *et al.*, 1992). In men, the most common cancers are lung (20.5%), non-melanoma skin cancers (14.9%), prostate (14.0%), stomach (4.6%), bladder (4.5%), larynx (4.4%) and colon (4.4%). These seven cancer sites constitute more than two-thirds of all male cancers. Among females, the breast was the most common cancer site (17.9%) followed by non-melanoma skin cancer (12.9%) and cancers of the uterine cervix (10.2%), lung (8.6%) and colon (5.7%). These cancers account for more than

half of all female cancers. There has been an increasing trend in the occurrence of lung and breast cancers.

Cancer health services

Cuba has developed a public health care system based on extended primary care and equality of access. At the community level, there is a family physician, supported by a nurse, for every 800 people and a dentist for every 1000 people. These medical staff live among the population they serve, providing basic health care. The general hospital services have been developed to cater for the need for specialized care for people referred from the primary health care services. Cancer diagnostic services and surgery are widely available throughout the country, with a total of 984 oncology beds and 162 specialists in oncology. Three comprehensive cancer centres located in three provinces (Havana City, Camagüey and Santiago de Cuba) provide specialized diagnostic facilities, radiotherapy and chemotherapy. Twelve general hospitals provide oncology services (five in Havana City, two in Granma and one each in Matanzas, Sancti-Spiritus, Ciego de Avila, Las Tunas and Guantánamo). Overall, there are 23 chemotherapy, 11 radiotherapy and eight paediatric oncology services throughout the country to facilitate the population's access to health services.

Cancer control programme

In Cuba, a comprehensive national cancer control programme was set up in 1987, with activities in prevention (anti-smoking programme), early diagnosis, screening, oncopaediatric health care and public health education.

Since 1968, a cervical cancer screening programme with cytology screening has been provided for sexually active women aged 20 years or over. Cytology is offered at two-year intervals. Just over one million smears are performed annually, and are processed in thirty regional cytology laboratories. More than 80% of women have been screened at least once. However, the incidence of and mortality from cervical cancer have not decreased since the introduction of the screening programme (Coleman et al., 1993; Fernandez Garrote et al., 1996; Sankaranarayanan & Pisani, 1997). On the contrary, small increases in incidence and mortality have been observed, particularly among young women. A recent evaluation stated that low coverage of high-risk groups and poor quality of cytology (taking, processing and reading smears) are probably responsible for the programme's lack of impact (Fernandez Garrote et al., 1996). Since 1997, the programme has covered women aged between 25 and 59 years, concentrating on women aged 35 or over, and the interval between screenings has been increased to three years.

An early detection programme for breast cancer was implemented in 1989. The objectives were to teach breast self-examination to all women aged 30 years or over, as well as encouraging them to have their breasts examined annually by their family physician. It had been intended to offer mammography once every two years to women aged 50–64 years, but economic difficulties have meant that this has not been done. Over the last six years, 452 508 women have been invited for mammography, of whom 211 258 (47%) complied, and 542 breast cancers have been detected.

An oral cancer screening programme was introduced in 1984, which required dentists to offer an annual visual inspection to all subjects aged 15 years and over to detect oral precancers and cancers (Fernandez Garrote et al., 1995). During the period 1984–90, 13 million examinations were carried out and 30 244 subjects with lesions were identified; however, the annual participation rate of the population and compliance with referral was only 28.8%. No reductions in incidence or mortality have been observed so far. At present, the target group for the programme is people aged 35 years and over.

A pain relief and palliative care programme is being developed and extended throughout the country. Hepatitis B vaccination is offered to high-risk population groups and to all neonates routinely as part of the extended immunization protocol.

There are active health education programmes to promote awareness of cancer risk factors and to encourage people with risk factors to remain vigilant in order to promote early detection of cancers.

Survival analysis

Subjects and methods

The cancer sites considered for the survival analysis were the tongue, oral cavity, oropharynx, colorectum, lung, female breast, cervix, corpus uteri, ovary and prostate, as well as lymphoid and haemopoietic malignancies. The total number of cases registered, the proportion of DCO registrations (which are mostly DCNs), the proportion with histological verification, and the number and proportion of cases included in the final survival analysis for these cancers are shown in Table 2.

We made an attempt to trace back the DCN cases in 1994 and 1995 after we began the survival study. We could trace back only 12% of DCO registrations in 1988 and 17% of those in 1989 (a total of 2570 cases). In Cuba, hospital medical records departments are not allowed to retain the clinical records of deceased persons for more than five years. For this reason, the records of many DCN registrations from 1988 and 1989 could not be traced.

A total of 24 601 cases were registered during 1988–89 for the sites considered for analysis. Of these 8 892 cases (36.1%) were based on DCNs and could not be traced back retrospectively in 1994–95. We have excluded all these cases. The other excluded cases were those with no follow-up information (N=2905, 11.8%) and eight cases with no information about the person's age. Thus a total of 11 805 (48.0%) cases were excluded and this left 12 796 cases (52.0% of the incident cases) for final analysis. The proportion of cases included in the final survival analysis varied from 36.5% for multiple myeloma to 74% for cervical cancer.

Table 1. Average annual cancer incidence per 100 000 person-years in Cuba, 1986

Site	MALES			FEMALES		
	Number	Crude rate	ASR	Number	Crude rate	ASR
Lip	138	2.7	2.6	22	0.4	0.4
Tongue	129	2.5	2.4	58	1.1	1.1
Salivary gland	41	0.8	0.8	24	0.5	0.4
Mouth	133	2.6	2.4	74	1.5	1.3
Oropharynx	97	1.9	1.8	20	0.4	0.4
Nasopharynx	35	0.7	0.7	16	0.3	0.3
Hypopharynx	47	0.9	0.9	11	0.2	0.2
Oesophagus	290	5.6	5.2	97	1.9	1.7
Stomach	562	10.9	9.8	278	5.5	5.0
Colon	533	10.3	9.4	572	11.2	10.2
Rectum	243	4.7	4.3	240	4.7	4.3
Liver	208	4.0	3.6	203	4.0	3.6
Gallbladder	90	1.7	1.6	146	2.9	2.7
Pancreas	308	6.0	5.4	222	4.4	3.8
Larynx	539	10.4	10.2	115	2.3	2.2
Lung	2499	48.4	44.3	861	16.9	15.7
Bone	106	2.1	1.9	69	1.4	1.3
Connective tissue	81	1.6	1.4	96	1.9	1.8
Melanoma of skin	63	1.2	1.2	47	0.9	0.9
Other skin	1816	35.2	33.2	1290	25.4	23.6
Breast	12	0.2	0.2	1787	35.1	35.0
Cervix uteri				1019	20.0	20.0
Corpus uteri				294	5.8	5.7
Ovary				294	5.8	5.7
Prostate	1714	33.2	27.3			
Testis	33	0.6	0.6			
Penis	102	2.0	1.9			
Bladder	555	10.8	9.7	159	3.1	2.8
Kidney	114	2.2	2.2	67	1.3	1.3
Brain	222	4.3	4.4	178	3.5	3.6
Thyroid	61	1.2	1.1	190	3.7	3.6
Hodgkin's disease	82	1.6	1.5	147	2.9	2.8
Non-Hodgkin lymphoma	171	3.3	3.3	201	4.0	3.9
Multiple myeloma	108	2.1	1.9	139	2.7	2.5
Lymphoid leukaemia	97	1.9	2.0	139	2.7	2.6
Myeloid leukaemia	137	2.7	2.5	141	2.8	2.6
All sites	12207	236.5	217.2	9964	195.9	187.2
All sites except skin	10391	201.3	184.0	8674	170.6	163.6

ASR: Age standardized incidence rate (world population)

Follow-up

In order to establish the vital status (alive/dead) of the cases up to the closing date of 31 December 1994, a mixed (passive and active) follow-up system was used. Incidence data files were matched with the files of the National Mortality Registry for 1988–94 to identify people who had died and establish their date and cause of death. A computerized record linkage procedure was used for this purpose. The remaining cases were then matched with the files of the National Identity Registry (a repository of citizens' names and identity numbers) by manual matching of the provincial, alphabetically arranged 'apparently alive cases' with the lists of subjects maintained in the provincial offices of the National Identity Registry. Other active follow-up methods were used to establish the vital status of people whose outcome could not be ascertained by the above methods, e.g. reply-paid postal enquiries were sent to their homes and employers. The vital status of the remaining cases was checked at their hospital of attendance, using the clinical record as the source.

Of the 12 796 cases included in the study, definite information about the vital status of 12 109 cases (94.6%) was available at the closing date. The rest (5.4%) were lost to follow-up prior to that; 3% at less than one year, 1.9% at 1–4 years and 0.5% five years or more from the date of diagnosis of cancer.

Analytical methodology (see Chapters 2, 3 and 5)

The index date for calculation of survival time was the incidence date. The survival time for each case was the time between the index date and the date of death *or* date of loss to follow-up *or* 31 December 1994. Cumulative observed and relative survival rates were calculated by Hakulinen's method (Hakulinen, 1982; Hakulinen *et al.*, 1994). The expected survival rate for a group of people in the general population similar to the patient population with respect to age, sex, and calendar period of observation was calculated using the national life tables for 1988–91 (National Statistics Office, 1995). Age-standardized relative survival (ASRS) was calculated for all ages and for the age group 0–74 years by directly standardizing the site-specific and age-specific relative survival to the site-specific age distributions of the estimated global incidence of major cancers in 1985, to facilitate comparison with survival results from other countries.

Results

The site-specific cumulative one-year, three-year and five-year observed and relative survival rates for both sexes combined and five-year survival by sex are shown in Table 3. A five-year relative survival in excess of 60% was observed for cancers of the breast and corpus uteri. Survival was less than 20% in lung cancer, multiple myeloma and myeloid leukaemia. Females had a notably higher survival rate than males in tongue, oral cavity and colon cancers. The differences were minimal for lymphomas and lymphatic leukaemia. The site-specific and age-specific number of cases and five-year relative survival, ASRS for all ages and ASRS in the age group 0–74 are shown in Table 4. Survival was generally higher in younger age groups, especially for cervical cancer and lymphomas. An increasing five-year relative survival with increasing age occurred in prostate cancer.

The five-year observed survival by clinical extent of disease for selected sites is shown in Table 5 and Figs. 3–8. Five-year observed survival rates indicate comparatively higher survival rates for localized cancers, particularly in the breast and cervix. This indicates that the information collected about extent of disease is valid and reflects the range of survival experience in early and advanced cancers to a certain extent. An inverse relationship between the extent of disease and survival is clearly seen.

Discussion

A major limitation of our study is the large proportion of DCO registrations, which were excluded from the analysis. There is justifiable concern about the quality of our data and the effects this may have had on our results. However, the plausible results obtained in the case of cancer sites included in the analysis indicate that the exclusions may not have resulted in a serious degree of selection bias. We believe that the cases selected for analysis represent a reasonable sample of all persons with cancer. The excluded cases represented a sample of all the registered cases and are unlikely exclusively or predominantly to represent cancers with a poor prognosis.

In most cancer registry settings, the DCO cases are most likely to be people with cancers with aggressive natural histories, elderly people and those of low social status who could not obtain adequate treatment when they were alive. However, this does not seem to be the case with our data from Cuba. If it were, we would have seen highly inflated survival rates. This conclusion is also supported by the results of an analysis of traced-back DCNs. Measures are now being implemented to improve coverage by registering patients soon after they are diagnosed and tracing patient records promptly after death certificate notifications. This will improve cancer registration in Cuba in the future.

In spite of Cuba's well organized health services, the impact of intervention programmes could not be measured satisfactorily from cancer registration and mortality data, owing to problems of documentation and information processing. The survival investigation is very important in this context and emphasizes the need to consider ways in which our information systems can be reorganized for valid evaluation of services. Even with their limitations, the data presented here reveal the importance of early detection in improving prognosis in cancers of the oral cavity, colorectum, breast and cervix.

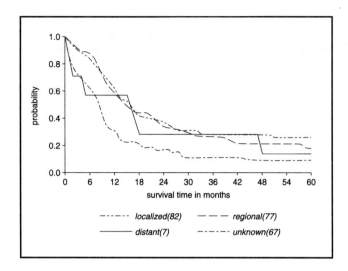

Figure 3. Survival from tongue cancer by clinical extent of disease in Cuba

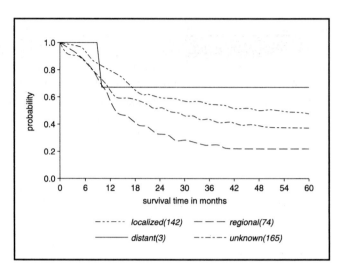

Figure 4. Survival from oral cavity cancer by clinical extent of disease in Cuba

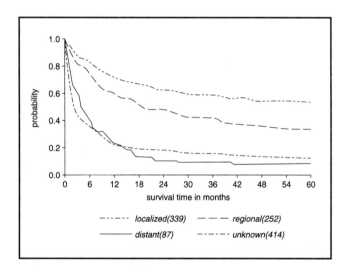

Figure 5. Survival from colon cancer by clinical extent of disease in Cuba

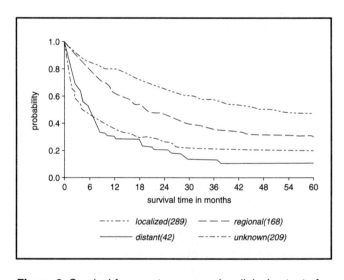

Figure 6. Survival from rectum cancer by clinical extent of disease in Cuba

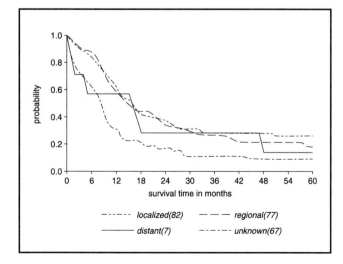

Figure 7. Survival from breast cancer by clinical extent of disease in Cuba

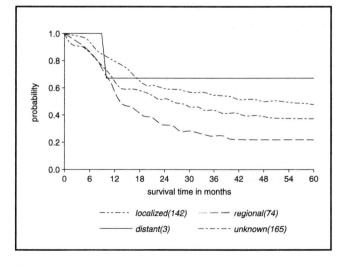

Figure 8. Survival from cervical cancer by clinical extent of disease in Cuba

Table 2. Cases of cancer registered and data quality indices, Cuba, 1988–89

Site	ICD 9	No. of cases registered	Data quality indices		Cases excluded from analysis		Cases included for survival analysis	
			% DCO	% HV	DCO	Others	No.	%
Tongue	141	341	21.7	75.1	74	34	233	68.3
Oral cavity	143–5	542	12.2	82.7	66	92	384	70.8
Oropharynx	146	178	18.5	76.4	33	34	111	62.4
Colon	153	2381	45.7	44.1	1089	200	1092	45.9
Rectum	154	1098	22.6	71.1	248	142	708	64.5
Colorectum	153–4	3479	38.4	52.6	1337	342	1800	51.7
Lung	162	6896	52.2	28.0	3597	520	2779	40.3
Breast	174	3501	19.1	73.8	668	458	2375	67.8
Cervix	180	2059	8.5	89.0	176	352	1531	74.4
Corpus uteri	182	553	8.3	88.6	46	105	402	72.7
Ovary	183	593	24.1	70.5	143	94	356	60.0
Prostate	185	3494	46.2	48.6	1614	484	1396	40.0
Hodgkin's lymphoma	201	465	26.5	73.5	123	58	284	61.1
Non-Hodgkin lymphoma	200,202	871	32.0	68.0	279	127	465	53.4
Multiple myeloma	203	480	50.4	49.6	242	63	175	36.5
Lymphatic leukaemia	204	455	34.3	65.5	156	77	222	48.8
Myeloid leukaemia	205	497	44.1	55.9	219	52	226	45.5
All leukaemia	204–8	1149	43.0	56.9	494	150	505	44.0

DCO : Death certificate only; HV : Histological verification

Implications

The major implication of this study is to show the need for a rapid improvement in coverage and the introduction of a systematic follow-up of cases, which would strengthen health information systems for a valid evaluation of cancer control measures. The existing early detection programmes also need to be made more effective. These are urgent requirements if we are to take advantage of the well developed diagnostic and therapeutic infrastructure of Cuba and sustain the progress already achieved in public health.

Acknowledgements

The authors gratefully acknowledge the award of an International Cancer Research Technology Transfer (ICRETT) fellowship by the International Union Against Cancer (UICC), Geneva, Switzerland to Mrs M. Graupera, which enabled her to study cancer survival analysis and perform a detailed analysis of our survival data at the Unit of Descriptive Epidemiology, International Agency for Research on Cancer, Lyon, France. We are grateful to IARC for the collaborative research agreement which made it easier for us to accomplish the tasks associated with this study. Thanks are due to Mayor Hilda Hernandez Soberon and the staff of the National Identity Registry for their assistance in following-up cases.

References

Coleman, M.P., Estève, J., Damiecki, P., Arslan, A. & Renard, H. (1993) *Trends in Cancer Incidence and Mortality* (IARC Scientific Publications No. 121). Lyon, International Agency for Research on Cancer

Fernandez Garrote, L., Sankaranarayanan, R., Lence Anta, J.J., Rodriguez Salva, A. & Parkin, D.M. (1995) An evaluation of the oral cancer control program in Cuba. *Epidemiology*, 6, 428–431

Fernandez Garrote, L., Lence Anta, J.J., Cabezas, E., Romero, T. & Camacho Rodriguez, R. (1996) Evaluation of the cervical cancer control program in Cuba. *Boletin OPS*, 21, 577–581

Graupera, M.C., Lence Anta, J.J., Caceres, C., Abascal, M.E. & Chacon, M. (1994) Survival rates of cancer in Cuba 1982. *Rev. Bras. Cancerol.*, 40, 135–139

Hakulinen, T. (1982) Cancer survival corrected for heterogeneity in patient withdrawal. *Biometrics*, 38, 933–942

Hakulinen, T., Gibberd, R., Abeywickrama, K.H. & Soderman, B. (1994) *A Computer Program Package for Cancer Survival Studies, Version 2.0.* Tampere, Finnish Cancer Registry/University of Newcastle, Australia

Table 3. Observed and relative survival by site and sex in Cuba, 1988-89

Site	ICD 9	Number included	All ages and both sexes combined Observed survival (OS)			Relative survival (RS)			% survival rate at 5 years by sex Male			Female		
			1 yr	3 yr	5 yr	1 yr	3 yr	5 yr	Number	OS	RS	Number	OS	RS
Tongue	141	233	52.3	23.1	19.0	56.6	27.9	25.5	172	15.8	21.8	61	28.2	35.1
Oral cavity	143–5	384	69.2	44.0	38.5	71.6	51.7	49.1	272	36.1	45.8	112	44.4	56.9
Oropharynx	146	111	65.3	31.9	27.0	70.8	37.3	33.7	89	28.7	36.3	22	19.8	23.6
Colon	153	1092	47.2	35.1	29.2	51.4	41.7	38.1	475	25.6	34.2	617	31.9	41.0
Rectum	154	708	59.5	38.2	31.7	64.8	45.6	41.7	354	30.1	40.7	354	33.4	42.6
Colorectum	153–4	1800	52.0	36.4	30.2	56.7	43.3	39.5	829	27.5	36.9	971	32.5	41.6
Lung	162	2779	23.7	10.6	8.4	25.5	12.4	10.7	2083	7.7	10.0	696	10.4	12.6
Breast	174	2375	81.1	64.6	54.0	83.8	69.5	60.8				2375	54.0	60.8
Cervix	180	1531	75.7	57.1	52.3	77.0	59.4	55.9				1531	52.3	55.9
Corpus uteri	182	402	78.4	59.3	51.7	81.6	65.5	60.9				402	51.7	60.9
Ovary	183	356	55.0	42.4	39.3	56.8	45.5	43.3				356	39.3	43.3
Prostate	185	1396	62.4	40.4	27.0	73.1	55.7	45.1	1396	27.0	45.1			
Hodgkin's lymphoma	201	284	70.3	58.5	51.0	71.9	61.2	54.9	167	50.4	54.0	117	51.9	56.2
Non-Hodgkin lymphoma	200,202	465	54.7	37.2	31.8	57.0	40.6	37.0	274	30.6	35.6	191	33.7	39.0
Multiple myeloma	203	175	40.1	21.5	14.9	41.8	23.8	17.9	104	13.7	16.7	71	17.0	19.8
Lymphatic leukaemia	204	222	49.0	33.1	27.0	51.0	36.0	30.7	137	25.6	29.1	85	29.1	33.4
Myeloid leukaemia	205	226	33.2	16.4	10.2	34.1	17.8	11.6	129	14.0	15.8	97	5.2	6.0
All leukaemia	204–8	505	40.0	24.2	18.5	41.5	26.6	21.3	299	19.3	22.3	206	17.3	20.0

Table 4. Site-specific and age-specific number of cases, five-year relative survival and ASRS in Cuba, 1988–89

Site	ICD 9	Number of cases by age group						% Relative survival (RS) at 5 years						RS	ASRS%	
		≤34	35–44	45–54	55–64	65–74	75+	≤34	35–44	45–54	55–64	65–74	75+	All ages	0–74	
Tongue	141	3	9	25	59	69	68	67.2	11.3	28.9	22.7	15.0	53.4	25.5	30.8	25.0
Oral cavity	143–5	9	18	60	83	120	94	52.9	36.1	41.9	38.7	47.0	91.6	49.1	52.4	42.4
Oropharynx	146	1	6	22	28	32	22	101.1	16.9	37.5	23.3	43.0	32.4	33.7	30.4	29.9
Colon	153	35	46	142	233	324	312	39.1	42.9	30.9	35.6	35.8	54.3	38.1	43.3	35.7
Rectum	154	14	36	85	157	199	217	36.0	33.0	34.0	43.8	41.5	50.1	41.7	43.9	39.7
Colorectum	153–4	49	82	227	390	523	529	38.3	38.6	32.1	38.9	37.9	52.6	39.5	43.5	37.2
Lung	162	27	175	387	637	849	704	26.0	12.0	13.2	7.9	9.0	15.2	10.7	11.8	10.2
Breast	174	100	400	591	553	441	290	53.7	62.1	57.9	55.7	58.7	104.0	60.8	67.2	57.9
Cervix	180	217	408	366	270	174	96	66.0	60.8	53.4	54.1	40.2	47.7	55.9	53.5	54.3
Corpus uteri	182	9	28	67	119	102	77	78.3	73.6	54.6	56.0	57.2	83.4	60.9	63.9	58.7
Ovary	183	45	51	80	85	64	31	60.3	46.8	42.0	26.2	41.4	92.5	43.3	50.1	41.1
Prostate	185	0	5	38	161	478	714	–	20.4	22.9	31.9	39.7	64.4	45.1	54.9	35.9
Hodgkin's lymphoma	201	136	38	33	38	19	20	63.8	65.5	61.0	29.1	6.3	46.8	54.9	54.3	54.8
Non-Hodgkin lymphoma	200,202	99	52	58	87	94	75	37.9	49.9	40.4	42.3	22.1	26.8	37.0	35.0	37.4
Multiple myeloma	203	0	8	24	50	56	37	–	12.7	22.8	8.6	22.9	24.3	17.9	14.9	12.2
Lymphatic leukaemia	204	104	11	13	28	36	30	38.8	39.5	7.9	39.3	13.4	8.1	30.7	26.6	31.1
Myeloid leukaemia	205	76	22	22	31	41	34	10.6	13.8	14.1	17.4	5.7	13.0	11.6	11.4	11.6
All leukaemia	204–8	200	39	37	62	91	76	27.0	20.1	11.2	25.8	9.4	19.8	21.3	21.0	21.3

– No cases; ASRS: Age-standardized relative survival

Table 5. Five-year observed survival by clinical extent of disease selected cancers in Cuba, 1988-89

Site	Clinical extent of disease classification			
	Localized	Regional	Distant	Unknown
Tongue	26.8	18.9	14.3	9.7
Oral cavity	47.8	22.0	66.7	37.7
Colon	52.4	33.0	8.4	12.1
Rectum	46.2	28.7	9.6	18.4
Breast	70.9	46.4	20.4	44.1
Cervix	70.9	34.2	24.2	41.0

National Statistics Office (1995) *Annual Statistics, 1995.* Havana, National Statistics Directorate

Parkin, D.M., Muir, C.S., Whelan, S.L., Gao, Y.-T., Ferlay, J. & Powell, J., eds. (1992) *Cancer Incidence in Five Continents,* Volume VI (IARC Scientific Publications No. 120). Lyon, International Agency for Research on Cancer

Sankaranarayanan, R. & Pisani, P. (1997) Prevention measures in the third world: are they practical? In: Franco, E. & Monsonego, J., eds., *New Developments in Cervical Cancer Screening and Prevention.* Oxford, Blackwell Science Publishers, pp. 70–83

Waterhouse, J.A.H., Muir, C.S., Correa, P. & Powell, J. (1976) *Cancer Incidence in Five Continents* Volume III (IARC Scientific Publications No. 15). Lyon, International Agency for Research on Cancer

Waterhouse, J., Muir, C., Shanmugaratnam, K. & Powell, J., eds. (1982) *Cancer Incidence in Five Continents,* Volume IV (IARC Scientific Publications No. 42). Lyon, International Agency for Research on Cancer

WHO (1976) *International Classification of Diseases for Oncology,* First Edition. Geneva, World Health Organization

WHO (1978) *International Classification of Diseases, Ninth Revision.* Geneva, World Health Organization

Chapter 9

Population-based survival from breast and cervical cancer and lymphoreticular malignancies in Bangalore, India

A. Nandakumar, N. Anantha, T.C. Venugopal

Coordinating Unit, National Cancer Registry Programme,
Indian Council of Medical Research and Population-Based Cancer
Registry, Kidwai Memorial Institute of Oncology,
Bangalore 560029, India

Introduction

Population-based cancer registration in the Bangalore urban agglomeration began in 1982 under the National Cancer Registry Programme of India, sponsored by the Indian Council of Medical Research. The registry, based at the Kidwai Memorial Institute of Oncology, covers a population of 4.5 million and an area of 191.2 km². Bangalore, the capital of Karnataka state in south India, is located at an altitude of 914 m above sea level, at latitude 12°58′N and longitude 77°38′E (Fig. 1). It is rapidly growing and is well known for high-technology industries, particularly computer software.

The registry has reported incidence data since 1982 in annual reports and in the reports published by the National Cancer Registry Programme.

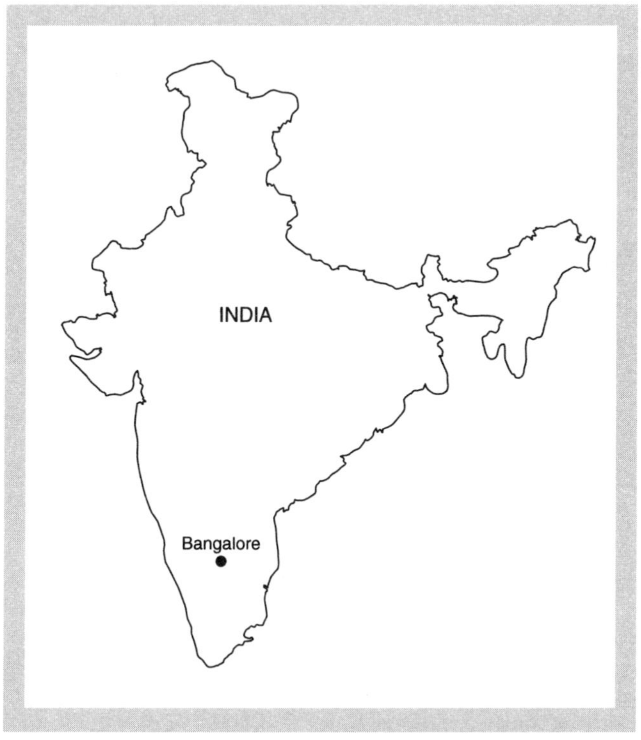

Figure 1. Map showing location of Bangalore

Incidence data were also published in Volumes V–VII of *Cancer Incidence in Five Continents* (Muir *et al.*, 1987; Parkin *et al.*, 1992, 1997). The registry has proved to be a valuable base for epidemiological and clinical investigations, as well as providing valid information for the Karnataka state cancer control programme.

The Coordinating Unit of the National Cancer Registry Programme, based at the Kidwai Memorial Institute of Oncology, and the Bangalore population-based cancer registry actively followed up cases of cancer in selected sites for the purposes of the survival study, once the routine registry operations concerning incident case-finding had stabilized. The survival experience of patients with breast cancer, uterine cervical cancer, Hodgkin's disease, non-Hodgkin lymphoma, multiple myeloma and leukaemia in our population are described in this report.

Cancer registration

Cancer registration is carried out by active case-finding carried out by 'social investigators' from the registry, who visit the various sources of data to identify incident cancer cases. The registry staff, who are university graduates in biological sciences or social sciences, have been trained or retrained in-house and in courses and workshops covering all aspects of cancer registration, organized by the National Cancer Registry Programme.

The social investigators collect information on a standard form, which is then returned to the registry for further processing. The registry has identified 30 large hospitals and 200 small hospitals as potential sources of data, and these are visited by the registry staff on a regular schedule. The Kidwai Memorial Institute of Oncology, where the registry is

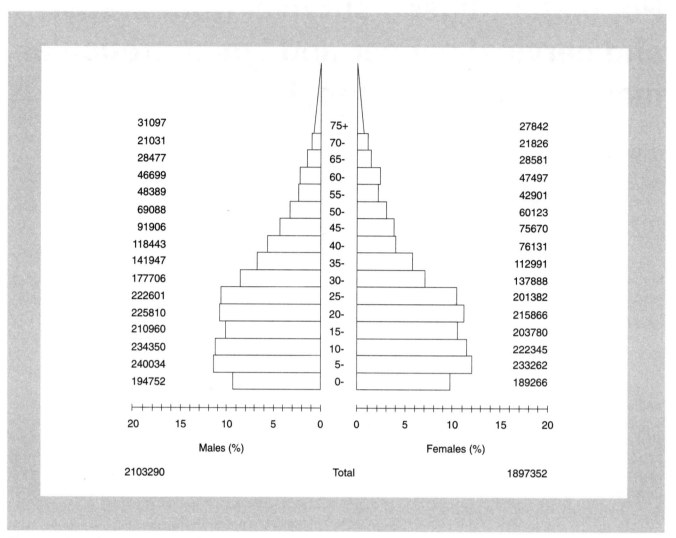

Males	Age	Females
31097	75+	27842
21031	70-	21826
28477	65-	28581
46699	60-	47497
48389	55-	42901
69088	50-	60123
91906	45-	75670
118443	40-	76131
141947	35-	112991
177706	30-	137888
222601	25-	201382
225810	20-	215866
210960	15-	203780
234350	10-	222345
240034	5-	233262
194752	0-	189266

Males (%) Females (%)

| 2103290 | Total | 1897352 |

Figure 2. Average annual population of Bangalore, 1988–92

based, is the largest source of data, accounting for two-thirds of registered cases. Records of deaths from all causes are scrutinized at 14 municipal corporation units and information on cancer deaths is abstracted. By means of personal data, these are matched with the incident cancer database. Efforts are made to trace back the unmatched cases to hospital records; if this is not successful, they are registered as 'death certificate only' (DCO) cases.

Information obtained from these various sources are processed and merged together in the registry. Data are coded using the manual of the National Cancer Registry Programme (National Cancer Registry Programme, 1987). The primary site and morphology are coded using the *International Classification of Diseases for Oncology*, First Edition (ICD-O) (WHO, 1976). The data are entered into the computer and further consistency checks and analyses are carried out in the registry. Internal quality control measures are regularly carried out. The registry staff are supervised by a medical officer, who is responsible for the quality of the data. The

data are reported using the *International Classification of Diseases, Ninth Revision* (ICD-9) codes (WHO, 1978). The data from the registry are reviewed annually in a review meeting of the National Cancer Registry Programme.

Cancer incidence in Bangalore

Table 1 gives the number of cases registered, average annual crude rates and age-standardized incidence rates for the period 1988–92 by sex and various cancer sites. Fig. 2 shows the age structure of the population, from which the incidence rates are calculated. The average annual crude and age-standardized incidence rates for all sites in males were 64.7 and 99.8 per 100 000 person-years; in females, they were 81.4 and 119.5 respectively.

The major cancer sites in males were the stomach (9.9%), oesophagus (8.3%), lung (7.4%), prostate (4.3%) and larynx (4.0%). Mouth and tongue cancer together accounted for 6.2% of the cases. Among females the common cancers were

Table 1. Annual cancer incidence per 100 000 person-years in Bangalore, India, 1988–92

Site	MALES			FEMALES		
	Number	Crude rate	ASR	Number	Crude rate	ASR
Lip	11	0.1	0.2	10	0.1	0.2
Tongue	228	2.2	3.5	70	0.7	1.2
Salivary gland	42	0.4	0.6	30	0.3	0.4
Mouth	188	1.8	2.8	534	5.6	8.9
Oropharynx	136	1.3	2.2	31	0.3	0.5
Nasopharynx	30	0.3	0.3	19	0.2	0.2
Hypopharynx	366	3.5	5.8	69	0.7	1.1
Oesophagus	557	5.3	8.8	501	5.3	8.5
Stomach	666	6.3	10.3	321	3.4	5.1
Colon	162	1.5	2.4	128	1.3	2.0
Rectum	212	2.0	3.1	172	1.8	2.8
Liver	185	1.8	2.7	80	0.8	1.3
Gallbladder	36	0.3	0.5	41	0.4	0.7
Pancreas	95	0.9	1.5	54	0.6	0.9
Larynx	267	2.5	4.3	37	0.4	0.6
Lung	495	4.7	8.1	103	1.1	1.7
Bone	97	0.9	1.0	81	0.9	0.9
Connective tissue	74	0.7	0.9	66	0.7	0.9
Melanoma of skin	21	0.2	0.3	14	0.1	0.2
Other skin	104	1.0	1.5	90	0.9	1.4
Breast	18	0.2	0.3	1381	14.6	21.3
Cervix uteri				1732	18.3	27.2
Corpus uteri				118	1.2	1.9
Ovary				293	3.1	4.3
Prostate	289	2.7	4.7			
Testis	50	0.5	0.5			
Penis	98	0.9	1.4			
Bladder	217	2.1	3.3	46	0.5	0.8
Kidney	78	0.7	1.2	45	0.5	0.7
Brain	262	2.5	3.1	132	1.4	1.6
Thyroid	92	0.9	1.1	233	2.5	3.2
Hodgkin's disease	122	1.2	1.3	52	0.5	0.6
Non-Hodgkin lymphoma	281	2.7	3.7	142	1.5	2.1
Multiple myeloma	43	0.4	0.7	36	0.4	0.6
Lymphoid leukaemia	103	1.0	1.1	54	0.6	0.7
Myeloid leukaemia	161	1.5	1.9	127	1.3	1.6
All sites	6808	64.7	99.8	7719	81.4	119.5
All sites except skin	6704	63.7	98.3	7629	80.4	118.1

ASR: Age-standardized incidence rate (world population)

uterine cervix (22.7%), breast (18.1%), mouth (7.0%), oesophagus (6.6%) and stomach (6.6%). The highest age-standardized incidence rate of mouth cancer and the second highest rate for oesophageal cancer in females in the world are observed in Bangalore. The male-to-female ratio of age-standardized incidence rates in Bangalore is 0.3:1 for mouth cancer and 0.97:1 for oesophageal cancer. There is a declining trend in the incidence of uterine cervical cancer (Nandakumar et al., 1995a). A slow but steady increase in female breast cancer has also been observed.

Cancer-related health services

Health services in Bangalore and in the state of Karnataka are predominantly provided by the health department of the state government of Karnataka. Recently, the private and voluntary sectors have participated increasingly in the provision of secondary and tertiary care, particularly in urban areas. Secondary and tertiary medical care in Bangalore are provided by 30 large hospitals and the teaching hospitals of the five medical schools. The Kidwai Memorial Institute of Oncology is the premier comprehensive cancer centre in the state, with responsibilities for cancer control. It has good facilities

Site	ICD 9	No. of cases registered	Data quality indices		Cases excluded from analysis		Cases included for survival analysis	
			% DCO	% HV	DCO	Others	No.	%
Breast	174	1514	2.4		34	119	1361	89.9
Cervix	180	2422	1.2	91.7	28	239	2155	89.0
Hodgkin's disease	201	230	1.7	96.1	4	20	206	89.6
Non-Hodgkin lymphoma	200,202	482	2.5	93.8	12	42	428	88.8
Multiple myeloma	203	100	2.0	91.0	2	1	97	97.0
Lymphatic leukaemia	204	187	2.1	95.2	4	12	171	91.4
Myeloid leukaemia	205	287	3.1	96.2	9	8	272	94.8
All leukaemia	204-8	586	5.0	91.5	29	23	534	91.1

Table 2. Cases of cancer registered and data quality indices, Bangalore, India, 1982–89

DCO: Death certificate only; HV: Histological verification

for cancer diagnosis and therapy and provides services for 10 000 new cancer patients per year. Facilities for cancer surgery exist in several hospitals in the city; radiotherapy is provided in six hospitals besides the Kidwai Memorial Institute of Oncology. Chemotherapy is also available in several hospitals.

Prevention and early detection activities

A state cancer control programme, following the recommendations of the World Health Organization, operates in the state of Karnataka. The emphasis is on health education, aimed at tobacco control, healthy diet and early detection of cervical, breast and oral cancer. Operational research into the implementation of specific cancer control measures is a major component of the programme. The introduction of anti-tobacco health education horizontally throughout the health services, using primary health care workers, was evaluated recently and the results showed an encouraging medium-term reduction in the prevalence of the tobacco habit (Anantha et al., 1995). Efforts are also under way to promote the early detection of cervical cancer, using female health workers in the primary health care sector of the health services. There are no organized screening programmes.

Survival analysis

Subjects

A total of 5334 cases were registered during the period 1982–89 for the following cancer sites/types, for which survival is described in this paper: breast (1514), uterine cervix (2422), lymphoma (712), multiple myeloma (100) and leukaemia (586) (Table 2). More than 90% of these patients had histological verification of their cancers.

The proportion of cases registered on a DCO basis ranged from 1.2% to 5.0% in different sites; a total of 109 DCO cases were excluded from the final analysis. Those without any follow-up information after diagnosis were also excluded. A total of 4781 cases (89.6% of incident cases) were thus eligible for survival analysis (Table 2).

Follow-up methods

The follow-up methods employed by the registry are described in detail elsewhere (Nandakumar, 1993; Nandakumar et al., 1995a, 1995b, 1995c). They involved both active and passive measures. The incident cases were first matched with death certificates mentioning cancer or tumour as cause of death. For the unmatched cases, information was obtained by active follow-up measures involving home visits, postal enquiries, enquiries in the workplace and scrutiny of case records based on listings for clinical follow-up in hospitals. For more than 85% of cases, follow-up information was obtained by active methods: matching with death certificates yielded information on only a few cases, because not all deaths were registered and certification of the cause of death was sometimes inadequate or incorrect. In most cases, the person's vital status was established by house visits by trained social workers. The closing date of the study was 31 December 1993.

			All ages and both sexes combined						% Survival rate at 5 years by sex					
			Observed survival (OS)			Relative survival (RS)			Male			Female		
Site	ICD 9	Number	1 yr	3 yr	5 yr	1 yr	3 yr	5 yr	Number	OS	RS	Number	OS	RS
		included												
Breast	174	1361	82.2	55.5	41.7	83.4	58.2	45.1				1361	41.7	45.1
Cervix	180	2155	76.4	50.5	37.6	77.5	52.8	40.4				2155	37.6	40.4
Hodgkin's disease	201	206	80.3	61.7	55.1	81.1	63.6	58.0	158	54.4	57.2	48	57.8	61.0
Non-Hodgkin lymphoma	200,202	428	59.7	42.2	31.6	60.8	44.5	34.5	289	29.5	32.4	139	36.0	38.7
Multiple myeloma	203	97	64.7	31.3	22.3	66.3	33.8	25.5	61	26.2	30.2	36	14.5	16.3
Lymphatic leukaemia	204	171	50.6	34.0	29.3	51.1	35.0	30.7	117	30.3	31.8	54	27.1	28.3
Myeloid leukaemia	205	272	52.4	30.9	20.5	52.9	31.8	21.5	145	14.2	14.9	127	27.9	29.0
All leukaemia	204-8	534	48.5	29.9	22.3	49.0	30.8	23.4	322	20.4	21.4	212	25.3	26.4

Table 3. Observed and relative survival by site and sex, Bangalore, India, 1982–89

Analytical methodology (see Chapters 2, 3 and 5)

The index date for calculation of survival time was the incidence date. The survival time for each case was the time between the index date and the date of death *or* date of loss to follow up *or* 31 December 1993. Cumulative observed and relative survival probabilities were calculated using Hakulinen's method (Hakulinen, 1982; Hakulinen *et al.*, 1994). The expected survival for a group of people in the general population similar to the patient population with respect to age, sex, and calendar period of observation were calculated using the abridged life tables of the urban Indian population (Registrar General of India, 1995). Age-standardized relative survival (ASRS) was calculated for all age groups and for the age group 0–74 years by directly standardizing site-specific and age-specific relative survival to the site-specific age distributions of the estimated global incidence of major cancers in 1985 for comparison with results from other countries.

Results

The one-year, three-year, and five-year observed and relative survival rates by site are given in Table 3. The one-year relative survival rate was over 75% for cancers of the breast and uterine cervix and for Hodgkin's disease. It was less than 60% for patients with leukaemia. The five-year relative survival rates were 45.1% for breast cancer; 40.4% for cervical cancer; 58% for Hodgkin's disease; 34.5% for non-Hodgkin lymphoma; 25.5% for multiple myeloma; 30.7% for lymphatic leukaemia; and 21.5% for myeloid leukaemia.

Higher five-year relative survival rates for lymphoma and myeloid leukaemia were observed among females as compared with males; lower rates were observed in females for multiple myeloma and lymphatic leukaemia (Table 3).

Declines in relative survival were observed with advancing age in the case of cancers of the breast and cervix and non-Hodgkin lymphoma (Table 4). Fig. 3 shows the observed survival by clinical extent of disease for breast cancer. For localized breast cancer, the five-year observed survival was 56.9%; for those with regional spread it was 37.6%; and for those with distant metastasis it was 13%.

Figs. 4 and 5 show the observed survival for cervical cancer patients by clinical extent of disease and by the different stages identified by the International Federation of Gynaecologists and Obstetricians (FIGO). The five-year observed survival rates were 49.5% for localized, 36.5% for regional and 19.3% for distant-spread categories of cervical cancer. The five-year observed survival rates for the various FIGO stages were as follows: stage I: 66%; stage II: 47.4%; stage III: 33.1%; stage IV: 6.2%; stage not categorized: 41.2% (Fig. 5).

Discussion

The relative survival rates experienced by our population for the cancer sites included in the study are rather low. The poor five-year survival in the case of breast and cervical cancers in our population is not surprising, since more than two-thirds of breast cancer patients, and four-fifths of cervical cancer patients for whom details of clinical extent of disease were available, presented at the time of diagnosis with non-localized cancers. The fact that one-quarter

Site	ICD 9	Number of cases by age group						% Relative survival (RS) at 5 years						RS	ASRS%	
		≤34	35–44	45–54	55–64	65–74	75+	≤34	35–44	45–54	55–64	65–74	75+	All ages	0–74	
Breast	174	151	344	387	280	143	56	49.5	50.1	44.3	44.1	36.3	25.6	45.1	40.4	44.1
Cervix	180	163	495	697	506	233	61	46.1	46.1	41.6	35.7	31.0	27.8	40.4	38.4	39.9
Hodgkin's disease	201	108	30	33	23	9	3	69.4	47.7	43.5	33.0	80.1	0.0	58.0	54.8	59
Non-Hodgkin lymphoma	200,202	164	48	73	73	49	21	42.1	35.0	37.1	28.2	20.3	0.0	34.5	25.4	32.8
Multiple myeloma	203	2	12	24	32	22	5	50.7	34.1	30.9	20.0	16.5	33.9	25.5	32.0	31.5
Lymphatic leukaemia	204	122	9	11	16	12	1	29.8	28.3	38.6	63.1	0.0	0.0	30.7	24.8	30.8
Myeloid leukaemia	205	129	42	53	34	12	2	13.2	28.6	36.4	22.3	22.6	0.0	21.5	16.6	20.6
All leukaemia	204-8	301	57	80	60	29	7	21.1	24.4	31.4	33.2	9.4	0.0	23.4	18.2	22.6

Table 4. Site-specific and age-specific number of cases by age group, five-year relative survival and ASRS, Bangalore, India, 1982–89

ASR: Age-standardized relative survival

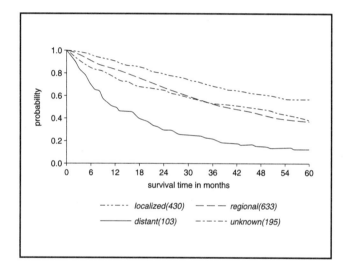

Figure 3. Survival from breast cancer by clinical extent of disease in Bangalore, India

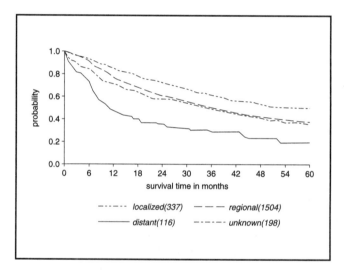

Figure 4. Survival from cervical cancer by clinical extent of disease in Bangalore, India

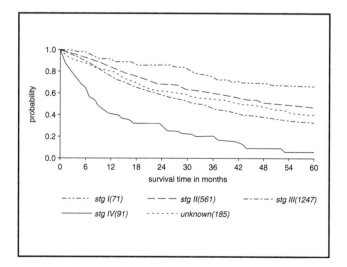

Figure 5. Survival from cervical cancer by stage of disease in Bangalore, India

of cancer patients either do not take up or do not complete their prescribed treatment at the Kidwai Memorial Institute of Oncology, the major cancer centre in the state, indicates that a good proportion of patients do not comply with treatment. This further explains the poor outcomes observed.

The age-standardized relative survival rates in our breast and cervical cancer patients (Table 4) are in the lower range of survival reported from developing countries (Sankaranarayanan *et al.*, 1996). The five-year relative survival for breast cancer observed in Bangalore is slightly lower than that reported from Madras, India (Gajalakshmi *et al.*, 1997) and from Khon Kaen, Thailand (Sriamporn *et al.*, 1995); that for cervical cancer in our population is lower than that reported from Khon Kaen, Thailand. The overall survival experience in both these sites in our population was far inferior to that in the population-based cancer registries belonging to the Surveillance Epidemiology End Results (SEER) programme of the National Cancer Institute, USA (Kosary *et al.*, 1995) and many cancer registries in Europe (Berrino *et al.*, 1995). Although there was a clear downward trend with advancing disease in both these sites, five-year survival in our localized patients was far lower than the experience reported from the SEER programme (Kosary *et al.*, 1995). Although some stage misclassifications might have accounted for the differences to some extent, the fact remains that outcomes could be further improved by changes in treatment-related factors.

Our results for Hodgkin's disease, non-Hodgkin lymphoma and leukaemia are comparable with those reported from the USA for the period 1967–73 (Axtell *et al.*, 1976). The figure for multiple myeloma is comparable with the survival reported from the SEER registries for the period 1974–86 (Ries *et al.*, 1990). Advances in treatment, particularly in the form of combination chemotherapy, have improved the outcome from these neoplasms over the last two decades. Our results for non-Hodgkin lymphoma and leukaemia are comparable with that reported from Khon Kaen, Thailand, for the period 1985–92 (Sriamporn *et al.*, 1995). The various difficulties involved in implementing such aggressive therapies in developing-country settings have led to a poor survival rate. The possibility that these neoplasms may have a different biology and natural history in developing countries cannot be entirely excluded.

The results are educative and provide valuable leads for improving outcome from these cancers. Early diagnosis and providing adequate therapy are fundamental in improving survival outcome from breast and cervical cancers. However, the vast potential for prevention in the case of cervical cancer as a means of reducing mortality and suffering from this major illness of women in developing countries should not be overlooked. Improvements in pathological categorization of lymphoreticular malignancies and adequate therapy are the main way of improving survival from lymphoreticular malignancies. Educating the public as well as reorienting the professionals involved in prevention and therapy are equally important.

Acknowledgements

The authors gratefully acknowledge the financial and technical support provided by the Indian Council of Medical Research for the Bangalore population-based cancer registry. We express our gratitude to all the staff of the Kidwai Memorial Institute of Oncology, other collaborating hospitals, laboratories and the municipal corporation of Bangalore for their kind cooperation. The contribution of all the social investigators in the cancer registry (Mr Rajanna, Mr N.M.S. Reddy, Mr Srinivas, Mr S. Swami, Ms Vinutha) by way of data collection is gratefully acknowledged.

References

Anantha, A., Nandakumar, A., Viswanath, N., Venkatesh, T., Pallad, Y.G., Manjunath, P., Kumar, D.R., Murthy, S.G.S., Shivashankariah, S. & Dayananda, C.S. (1995) Efficacy of an anti-tobacco community education program in India. *Cancer Causes Control*, 6, 119–129

Axtell, L.M., Asire, A.J., Myers, M.H. (1976) *Cancer Patient Survival; Report No. 5.* (DHEW Publication No. (NIH) 77-992). Bethesda, MD, National Cancer Institute

Berrino, F., Sant, M., Verdecchia, A., Capocaccia, R., Hakulinen, T. & Estève, J., eds. (1995) *Survival of Cancer Patients in Europe: the EUROCARE Study* (IARC Scientific Publications No. 132). Lyon, International Agency for Research on Cancer

Gajalakshmi, C.K., Shanta, V., Swaminathan, R., Sankaranarayanan, R. & Black, R.J. (1997) A population based survival study from female breast cancer in Madras, India. *Br. J. Cancer*, 75, 771–775

Hakulinen, T. (1982) Cancer survival corrected for heterogeneity in patient withdrawal. *Biometrics*, 38, 933–942

Hakulinen, T., Gibberd, R., Abeywickrama, K.H. & Soderman, B. (1994) *A Computer Program Package for Cancer Survival Studies, Version 2.0.* Tampere, Finnish Cancer Registry/University of Newcastle, Australia

Kosary, C.L., Ries, L.A.G., Miller, B.A., Hankey, B.F., Harras, A. & Edwards, B.K., eds. (1995) *SEER Cancer Statistics Review, 1973-1992: Tables and Graphs* (NIH Publication No. 96-2789). Bethesda, MD, National Cancer Institute

Muir, C., Waterhouse, J., Mack, T., Powell, J. & Whelan, S., eds. (1987) *Cancer Incidence in Five Continents*, Volume V (IARC Scientific Publications No. 88). Lyon, International Agency for Research on Cancer

Nandakumar, A. (1993) *Strategy for Active Follow-up in the Conduct of Survival Studies. Status report.* Bangalore, Coordinating Unit of National Cancer Registry Programme of India

Nandakumar, A., Anantha, N. & Venugopal, T.C. (1995a) Incidence, mortality and survival in cancer of the cervix in Bangalore, India. *Br. J. Cancer*, 71, 1348–1352

Nandakumar, A., Anantha, N., Venugopal, T.C., Sankaranarayanan, R., Thimmasetty, K. & Dhar, M. (1995b) Survival in breast cancer: A population-based study in Bangalore, India. *Int. J. Cancer*, 60, 593–596

Nandakumar, A., Anantha, N., Venugopal, T., Reddy, S., Padmanabhan, P., Swamy, K., Doval, D. & Ramarao, C. (1995c) Descriptive epidemiology of lymphoid and haemopoietic malignancies in Bangalore, India. *Int. J. Cancer*, **63**, 37–42

National Cancer Registry Programme (1987) *Code Manual For Population Based Cancer Registry*. New Delhi, Indian Council of Medical Research

Parkin, D.M., Muir, C.S., Whelan, S.L., Gao, Y.-T., Ferlay, J. & Powell, J., eds. (1992) *Cancer Incidence in Five Continents, Volume VI* (IARC Scientific Publications No. 120). Lyon, International Agency for Research on Cancer

Parkin, D.M., Whelan, S.L., Ferlay, J., Raymond L. & Young J., eds. (1997) *Cancer Incidence in Five Continents, Volume VII* (IARC Scientific Publications No. 143). Lyon, International Agency for Research on Cancer

Registrar General of India (1995) *SRS based abridged life tables 1988-92. Occasional Paper No. 4 of 1995.* New Delhi, Office of the Registrar General

Ries, L.A.G., Hankey, B.F., Edwards, B.K. (1990) *SEER Cancer Statistics Review, 1973-87* (NIH Publication No. 90-2789). Bethesda, MD, National Cancer Institute

Sankaranarayanan, R., Swaminathan, R. & Black, R.J. (for Study Group on Cancer Survival in Developing Countries) (1996) Global variations in cancer survival. *Cancer*, **78**, 2461–2464

Sriamporn, S., Black, R., Sankaranarayanan, R., Kamsa-ad, S., Parkin, D.M. & Vatanasapt, V. (1995) Cancer survival in Khon Kaen province, Thailand. *Int. J. Cancer*, **61**, 296–300

WHO (1976) *International Classification of Diseases for Oncology,* First Edition. Geneva, World Health Organization

Chapter 10

Survival from cervical cancer in Barshi registry, rural India

K. Jayant, B.M. Nene, K.A. Dinshaw, A.M. Budukh, P.S. Dale

Rural Cancer Registry
Tata Memorial Centre Rural Cancer Project
Nargis Dutt Memorial Cancer Hospital
Agalgaon Road, Barshi, India

Introduction

The first rural population-based cancer registry in India was established in 1987 in Barshi, in the state of Maharashtra in western India, as part of the National Cancer Registry Programme of the Indian Council of Medical Research, Government of India. The need for data on cancer incidence from rural areas of India had long been recognized, as more than 75% of the Indian population lives in rural areas. A realistic estimate of the national cancer burden is therefore possible only if rural cancer incidence is documented. Before the establishment of the Barshi registry, the incidence of cancer in rural areas of the country was estimated by undertaking ad hoc surveys in selected areas, at considerable cost in both money and time (Wahi, 1968; Jayant *et al.*, 1975; 1976; Gupta *et al.*, 1980). In recent years, more

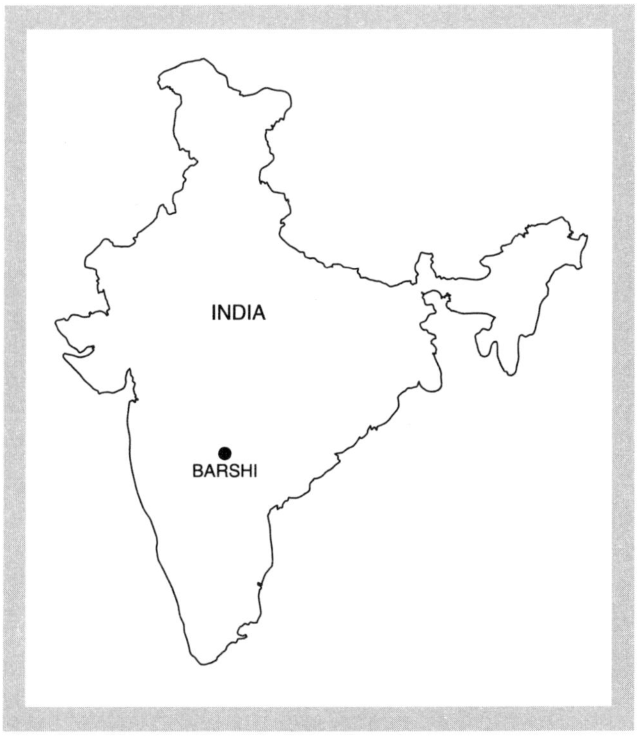

Figure 1. Map showing location of Barshi

rural cancer registries have been, or are now being, established in different parts of the country.

The Barshi cancer registry covers the rural areas of Barshi, Paranda and Bhum *tahsils* (a *tahsil* is an administrative structure equivalent to a subdistrict), with 346 villages spread over an area of 3713.4 km² in Maharashtra state, about 600 m above sea level and 400 km south-east of Bombay (Fig. 1). The village is the basic administrative unit in nonurban areas of India. Barshi *tahsil* is in Solapur district, and Paranda and Bhum *tahsils* are in Osmanabad district. The literacy level ranges from 30% to 44% in different regions of the registry area, although efforts are being made to improve it, with primary schools now established in every village.

In this chapter, we describe the population-based survival experience of cervical cancer patients in Barshi registry, and discuss the implications of the results in the context of cancer control.

Cancer registration in Barshi registry

Cancer registration in rural areas of India poses a number of challenges. Lack of medical facilities, a low literacy rate, lack of cancer awareness, poor referral practices, poor quality of records and a number of other constraints make it difficult to achieve adequate coverage of cases. We have developed a unique method of case-finding to overcome these deficiencies (Jayant *et al.*, 1989, 1991, 1995).

Case identification is undertaken by trained investigators, who visit the allotted villages at least once every six months to collect information on proven/likely cases as well as chronically ill persons. They contact all medical practitioners in the area and meet health workers from the local primary health centres at their monthly meetings. They hold group meetings to improve cancer awareness among the villagers. They also visit every tenth household in the

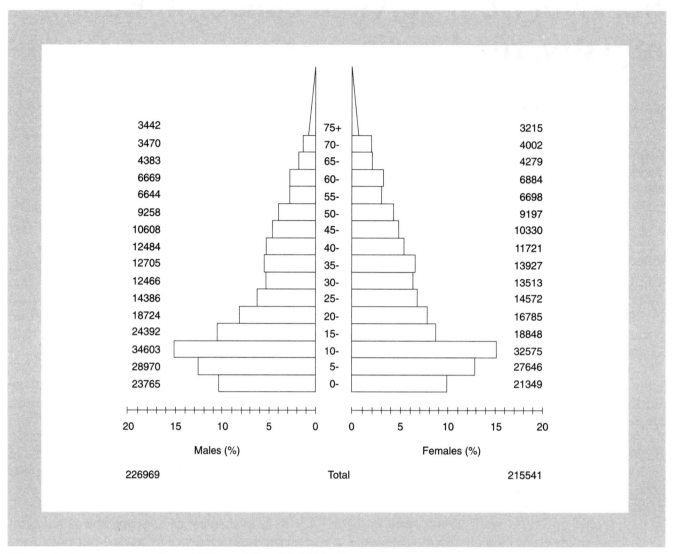

Males	Age	Females
3442	75+	3215
3470	70-	4002
4383	65-	4279
6669	60-	6884
6644	55-	6698
9258	50-	9197
10608	45-	10330
12484	40-	11721
12705	35-	13927
12466	30-	13513
14386	25-	14572
18724	20-	16785
24392	15-	18848
34603	10-	32575
28970	5-	27646
23765	0-	21349

Males (%) 20 15 10 5 0   Females (%) 0 5 10 15 20

| 226969 | Total | 215541 |

Figure 2. Average annual population of Barshi, 1988–92

village to enquire about proven or likely cancer cases. They give a referral card to any people with suspected cancer and ask them to attend the cancer hospital at Barshi quickly or to visit the opportunistic cancer detection clinics conducted in their vicinity at regular intervals. People who do not comply are revisited to ascertain whether the symptoms have persisted and to encourage them to seek medical attention.

The registry staff regularly visit hospitals within and outside the registry area (N=35), all the primary health centres in the registry area (N=15), and the cancer registries of Bombay, Pune and Aurangabad to collect information on cancer cases actively and in a standard format. Deaths are registered in the respective block development and panchayath offices attached to specific villages. Registry staff visit these offices to collect death information in a standard format.

The data collected are checked for completeness, duplicates are eliminated by visual inspection of registry lists, and the data are coded using the National Cancer Registry Programme manual (National Cancer Registry Programme, 1987). The primary site and histology are coded using the *International Classification Of Diseases For Oncology,* First Edition codes (WHO, 1976). *International Classification of Diseases, Ninth Revision* (ICD-9) codes are used for reporting purposes (WHO, 1978).

The population of each village in the registry area by sex is listed in the ten-yearly census reports issued by the state of Maharashtra. Age-sex distributions are estimated on the basis of sample surveys in each district. The population structure of the registry for the mid-period of 1988–92 is shown in Fig. 2. The total population is 0.4 million and the sex ratio is 950 females to every 1000 males. The proportion of people under 15 years of age is 38.2%, and that of people over 64 years is 5.2%.

The incidence data from the registry have been published in annual reports (Jayant *et al.*, 1989, 1991,

Table 1. Annual average cancer incidence per 100 000 person-years in Barshi registry, India, 1988–92

Site	MALES			FEMALES		
	Number	Crude rate	ASR	Number	Crude rate	ASR
Lip	3	0.3	0.3	0		
Tongue	19	1.7	2.3	3	0.3	0.3
Salivary gland	4	0.4	0.5	1	0.1	0.1
Mouth	33	2.9	3.8	7	0.6	0.8
Oropharynx	6	0.5	0.8	1	0.1	0.1
Nasopharynx	0			0		
Hypopharynx	56	4.9	6.7	5	0.5	0.5
Oesophagus	49	4.3	5.8	16	1.5	1.9
Stomach	7	0.6	0.8	8	0.7	0.9
Colon	6	0.5	0.7	4	0.4	0.4
Rectum	23	2.0	2.6	10	0.9	1.1
Liver	15	1.3	1.8	6	0.6	0.7
Gallbladder	1	0.1	0.1	2	0.2	0.2
Pancreas	4	0.4	0.5	2	0.2	0.2
Larynx	21	1.9	2.5	0		
Lung	11	1.0	1.3	3	0.3	0.3
Bone	4	0.4	0.3	5	0.5	0.5
Connective tissue	6	0.5	0.5	2	0.2	0.2
Melanoma of skin	0			1	0.1	0.1
Other skin	12	1.1	1.4	10	0.9	1.1
Breast	0			78	7.2	8.7
Cervix uteri				252	23.4	27.4
Corpus uteri				3	0.3	0.3
Ovary				12	1.1	1.2
Prostate	12	1.1	1.4			
Testis	3	0.3	0.3			
Penis	29	2.6	3.3			
Bladder	9	0.8	1.0	0		
Kidney	4	0.4	0.4	1	0.1	0.1
Brain	4	0.4	0.4	2	0.2	0.2
Thyroid	5	0.4	0.5	2	0.2	0.2
Hodgkin's disease	5	0.4	0.4	0		
Non-Hodgkin lymphoma	9	0.8	1.0	5	0.5	0.6
Multiple myeloma	1	0.1	0.1	1	0.1	0.1
Lymphoid leukaemia	9	0.8	0.7	6	0.6	0.5
Myeloid leukaemia	10	0.9	1.1	5	0.5	0.4
All sites	453	39.9	51.8	502	46.6	55.0
All sites except skin	441	38.9	50.4	492	45.7	53.9

ASR: Age-standardized incidence rate (world population)

1996a), in reports of the Indian Council of Medical Research (National Cancer Registry Programme, 1992) and in Volume VII of *Cancer Incidence in Five Continents* (Parkin *et al.*, 1997). A preliminary report on the observed survival of cervical cancer patients registered during the period 1988–91 was published recently (Jayant *et al.*, 1996b).

Cancer incidence in Barshi registry

In terms of overall cancer incidence, 453 cases among males and 502 cases among females were registered in the period 1988–92. The average annual age-standardized incidence rates per 100 000 population were 51.8 for males and 55.0 for females (Table 1). These are less than half the rates observed in urban populations in India (Parkin *et al.*, 1997). Though underdiagnosis and under-registration may account for the lower rates, a genuine low risk for many cancer sites is a distinct possibility, given the differences in lifestyle and other exposures.

Among males, cancers of the hypopharynx, oesophagus, mouth and penis have the highest incidence rates, accounting for more than one-third

Table 2. Cases of cancer registered and data quality indices, Barshi registry, India, 1988–92

Site	ICD 9	No. of cases registered	Data quality indices		Cases excluded from analysis		Cases included for survival analysis	
			% DCO	% HV	DCO	Others	No.	%
Cervix	180	252	0.0	92.5	0	5	247	98.0

DCO : Death certificate only; HV : Histological verification

Table 3. Observed and relative survival by site and sex, Barshi registry, India, 1988–92

Site	ICD 9	Number included	All ages					
			Observed survival			Relative survival		
			1 yr	3 yr	5 yr	1 yr	3 yr	5 yr
Cervix	180	247	62.8	36.2	30.9	63.7	37.9	33.3

of all cancers. There is a high risk of hypopharyngeal cancer in western India, as indicated by high rates in Bombay (Parkin *et al.*, 1997) and Ahmedabad (Parkin *et al.*, 1992).

Among females, there is a high risk of cervical cancer (age-standardized incidence rate (ASR) 27.4/100 000), accounting for half of all female cancers. It is likely that these are underestimates of the true risk, because of underdiagnosis and some incompleteness in registration. Preliminary results from a rural cancer registry at Ambilikkai, in South India, indicate an even higher risk of cervical cancer (ASR 47.1/100 000 in 1995–96) among women in rural areas of India (Cherian and Rajkumar, 1997).

Health services

Primary health care delivery is administered through primary health centres and rural hospitals. There is one primary health centre with a medical officer and support staff for about 30 000 people. Under each primary health centre, there are several subcentres in the charge of an auxiliary nurse-midwife and a multipurpose health worker. Besides these workers, there is one community health worker for every 1000 people. There is a total of 15 primary health centres, 18 rural hospitals, 76 subcentres, 140 medical practitioners and 550 health workers in the registry area.

A voluntary body (the Ashwini Rural Cancer Research and Relief Society) took the initiative of setting up a comprehensive cancer hospital (Nargis Dutt Memorial Cancer Hospital), in the rural environs of Barshi, to serve the needs of the rural population. This hospital is now fully equipped to carry out histopathological, cytological, radiological and surgical procedures for cancer diagnosis and provides cancer surgery, radiotherapy, chemotherapy and palliative care.

Early detection

As already indicated, one of the registry's methods of case-finding is to promote awareness of cancer risk factors and symptoms among the rural population and to encourage early detection behaviours. The registry area is divided into 12 zones, each covering approximately 30 villages. Opportunistic detection clinics are conducted twice a year in each zone, soon after completion of village visits by the registry staff. To facilitate referrals, a complete list of dates and locations of these detection clinics is given to all medical practitioners, hospitals and primary health centres in the area. The detection clinics are conducted by fully qualified oncologists. Cervical cytology is offered to women attending the clinics.

The results of a pilot population-based study to evaluate the performance of visual inspection in the early detection of cervical cancer, involving the female population of Agalgaon primary health centre area, have been published (Nene *et al.*, 1996).

Survival analysis

Subjects

A total of 252 cervical cancer cases were registered during the period 1988–92 (Table 2). Of these, 92.5% cases had histological verification. Four cases without any follow-up information and one case

Site	ICD 9	Number of cases by age group						% Relative survival (RS) at 5 years						RS	ASRS%
		≤34	35–44	45–54	55–64	65–74	75+	≤34	35–44	45–54	55–64	65–74	75+	All ages	0–74
Cervix	180	16	67	68	74	18	4	31.8	39.4	34.5	24.7	28.5	84.7	33.3	38.5 32.0

Table 4. Age-specific number of cases, five-year relative survival and ASRS, Barshi registry, India, 1988–92

ASRS: Age-standardized relative survival

without date of diagnosis were excluded, leaving 247 cases for final analysis. Since there was a focus on studies of cervical cancer in this rural population, particular attention was paid to collecting details of histology, staging (using the International Federation of Gynaecologists and Obstetricians (FIGO) system) and treatment.

The distribution of histology was as follows:
- squamous cell carcinoma 219 cases (88.7%)
- adenocarcinoma 10 cases (4.0%)
- histology unknown 18 cases (7.3%).

The stage distribution was as follows:
- stage I 47 cases (19.0%)
- stage II 44 cases (17.8%)
- stage III 113 cases (45.7%)
- stage IV 5 cases (2.0%)
- unknown 38 cases (15.5%).

The treatment details were as follows:
- 104 people (42.1%) had completed prescribed treatment
- 26 people (10.5%) had only partial treatment
- 117 people (47.4%) had no treatment.

Follow-up
The vital status of subjects was mainly established by house visits. At the closing date for follow-up (31 December 1995), 171 (69.2%) subjects were known to be dead, 66 (26.7%) were alive; and 10 (4.1%) had been lost to follow-up.

Analytical methodology (see Chapters 2, 3 and 5)
The index date for calculation of survival time was the incidence date. The survival time for each case was the time between the index date and the date of death *or* date of loss to follow-up *or* 31 December 1995. Cumulative observed and relative survival probabilities were calculated using Hakulinen's method (Hakulinen, 1982; Hakulinen *et al.*, 1994). The expected survival for a group of people in the general population similar to the patient population with respect to age, sex, and calendar period of

observation was calculated using the abridged life tables of the rural Indian population (Registrar General of India, 1995). Age-standardized relative survival (ASRS) rates were calculated for all age groups and for the age group 0–74 years by directly standardizing site-specific and age-specific relative survival to the site-specific age distributions of the estimated global incidence of major cancers in 1985 for comparison with results from other countries.

Since we had reliable information on age, stage and histology, we wished to examine the prognostic importance of these variables for survival. We also divided the period of observation into two periods: 1988–89 and 1990–92. The log rank test (Mantel, 1966) was used to identify significant factors on univariate analysis. These were then entered stepwise into a proportional hazards regression model (Cox, 1972) to identify independent predictors of survival outcome.

Results
The one-year, three-year and five-year observed and relative survival from cervical cancer are shown in Table 3. One-third of patients had survived five years from diagnosis. The age-specific five-year relative survival rates do not indicate any impact of age on survival (Table 4). Table 5 shows observed survival by stage, histology, registration period and treatment, and Figs. 3–5 show the survival outcome until five years from diagnosis according to histology, stage of disease and period of registration, respectively. The five-year survival by histology was 32.1% for squamous cell carcinoma, 20% for adenocarcinoma and 24.7% for those without a histological diagnosis (Fig. 3); survival by FIGO stages was 59.6% for stage I, 31.5% for stage II, 11.6% for stage III, 20% for stage IV and 54.8% for unstaged cancers (Fig. 4). The observed five-year survival was higher for cases diagnosed in 1990–92 than for cases from 1988–89 (Fig. 5).

On univariate analysis, stage, histology and period of registration emerged as significant variables affecting survival outcome. The results of multifactorial analysis, after adjustment for any residual effect of age at incidence date, are given in

Factor	Number	%	Survival %		
			1 year	3 years	5 years
Stage					
I	47	19.0	95.7	68.1	59.6
II	44	17.8	70.5	43.0	31.5
III	113	45.7	44.2	15.0	11.6
IV	5	2.0	40.0	20.0	20.0
Unknown	38	15.5	71.1	54.8	54.8
Histology					
Squamous cell carcinoma	219	88.7	64.4	37.4	32.1
Adenocarcinoma	10	4.0	40.0	20.0	20.0
Unknown	18	7.3	55.6	32.9	24.7
Registration period					
1988–89	78	31.6	52.6	26.9	24.4
1990–92	169	68.4	67.5	40.6	33.1
Treatment					
Complete	104	42.1	90.4	65.3	54.8
Partial/no details	26	10.5	61.5	17.6	17.6
No treatment & treatment details not known	117	47.4	38.5	14.3	12.6

Table 5. Observed survival by stage, histology, registration period and treatment, Barshi registry, India, 1988–92

Table 6. Advanced stage of disease and adenocarcinoma emerged as poor prognostic factors. Cases registered during 1990–92 demonstrated a significantly lower relative risk of death than cases from 1988–89.

Discussion

This is the first comprehensive report of cervical cancer survival in an entirely rural population in India. Every effort has been made to improve opportunities for diagnosis, and to register all diagnosed cases in the population. We are confident that more than 90% of the diagnosed cases of cervical cancer from the area are in our database. Our unique method of active coverage and the rudimentary death registration system in the region explain the absence of DCO cases.

We began to observe a stage shift in diagnosed cases as registration activity progressed, possibly because our case-finding mechanism involved cancer-related health education and early detection initiatives (Jayant et al., 1995). Because of this, we wished to examine the survival of cancer patients registered during 1988–89 and 1990–92, to see whether there were any differences in survival between the two periods (Fig. 5). It is interesting to note that the five-year observed survival for the second period was significantly higher than for the first: 33.1% versus 24.4% ($p < 0.05$). When this was adjusted for stage distribution, histology and age in a Cox proportional hazards regression analysis, the observed survival difference remained significant (Table 6).

Cases diagnosed during the second period had a favourable stage distribution, and there were differences in treatment as well (Table 7). Sixty percent of patients diagnosed during the first period did not begin or complete treatment, compared with 42% of patients during the second period. It is obvious that health education, plus the opportunities for early detection provided by the unique case-finding mechanism of our registry, improved both stage distribution and compliance with treatment. This seems to be responsible for the better prognosis observed during the second period. Compliance with treatment had a major impact on survival, as shown in Table 5 and Fig. 6.

The five-year observed survival among cervical cancer patients in Barshi (30.9%) is a little lower than that observed in Bangalore (34.4%) (Nandakumar et al., 1995). It is much lower than that reported in a hospital-based study from Trivandrum, India (47.4%) (Sankaranarayanan et al., 1995). Age-standardized relative survival from cervical cancer in Barshi is in the lower half of the

Table 6. Multifactorial analysis of prognostic factors for cervical cancer in Barshi registry, India

Factor	Hazard ratio[1]	95% CI	χ^2 value	*p* value
Stage			58.1	<0.0001
I	1.0			
II	2.6	1.4–4.6		
III	5.9	3.4–10.0		
IV	4.4	1.2–15.3		
Histology			5.6	<0.05
Squamous cell carcinoma	1.0			
Adenocarcinoma	2.8	1.3–5.9		
Period of registration			4.9	<0.05
1988–89	1.0			
1990–92	0.7	0.4–0.9		

[1]After age adjustment

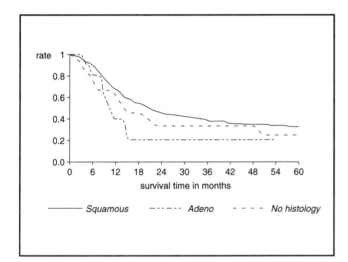

Figure 3. Survival from cervical cancer by histology in Barshi registry, India

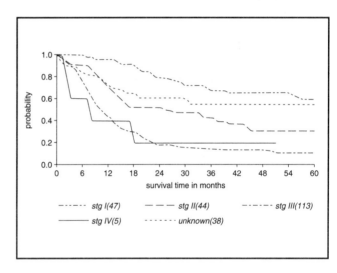

Figure 4. Survival from cervical cancer by stage of disease in Barshi registry, India

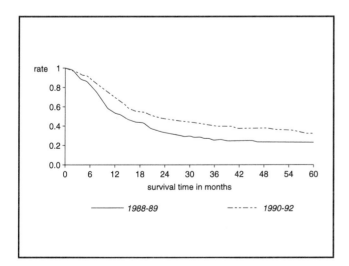

Figure 5. Survival from cervical cancer by period of registration in Barshi registry, India

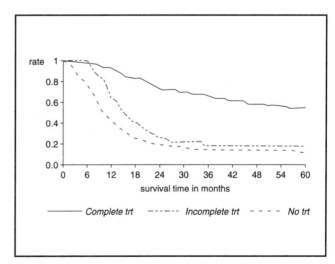

Figure 6. Survival from cervical cancer by treatment in Barshi registry, India

Table 7. Stage and treatment of disease by registration period, Barshi registry, India

Stage (FIGO)	1988-89 (%)	1990-92 (%)	Total (%)
I	12 (15.4)	35 (20.7)	47 (19.0)
II	13 (16.7)	31 (18.3)	44 (17.8)
III	39 (50.0)	74 (43.8)	113 (45.8)
IV	3 (3.8)	2 (1.2)	5 (2.0)
Unknown	11 (14.1)	27 (16.0)	38 (15.4)
Treatment			
Surgery	11 (14.1)	21 (12.4)	32 (13.0)
Radiotherapy			
Completed	10 (12.8)	52 (30.8)	62 (25.1)
Partial	5 (6.4)	9 (5.3)	14 (5.7)
No details	4 (5.1)	4 (2.4	8 (3.2)
Surgery + Radiotherapy			
Completed	2 (2.6)	8 (4.7)	10 (4.0)
Incomplete	0	4 (2.4)	4 (1.6)
No treatment & treatment details not known	46 (60.0)	71 (42.0)	117 (47.4)

range reported from developing countries, the USA in the 1960s (Sankaranarayanan et al., 1996). and Europe (Berrino et al., 1995).

Our results have important implications for cervical cancer control in the developing world. Our studies, as well as the experience in Sweden in the precytology era (Pontén et al., 1995), indicate that a programme of health education motivating women to seek early diagnosis and treatment and improving opportunities for early diagnosis and therapy can lead to improved survival outcome from cervical cancer.

Acknowledgements

The authors gratefully acknowledge the International Cancer Research Technology Transfer (ICRETT) fellowship awarded to A.M. Budukh by the International Union Against Cancer (UICC), Geneva, Switzerland, which made possible the detailed analysis of these data at the Unit of Descriptive Epidemiology, International Agency for Research on Cancer, Lyon, France. The authors thank the Indian Council of Medical Research, New Delhi, India, for its continuing assistance to the registry.

References

Berrino, F., Sant, M., Verdecchia, A., Capocaccia, R., Hakulinen, T. & Estève, J., eds. (1995) *Survival of Cancer Patients in Europe: the EUROCARE Study* (IARC Scientific Publications No. 132). Lyon, International Agency for Research on Cancer

Cherian, J. & Rajkumar, R. (1997) *Annual Report 1995, Ambilikkai Population Based Cancer Registry*. Ambilikkai, Tamil Nadu, India, Christian Fellowship Community Health Centre

Cox, D.R. (1972) Regression models and life tables. *J. R. Stat. Soc.*, **34**, 187–220

Gupta, P.C., Mehta, F.S., Daftary, D.K., Pindborg, J.J., Bhonsle, R.B., Jalnawalla, P.N., Sinor, P.N., Pitkar, V.K., Murti, P.R., Irani, R.R., Shah, H.T., Kadam, P.M., Iyer, K.S.S., Iyer, H.M., Hegde, A.K., Chandrasekhar, G.K., Shroff, B.C., Sahiar, B.E. & Mehta, M.N. (1980) Incidence of oral cancer and natural history of oral precancerous lesions in a 10-year follow-up study of Indian villagers. *Community Dent. Oral Epidemiol.*, **8**, 287–333

Hakulinen, T. (1982) Cancer survival corrected for heterogeneity in patient withdrawal. *Biometrics*, **38**, 933–942

Hakulinen, T., Gibberd, R., Abeywickrama, K.H. & Soderman, B. (1994) *A Computer Program Package for Cancer Survival Studies, Version 2.0*. Tampere, Finnish Cancer Registry/University of Newcastle, Australia

Jayant, K., Potdar, G.G., Paymaster, J.C., Sanghvi, L.D., Gangadharan, P., Sirsat M.V. & Jussawalla, D.J. (1975) Methodology for the study of cancer in a rural population in India. *Ind. J. Cancer*, **12**, 243–251

Jayant, K., Potdar, G.G., Paymaster, J.C., Sanghvi, L.D., Sirsat, M.V., Gangadharan, P. & Jussawala, D.J. (1976) Feasibility of undertaking cancer incidence studies in rural areas of India. *Bull. WHO*, **54**, 11–18

Jayant, K., Rao, R.S., Nene, B.M. & Dale, P.S. (1989) *Population-based Rural Cancer Registry, Annual Report 1987-88*. Bombay, Tata Memorial Centre

Jayant, K., Rao, R.S., Nene, B.M. & Dale, P.S. (1991) *A Report of the Rural Cancer Registry*. Bombay, Tata Memorial Centre

Jayant, K., Rao, R.S., Nene, B.M. & Dale, P.S. (1995) Improved stage at diagnosis of cervical cancer with increased cancer awareness in a rural Indian population. *Int. J. Cancer*, **63**, 161–163

Jayant, K., Rao, R.S., Nene, B.M. & Dale, P.S. (1996a) *A Report of the Rural Cancer Registry*. Bombay, Tata Memorial Centre

Jayant, K., Rao, R.S., Nene, B.M., Dale, P.S. & Nandakumar, A. (1996b) Improved survival in cervical cancer cases in a rural population. *Br. J. Cancer*, **74**, 285–287

Mantel, N. (1966) Evaluation of survival data and two new rank order statistics arising in its consideration. *Cancer Chemother. Rep.*, **50**, 163–170

Nandakumar, A., Anantha, N. & Venugopal, T.C. (1995) Incidence, mortality and survival in cancer of the cervix in Bangalore, India. *Br. J. Cancer*, **71**, 1348–1352

National Cancer Registry Programme (1987) *Code Manual For Population-based Cancer Registry*. New Delhi, Indian Council of Medical Research

National Cancer Registry Programme (1992) *Biennial Report 1988-89*. New Delhi, Indian Council of Medical Research

Nene, B.M., Deshpande, S., Jayant, K., Budukh, A.M., Dale, P.S., Deshpande, D.A., Chiwate, A.S., Malvi, S.G., Deokar, S., Parkin, D.M. & Sankaranarayanan, R. (1996) Early detection of cervical cancer by visual inspection: a population-based study in rural India. *Int. J. Cancer*, **68**, 770–773

Parkin, D.M., Muir, C.S., Whelan, S.L., Gao, Y.-T., Ferlay, J. & Powell, J., eds. (1992) *Cancer Incidence in Five Continents, Volume VI* (IARC Scientific Publications No. 120). Lyon, International Agency for Research on Cancer

Parkin, D.M., Whelan, S.L., Ferlay, J., Raymond L. & Young J., eds. (1997) *Cancer Incidence in Five Continents, Volume VII* (IARC Scientific Publications No. 143). Lyon, International Agency for Research on Cancer

Pontén, J., Adami, H.O., Bergström, R., Dillner, J., Friberg, J., Gustafsson, L., Miller, A.B., Parkin, D.M., Sparén, P. & Trichopoulos, D. (1995) Strategies for global control of cervical cancer. *Int. J. Cancer*, **60**, 1–26

Registrar General of India (1995) *SRS-based Abridged Life Tables 1988-92. Occasional Paper No. 4 of 1995*. New Delhi, Office of the Registrar General

Sankaranarayanan, R., Krishnan Nair, M., Jayaprakash, P.G., Stanley, G., Varghese, C., Ramadas, V., Padmakumary, G. & Padmanabhan, T.K. (1995) Cervical cancer in Kerala: a hospital registry-based study on survival and prognostic factors. *Br. J. Cancer*, **72**, 1039–1042

Sankaranarayanan, R., Swaminathan, R. & Black, R.J. (for Study Group on Cancer Survival in Developing Countries) (1996) Global variations in cancer survival. *Cancer*, **78**, 2461–2464

Wahi, P.N. (1968) The epidemiology of oral and oropharyngeal cancer, a report of the study in Mainpuri district, Uttar Pradesh, India. *Bull. WHO*, **38**, 495–521

WHO (1976) *International Classification of Diseases for Oncology*, First Edition, Geneva, World Health Organization

WHO (1978) *International Classification of Diseases, Ninth Revision*. Geneva, World Health Organization

Chapter 11

Survival from breast and cervical cancer in Mumbai (Bombay), India

B.B. Yeole, D.J. Jussawalla, S.D. Sabnis, Lizzy Sunny

Bombay Cancer Registry,
Indian Cancer Society, Mumbai (Bombay)

Introduction

The Bombay cancer registry was the first population-based cancer registry in India, established as a unit of the Indian Cancer Society in 1963, with assistance from the Biometry Branch of the National Cancer Institute, USA. The Department of Science and Technology, Government of India, supported this initiative from 1976 to 1980, and since 1981 it has been partially funded by the Indian Council of Medical Research through the National Cancer Registry Programme of India. The registry covers a population of more than 10 million residents in the entire urban area of Mumbai (Bombay) (603 km²), which is the most important commercial and industrial centre in India. It is the capital of state of Maharashtra and is located on the west coast of India between latitudes 18°54′N and 19°16′ N and longitudes 70°47′E and 73°E (Fig. 1). Mumbai is the only district in India with a 100% urban population.

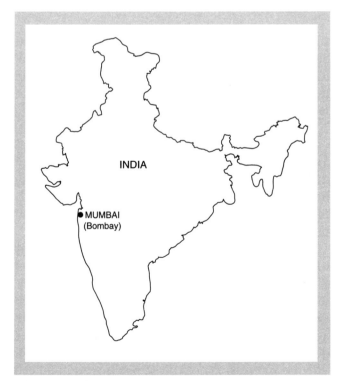

Figure 1. Map showing location of Mumbai (Bombay)

This registry has reported incidence data without a break since 1964, in Volumes II–VII of *Cancer Incidence in Five Continents* (Doll *et al.*, 1970; Waterhouse *et al.*, 1976, 1982; Muir *et al.*, 1987; Parkin *et al.*, 1992, 1997). It is one of the few cancer registries in the developing world with an incidence database spanning over 30 years to allow the study of trends in cancer incidence.

In this chapter we report the survival experience of breast and cervical cancer patients registered during 1982–86 in Bombay Cancer Registry.

Cancer registration

Information is obtained from 168 hospitals and clinics in the public and private sector using a structured form. The registry staff visit the data sources to abstract data on resident cancer cases. They interview cancer patients personally and then review records maintained by various services concerned with cancer diagnosis and management. The major source of data is the Tata Memorial Centre, the premier cancer hospital in Maharashtra state, where outpatient records are also scrutinized. Copies of death certificates mentioning cancer or tumour as the cause of death are obtained from the Vital Statistics Division of the municipal death register. These are matched with the registry cancer database. The unmatched cases are traced back to hospitals and residences. If this cannot be done, the cases are registered as 'death certificate only' (DCO).

The information obtained from these sources is merged together in the registry in order to complete the records and eliminate any duplicates. The forms containing the information are classified into three groups: resident, residence status not known and nonresident. People whose residence status is not known are checked against the electoral rolls, and if they are found they are treated as resident cases.

Data are coded using the manual of the National Cancer Registry Programme (National Cancer Registry Programme, 1987). The primary site and histology are coded using the *International Classification of Diseases for Oncology*, First Edition (WHO, 1976). The data are

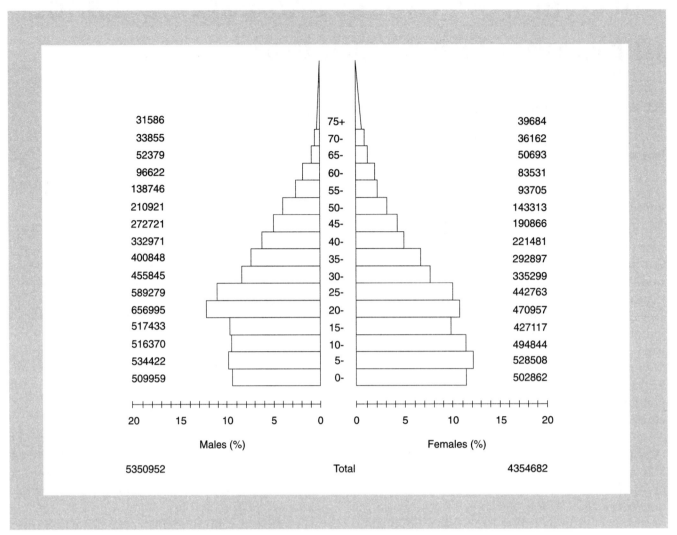

Males	Age	Females
31586	75+	39684
33855	70-	36162
52379	65-	50693
96622	60-	83531
138746	55-	93705
210921	50-	143313
272721	45-	190866
332971	40-	221481
400848	35-	292897
455845	30-	335299
589279	25-	442763
656995	20-	470957
517433	15-	427117
516370	10-	494844
534422	5-	528508
509959	0-	502862

Males (%)   Females (%)

5350952   Total   4354682

Figure 2. Average annual population of Mumbai (Bombay), 1988–92

reported using the *International Classification of Diseases, Ninth Revision* (ICD-9) codes (WHO, 1978). For several years, data were processed manually, but personal computers are now used. Internal quality control measures are regularly applied to ensure completeness and reliability of the collected data (Yeole & Jussawalla, 1988). Incidence data from the registry are reviewed annually in a review meeting of the National Cancer Registry Programme and any discrepancies are rectified.

The registry is supervised by a deputy director, and the registry staff include a biostatistician, a programmer, a computing assistant, 12 medical social workers, six research assistants and three clerks. The registry staff regularly attend the training programmes conducted by the National Cancer Registry Programme in various locations in India.

Cancer incidence in Bombay

Details on cancer incidence during the period 1988–92 are given in Table 1. Fig. 2 shows the age structure of the resident population. The average annual crude and age-adjusted incidence rates for all sites during the above period in males were 70.7 and 133.1/100 000 person-years, respectively; the corresponding rates in females were 77.1 and 126.6, respectively.

The major cancer sites among males were lung, oesophagus, hypopharynx, larynx, stomach, mouth and tongue, which together accounted for 45% of all male cancers. Among females, cancers of the breast, uterine cervix, ovary, oesophagus and mouth predominated. Annual reports on cancer incidence are published.

Because data have been available since 1964, it has been possible to study time trends in incidence. There has been a significant increase in breast cancer incidence (Yeole *et al.*, 1990; Coleman *et al.*, 1993; Parkin, 1994). The average annual increase in the age-standardized incidence rate for breast cancer during the period 1964–87 was 1.2% (Parkin, 1994). The rise in breast cancer incidence is seen in all age groups, except in the very old. A small but steady decline is observed in the incidence of cancers of the cervix, tongue, hypopharynx, colorectum and larynx (Jayant & Yeole, 1987; Yeole *et al.*, 1989; Coleman *et al.*, 1993; Parkin, 1994). Higher age at marriage, fewer childbirths and improvements in socioeconomic status have largely contributed to the decline in cervical cancer incidence and the increase in breast cancer rates. Lung cancer rates have remained fairly stable and the risk is still low compared with that in the developed world. There has even been a nonsignificant decrease in incidence in females (Coleman *et al.*, 1993).

Health services

The state government of Maharashtra and the Bombay Municipal Corporation are mainly responsible for the organization of public health and medical services in the city. More than 100 hospitals in Bombay, which include the Tata Memorial Centre (the premier comprehensive cancer centre in the country) and four medical schools, have the infrastructure for diagnostic facilities for cancer. However, both diagnostic and treatment facilities are concentrated in certain hospitals. Cancer surgery is undertaken in all the major public and private hospitals. Megavoltage radiotherapy using cobalt machines or linear accelerators is available in six hospitals; orthovoltage deep X-ray therapy in 10 hospitals, and brachytherapy in six hospitals. Cancer chemotherapy is administered in over 10 hospitals. Hospices and palliative care facilities are widely available. There is a focus on psychological and vocational rehabilitation of cancer patients, under the leadership of the Indian Cancer Society. Support services, such as ostomy care, counselling, homecare and hospices, have been widely developed under the patronage of dedicated organizations.

Early detection activities

There are no organized screening programmes in Bombay. However, the Indian Cancer Society and the Preventive Oncology Division of the Tata Memorial Centre have early detection clinics. Cytology services are widely available on demand. There are programmes to improve professional awareness of cancer diagnosis and therapy.

Survival analysis

Subjects

A total of 2973 breast and 2426 cervical cancer cases were registered during the period 1982–86

(Table 2), four-fifths of which had histological confirmation. A number of cases were excluded from the final survival analysis: 168 cases which were registered as DCOs, three cases with invalid ICD-9 codes and two cases without information on age. This left 2872 breast cancer cases (96.6% of the incident cases) and 2354 cervical cancer cases (97.0% of the incident cases) for survival analysis. Details on marital status, mother tongue, religion, education and clinical extent of disease were available for these cases.

Follow-up methods

The closing date for follow-up was 31 December 1993. The incident cases were matched with death certificates mentioning cancer or tumour as cause of death up to 1993. For the unmatched cases, telephone enquiries were made for those with telephone numbers, and reply-paid letters sent to the remainder. If no reply was received, home visits were carried out. When home visits were not successful, the case-records from reporting hospitals were scrutinized to determine the date of the last visit and the person's vital status (alive/dead).

The outcome of follow-up is given in detail for both sites in Table 3. Vital status was known for 69.0% of breast cancers and 72.4% of cervical cancers. For cases lost to follow-up before the closing date, partial information was available for varying periods of time from the diagnosis date. Overall, complete information on vital status was available for three-quarters of the subjects five years after diagnosis.

Analytical methodology (see Chapters 2, 3 and 5)

The index date for calculation of survival time was the incidence date. The survival time for each case was the time between the index date and the date of death *or* date of loss to follow-up *or* 31 December 1993. Cumulative observed and relative survival probabilities were calculated using Hakulinen's method (Hakulinen, 1982; Hakulinen *et al.*, 1994). The expected survival for a group of people in the general population similar to the patient population with respect to age, sex, and calendar period of observation was calculated using the abridged life tables of the urban Indian population (Registrar General of India, 1995). Age-standardized relative survival (ASRS) was calculated for all age groups and for the age group 0–74 years by directly standardizing site-specific and age-specific relative survival to the site-specific age distributions of the estimated global incidence of major cancers in 1985 for comparison with results from other countries.

Table 1. Annual average cancer incidence per 100 000 person-years in Mumbai (Bombay), India, 1988–92						
	MALES			FEMALES		
Site	Number	Crude rate	ASR	Number	Crude rate	ASR
Lip	54	0.2	0.4	37	0.2	0.3
Tongue	950	3.6	6.5	287	1.3	2.3
Salivary gland	97	0.4	0.6	48	0.2	0.3
Mouth	1023	3.8	6.2	584	2.7	4.6
Oropharynx	482	1.8	3.5	57	0.3	0.5
Nasopharynx	120	0.4	0.7	39	0.2	0.3
Hypopharynx	1167	4.4	8.3	262	1.2	2.0
Oesophagus	1383	5.2	10.8	962	4.4	8.3
Stomach	1010	3.8	7.7	462	2.1	3.8
Colon	522	2.0	3.7	354	1.6	3.0
Rectum	537	2.0	3.9	330	1.5	2.7
Liver	506	1.9	3.9	226	1.0	1.9
Gallbladder	249	1.1	2.3	324	1.5	2.7
Pancreas	302	1.1	2.3	214	1.0	1.8
Larynx	1093	4.1	8.2	163	0.7	1.4
Lung	1867	7.0	14.5	432	2.0	3.7
Bone	200	0.7	0.8	105	0.5	0.6
Connective tissue	239	0.9	1.3	156	0.7	1.0
Melanoma of skin	53	0.2	0.4	43	0.2	0.3
Other skin	244	0.9	1.7	159	0.7	1.2
Breast	75	0.3	0.6	3864	17.7	28.2
Cervix uteri				2828	12.9	20.2
Corpus uteri				296	1.4	2.5
Ovary				989	4.5	7.2
Prostate	764	2.9	7.9			
Testis	229	0.9	0.9			
Penis	219	0.8	1.5			
Bladder	554	2.1	4.8	132	0.6	1.2
Kidney	301	1.1	2.0	130	0.6	0.9
Brain	660	2.5	3.3	357	1.6	2.2
Thyroid	133	0.5	0.8	326	1.5	2.1
Hodgkin's disease	283	1.1	1.3	107	0.5	0.6
Non-Hodgkin lymphoma	696	2.6	4.1	377	1.7	2.7
Multiple myeloma	158	0.6	1.2	103	0.5	0.9
Lymphoid leukaemia	324	1.2	1.6	194	0.9	1.1
Myeloid leukaemia	416	1.6	2.0	254	1.2	1.5
All sites	18904	70.7	133.1	16785	77.1	126.6
All sites except skin	18660	69.7	131.4	16626	76.4	125.4

ASR: Age-standardized incidence rate (world population)

Table 2. Cases of cancer registered and data quality indices, Mumbai (Bombay), India, 1982–86

Site	ICD 9	No. of cases registered	Data quality indices		Cases excluded from analysis		Cases included for survival analysis	
			% DCO	% HV	DCO	Others	No.	%
Breast	174	2973	3.3	78.5	99	2	2872	96.6
Cervix	180	2426	2.8	83.0	69	3	2354	97.0

DCO : Death certificate only; HV : Histological verification

Table 3. Details of outcome of follow-up of cases in Mumbai (Bombay)

Site	Vital status known	Cases with partial follow-up information		
		≤ 1 year	2–4 years	≥ 5 years
Breast	1981 (69.0%)	179 (6.2%)	533 (18.6%)	179 (6.2%)
Cervix	1704 (72.4%)	181 (7.7%)	447 (19.0%)	22 (0.9%)

Table 4. Cumulative observed and relative survival, Mumbai (Bombay), India, 1982–86

Site	ICD 9	Number included	Observed survival			Relative survival		
			1 yr	3 yr	5 yr	1 yr	3 yr	5 yr
Breast	174	2872	84.2	61.9	51.1	85.5	64.7	55.1
Cervix	180	2354	81.0	56.0	47.7	82.0	58.0	50.7

Table 5. Site-specific and age-specific number of cases, five-year relative survival and ASRS, Mumbai (Bombay), India, 1982–86

Site	ICD 9	Number of cases by age group						% Relative survival (RS) at 5 years						RS	ASRS%
		≤34	35–44	45–54	55–64	65–74	75+	≤34	35–44	45–54	55–64	65–74	75+	All ages	0–74
Breast	174	281	744	837	589	307	114	59.5	56.1	53.7	53.7	55.8	49.6	55.1	54.0	55.1
Cervix	180	253	624	735	511	181	50	66.5	57.4	42.3	46.3	44.5	20.9	50.7	46.0	49.5

ASRS: Age-standardized relative survival

The Cox proportional hazard model was used to elicit the main effects in univariate and multivariate analysis of risk factors (Cox, 1972).

Results

The one-year, three-year and five-year observed and relative survival rates and the five-year relative survival rates by age group are shown in Tables 4 and 5, respectively. The five-year relative survival was 55% for breast cancer and 51% for cervical cancer. There was a decreasing trend in relative survival with age in cervical cancer; no effect of age was evident in the case of breast cancer.

Figs. 3 and 4 show the observed survival until five years from diagnosis by different categories of clinical extent of disease for breast and cervical cancers, respectively. The information on clinical extent of disease was available for 91.1% of breast cancers and 94.8% of cervical cancers. An inverse relationship between clinical extent of disease and survival is observed.

Table 6 shows the five-year observed survival for breast and cervical cancers according to age group, religion, marital status and clinical extent of disease. On univariate analysis, age group ($p < 0.001$), marital

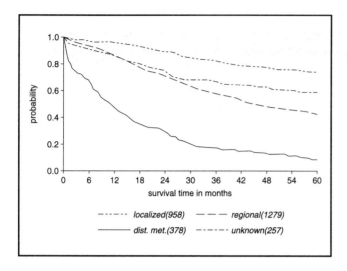

Figure 3. Survival from breast cancer by clinical extent of disease in Mumbai (Bombay), India

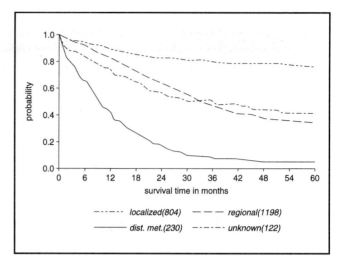

Figure 4. Survival from cervical cancer by clinical extent of disease in Mumbai (Bombay), India

status ($p < 0.001$) and clinical extent of disease ($p < 0.001$) emerged as significant factors affecting survival in breast and cervical cancer. On multivariate analysis, all of these emerged as independent predictors of survival for breast cancer (Table 7). For cervical cancer, age group ($p < 0.001$), and clinical extent of disease ($p < 0.001$) were independent predictors of survival with both the factors showing an inverse relationship (Table 8). The most important prognostic factor for both cancers seems to be the clinical extent of disease at presentation. The risk of dying was three times higher for regional disease and 10 times higher for distant metastatic disease compared with localized disease in breast cancer. The relative risk of death was 3–4 times higher for regional and 11–12 times higher for distant metastasis compared with localized disease in cervical cancer. The relationship of age with survival from breast cancer did not reveal any trend, although people aged 75 years and over had a significantly lower survival rate than those aged under 35 years. On the other hand, an increasing hazard with age was evident among cervical cancer cases.

Discussion

The results of our analysis represent an average prognosis from breast and cervical cancers in Bombay, in view of the very low number of cases excluded from the final analysis. Information on prognostic factors such as clinical extent of disease was available for over 90% of the cases. Every effort was taken to obtain information on the vital status of patients, and complete follow-up information was available for over 70% of patients at the closing date.

The clear downward gradient in survival with advanced disease indicates that the classification of the clinical extent of disease was reasonably accurate. It is generally recognized that it is often not possible for population-based registries to obtain reliable information on various clinically important factors such as stage, clinical extent of disease and treatment in view of the variety of sources from which data are obtained and the wide variation in staging and treatment practices, as well as record-keeping and accessibility, between these centres. Moreover, a reasonably well developed health care infrastructure is essential for the various investigations which are required for accurate staging. Despite these difficulties, we were able to collect information on clinical extent of disease from several sources and classify it according to the categories defined by the manual of the National Cancer Registry Programme (National Cancer Registry Programme, 1987). Our results indicate that, if the lesions are diagnosed at an early stage and appropriate treatment can be ensured, satisfactory survival can be achieved in developing-country settings.

Marital status emerged as an independent predictor of survival for breast cancer in our study. This can be considered as a surrogate for socioeconomic status. The poor survival observed among widowed or divorced or separated women indicates the influence of socioeconomic factors and their bearing on general health, nutritional status, attitudes and health behaviour. The adverse effect of poor socioeconomic status on cancer survival has been well established (Kogevinas *et al.*, 1991; Mackillop *et al.*, 1997). Religion did not contribute to differences in survival.

The five-year age-adjusted relative survival observed for breast cancer in our population is on the

Table 6. Five-year observed survival by selected patient and disease characteristics in Mumbai (Bombay), India, 1982–86

Factor	Breast cancer % (no. of cases)		Cervical cancer % (no. of cases)	
Age group				
< 35 years	59.0	(281)	65.9	(253)
35–44	55.0	(744)	56.6	(624)
45–54	51.3	(837)	40.9	(735)
55–64	48.6	(589)	42.4	(511)
65–74	43.3	(307)	34.4	(181)
75+	29.3	(114)	12.4	(50)
Religion				
Hindu	51.0	(1974)	47.3	(1871)
Muslim	49.9	(399)	51.0	(240)
Christian	54.1	(239)	57.4	(88)
Parsi/ neo-Buddhist	48.2	(132)*	36.6	(101)**
Others	54.5	(121)	52.0	(46)
Marital status				
Married	53.6	(1959)	49.0	(1557)
Widowed/divorced/separated	44.6	(468)	40.0	(566)
Single	49.4	(108)	63.2	(15)
Unknown	45.4	(337)	57.2	(216)
Clinical extent of disease				
Localized	74.4	(958)	77.4	(804)
Regional	43.0	(1279)	35.0	(1198)
Distant metastasis	9.5	(378)	5.6	(230)
Unknown	59.5	(257)	41.8	(122)

* Parsi only; ** neo-Buddhist only

higher side of the range of survival rates reported from India and other developing countries (Gajalakshmi *et al.*, 1997; Nandakumar *et al.*, 1995a; Sankaranarayanan *et al.*, 1996). The corresponding rate for cervical cancer is higher than in Bangalore, India (Nandakumar *et al.*, 1995b) and is in the middle of the range from developing countries (Sankaranarayanan *et al.*, 1996). The figures for both cancers were lower than for the whole of Europe (Berrino *et al.*, 1995) and the USA in the late 1960s (Sankaranarayanan *et al.*, 1996). Bombay has a level of health services which allows patients reasonable access to diagnostic and therapeutic services. Moreover, one-third of patients in both cancer sites presented at localized clinical stages. These two factors may have contributed to the good survival observed in Bombay. However, there is considerable scope for improving the outcome by early diagnosis and treatment, and it would be prudent to consider ways of achieving this at minimal cost. With the prevailing incidence rates of breast cancer, it is unlikely that an organized screening programme would prove cost-effective, given the infrastructure needed and the cost of mammography. The incidence

of cervical cancer is slowly, but steadily, declining owing to changes in socioeconomic status and childbearing practices. It seems, for both cancers, that a programme of health education to improve awareness and to promote early detection among high-risk groups is the most feasible approach to control.

Acknowledgements

The authors gratefully acknowledge the assistance provided by the US National Cancer Institute, the Department of Science and Technology, Government of India, and the Indian Council of Medical Research, New Delhi, to the Bombay Cancer Registry. We are grateful to the Finnish Cancer Society, Helsinki, the International Agency for Research on Cancer, Lyon, France and the Association for International Cancer Research, St. Andrews, Scotland, for their assistance in studying cancer survival in Bombay. The continuing assistance by the Indian Council of Medical Research, New Delhi, in cancer registration in Mumbai is gratefully acknowledged.

Table 7. Independent predictors of survival from breast cancer in Mumbai (Bombay), India

Factor	Hazard ratio	95% CI	χ^2 value	p value
Marital status			7.6	<0.05
Married	1.00			
Widowed/divorced/separated	1.24	1.05–1.45		
Single	1.19	0.89–1.57		
Age group			19.26	<0.005
<35 years	1.00			
35–44	0.87	0.69–1.09		
45–54	0.98	0.78–1.23		
55–64	0.97	0.76–1.23		
65–74	1.10	0.84–1.44		
75+	1.79	1.26–2.53		
Clinical extent of disease			604.1	<0.0001
Localized	1.00			
Regional	2.98	2.55–3.47		
Distant	9.93	8.28–11.90		

CI: Confidence interval

Table 8. Independent predictors of survival from cervical cancer in Mumbai (Bombay), India

Factor	Hazard ratio	95% CI	χ^2 value	p value
Age group			37.55	<0.001
<35 years	1.00			
35–44	1.29	1.00–1.67		
45–54	1.68	1.31–2.16		
55–64	1.62	1.25–2.10		
65–74	1.97	1.46–2.68		
75+	2.38	1.59–3.56		
Clinical extent of disease			516.45	<0.0001
Localized	1.00			
Regional	3.43	2.89–4.07		
Distant	11.62	9.40–14.36		

CI: Confidence interval

References

Berrino, F., Sant, M., Verdecchia, A., Capocaccia, R., Hakulinen, T. & Estève, J., eds. (1995) *Survival of Cancer Patients in Europe: the EUROCARE Study* (IARC Scientific Publications No. 132). Lyon, International Agency for Research on Cancer

Coleman, M.P., Estève, J., Damiecki, P., Arslan, A. & Renard, H. (1993) *Trends in Cancer Incidence and Mortality* (IARC Scientific Publications No. 121). Lyon, International Agency for Research on Cancer

Cox, D.R. (1972) Regression models and life tables. *J. R. Stat. Assoc.*, **34**, 187–220

Doll, R., Muir, C.S. & Waterhouse, J. (1970) *Cancer Incidence in Five Continents*, Volume II. Berlin, Springer-Verlag

Gajalakshmi, C.K., Shanta, V., Swaminathan, R., Sankaranarayanan, R. & Black, R.J. (1997) A population based survival study from female breast cancer in Madras, India. *Br. J. Cancer*, **75**, 771–775

Hakulinen, T. (1982) Cancer survival corrected for heterogeneity in patient withdrawal. *Biometrics*, **38**, 933–942

Hakulinen, T., Gibberd, R., Abeywickrama, K.H. & Soderman, B. (1994) *A Computer Program Package for Cancer Survival Studies, Version 2.0*. Tampere, Finnish Cancer Registry/University of Newcastle, Australia

Jayant, K. & Yeole, B.B. (1987) Cancers of the upper alimentary and respiratory tracts in Bombay, a study of incidence over two decades. *Br. J. Cancer*, **56**, 847–852

Kogevinas, M., Marmot, M.G., Fox, A.J. & Goldblatt, P.O. (1991) Socio-economic differences in cancer survival. *J. Epidemiol. Community Health*, **45**, 216–219

Mackillop, W.J., Zhang-Solomons, J., Groome, P.A., Paszat, L. & Holowaty, E. (1997) Socioeconomic status and cancer survival in Ontario. *J. Clin. Oncology*, **15**, 1680–1689

Muir, C., Waterhouse, J., Mack, T., Powell, J. & Whelan, S., eds. (1987) *Cancer Incidence in Five Continents, Volume V* (IARC Scientific Publications No. 88). Lyon, International Agency for Research on Cancer

Nandakumar, A., Anantha, N., Venugopal, T.C., Sankaranarayanan, R., Thimmasetty, K. & Dhar, M. (1995a) Survival in breast cancer: A population-based study in Bangalore. *Int. J. Cancer*, **60**, 593–596

Nandakumar, A., Anantha, N. & Venugopal, T.C. (1995b) Incidence, mortality and survival in cancer of the cervix in Bangalore, India. *Br. J. Cancer*, **71**, 1348–1352

National Cancer Registry Programme (1987) *Code Manual for Population Based Cancer Registry*. New Delhi, Indian Council of Medical Research

Parkin, D.M. (1994) Cancer in developing countries. In: Doll, R., Fraumeni, J.F. and Muir, C.S., eds., Trends in cancer incidence and mortality. *Cancer Surveys*, **19/20**, 519–561

Parkin, D.M., Muir, C.S., Whelan, S.L., Gao, Y.-T., Ferlay, J. & Powell, J., eds. (1992) *Cancer Incidence in Five Continents, Volume VI* (IARC Scientific Publications No. 120). Lyon, International Agency for Research on Cancer

Parkin, D.M., Whelan, S.L., Ferlay, J., Raymond L. & Young J., eds. (1997) *Cancer Incidence in Five Continents, Volume VII* (IARC Scientific Publications No. 143). Lyon, International Agency for Research on Cancer

Registrar General of India (1995) *SRS based abridged life tables 1988-92. Occasional Paper No. 4 of 1995*. New Delhi, Office of the Registrar General

Sankaranarayanan, R., Swaminathan, R. & Black, R.J. (for Study Group on Cancer Survival in Developing Countries) (1996) Global variations in cancer survival. *Cancer*, **78**, 2461–2464

Waterhouse, J.A.H., Muir, C.S., Correa, P. & Powell, J., eds. (1976) *Cancer Incidence in Five Continents*, Volume III (IARC Scientific Publications No. 15). Lyon, International Agency for Research on Cancer

Waterhouse, J., Muir, C., Shanmugaratnam, K. & Powell, J., eds. (1982) *Cancer Incidence in Five Continents, Volume IV* (IARC Scientific Publications No. 42). Lyon, International Agency for Research on Cancer

WHO (1976) *International Classification of Diseases for Oncology*, First Edition. Geneva, World Health Organization

WHO (1978) *International Classification of Diseases, Ninth Revision*. Geneva, World Health Organization

Yeole, B.B. & Jussawalla, D.J. (1988) An assessment of reliability and completeness of Bombay Cancer Registry data. *Indian J. Cancer*, **25**, 177–190

Yeole, B.B., Jayant, K. & Jussawalla, D.J. (1989) Declining trend in cervical cancer incidence in Bombay, India (1964-1985). *J. Surg. Oncol.*, **42**, 267–271

Yeole, B.B., Jayant, K. & Jussawalla, D.J. (1990) Trends in breast cancer incidence in Greater Bombay: an epidemiological assessment. *Bull. WHO*, **68**, 245–249

Chapter 12

Cancer survival in Chennai (Madras), India

V. Shanta, C.K. Gajalakshmi, R. Swaminathan

Cancer Institute (WIA), Adyar
Chennai (Madras) 600020, India

Introduction

Chennai (Madras), the capital of the state of Tamil Nadu in the Indian Union, is the fourth largest city in India. It is the commercial and industrial centre of south India, located on the south-east coast at latitude 13°04´N and longitude 80°17´E (Fig. 1). It has a well developed health care infrastructure, consisting of various facilities provided by the Government, voluntary and private sectors. Cancer incidence in Madras is monitored by the Madras Metropolitan Tumour Registry, which is a population-based cancer registry, covering the population (4.1 million in 1995) of an area of 170 km² within the boundaries of the Corporation of Madras.

The registry was established in 1982 as part of the National Cancer Registry Programme of the Indian Council of Medical Research, Government of India. It is located in the Cancer Institute (WIA), Adyar, Madras, which is a regional cancer centre, recognized by the Government of India. The first report on the incidence of cancer in Madras registry was published in 1983 (National Cancer Registry Programme, 1983). Following this, regular annual

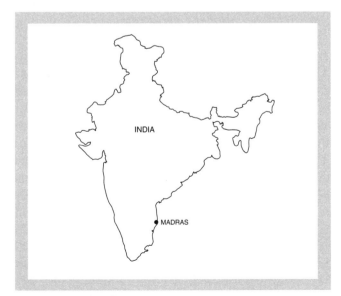

Figure 1. Map showing location of Chennai (Madras)

reports have been published. Data from this registry have been published in Volumes V–VII of *Cancer Incidence in Five Continents* (Muir *et al.*, 1987; Parkin *et al.*, 1992, 1997).

Since 1985, the registry has emphasized follow-up of registered patients, in order to establish their vital status over time. Initially, follow-up was confined to selected cancer sites with a good prognosis (e.g. cervix, breast) and a poor prognosis (e.g. lung, oesophagus and stomach). This was extended to cover all sites in 1991.

Cancer registration in Madras

Cancer is not a notifiable disease in India, so case registration is carried out actively. The cancer registration methodology of the Madras Metropolitan Tumour Registry has been described elsewhere (Shanta *et al.*, 1994). Data sources, besides the Cancer Institute, include 31 Government hospitals, 167 voluntary/private hospitals, nursing homes, pathology laboratories, imaging centres and the Vital Statistics Division of the Madras Corporation. Data are collected by investigators who visit six major government hospitals every day and personally interview patients attending them, and by reviewing medical records from other hospitals. The frequency with which each data source is visited depends upon the number of cases registered there. The data collected include sociodemographic characteristics (age at incidence date, sex, place of residence with duration of stay, place of birth, marital status, mother tongue, religion and literacy level), incidence date, most valid basis of cancer diagnosis, clinical extent of disease before treatment/tumour stage, primary and secondary sites of cancer, laterality, sequence of cancer, morphology, type of treatment given and vital status. One criterion for registration of cases at the registry is that the person should have lived in Madras for at least one year before the date of incidence of cancer. Postal enquiries, field visits and

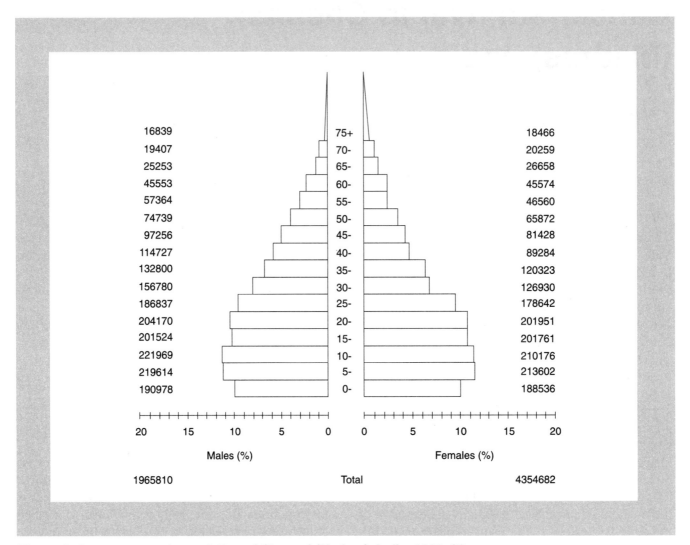

Figure 2. Average annual population of Chennai (Madras), India, 1988–92

scrutiny of population registers and the voters' list are conducted to check the person's residential status, if necessary.

Information on mortality is collected from the Vital Statistics Division and hospital death registers. There are 155 divisional offices of the Vital Statistics Division in the city of Madras, each of which maintains a divisional death register. Social investigators abstract the mortality data from these for all people whose permanent addresses are within Madras city, regardless of the stated cause of death. Trace-back procedures, in the form of house visits, are regularly performed to collect more details of cancer cases which first become known to the registry through death certificate notifications (DCN). If no additional details are forthcoming, these cases are registered on the basis of death certificate only (DCO).

The completed forms are checked by statisticians in the registry office for coding errors, inconsistencies and missing information. Duplicates are eliminated using specially developed computer programs and visual scrutiny to detect identical names, ages, sex, addresses and site of cancer. The *International Classification of Diseases, Ninth Revision* (ICD-9) and the *International Classification of Diseases for Oncology*, First Edition (ICD-O) are used to code cancer sites and histology (WHO, 1976, 1978). The forms are then scrutinized for inconsistencies by a medical officer. Data are entered twice into the computer by different operators, so that errors in data entry can be detected using a specially developed program. The data are then subjected to various consistency checks developed by the registry, as well as the CHECK program (Parkin *et al.*, 1994).

The registry, besides the project chief and a co-investigator, has a medical officer, two statisticians, a computer programmer, nine social investigators, three field staff and a typist. Annual reports are published. A comprehensive analysis of incidence data for the period 1982–91 has been published (Shanta *et al.*, 1993).

Cancer incidence in Madras

Table 1 gives the average annual crude and age-standardized incidence rates for various cancer sites in both sexes in Madras during the period 1988–92. Fig. 2 shows the age structure of the population during this period. The population sex ratio is 934 females to 1000 males; the proportion of subjects under 15 years of age is 32.7% and the proportion of people aged 65+ years is 3.3%. Among males, the major cancer sites are the stomach, lung, oral cavity and oesophagus. Tobacco-related cancers (oral cavity, oropharynx, hypopharynx, oesophagus, pancreas, larynx, lung and urinary bladder) account for 45% of the total cancer burden in males. Among females, cancers of the uterine cervix, breast, oral cavity, stomach, oesophagus and ovary predominate, accounting for 70% of all female cancers. Tobacco-related cancers account for 18% of all cancers in females.

Madras is one of the areas with the highest incidence of cancer of the cervix in the world, especially in the age group 35–64 years. However, a slow but steady decline in the incidence of cervical cancer has been observed since 1986 (Shanta et al., 1993). The higher incidence of cancer in females compared with males is due to the high risk of cervical cancer among females. A steady increase in breast cancer risk has also been observed. It is likely that socioeconomic changes leading to changes in lifestyle, particularly in age at marriage and childbearing patterns (Gajalakshmi & Shanta, 1991), partly explain the above trends. Changes in diagnostic practices might be a possible reason for the increase in ovarian cancer incidence.

The high risk of oral cancer in both sexes has been well documented in Madras. Case-control studies have identified *pan* tobacco chewing and *bidi* smoking as major risk factors (Shanta & Krishnamurthi, 1963). A general increasing trend of tobacco-related cancers has been observed (Gajalakshmi et al., 1996a).

The highest incidence of stomach cancer in India has been observed in Madras (National Cancer Registry Programme, 1992). This moderately increased risk may be attributed to the use of fried food, consumption of a more-than-moderate amount of chillies and tobacco smoking (Gajalakshmi & Shanta, 1996a, 1996b; Nagarajan, 1996). Incidence rates have remained more or less stable. There has been an increase in the incidence of lung cancer, from fifth place in 1982 to second place in 1994 among males. An increasing trend in oesophageal cancer has also been observed. Overall, there has been an increase in age-standardized incidence rates for all sites together, which is greater in men than in women.

Health services in Madras

Madras has a well developed health care infrastructure supported by Government, voluntary and private organizations. Primary health care is provided through dispensaries and general practitioners. Secondary care is available in over 60 hospitals and tertiary care in over 30 hospitals. There are three medical schools within the boundaries of the Corporation of Madras, and one in the suburbs.

Cancer diagnostic services are widely available in secondary care facilities. Madras has probably one of the largest concentrations of advanced diagnostic facilities in the country. Pathology, radiology, immunology, non-invasive imaging, endoscopy and nuclear medicine facilities are distributed among the various secondary and tertiary care facilities.

Surgical specialties are extremely well developed. Cancer surgery is carried out in more than 50 hospitals in Madras. Madras has the most radiotherapy equipment and the highest number of specialists in the country. Radiotherapy services are available in nine hospitals. Chemotherapy is provided in all tertiary care centres. The Cancer Institute, Adyar, is a comprehensive cancer centre, with major responsibility for cancer control in the region.

Early detection activities

There is an official district-level cancer control programme funded by the Government of India and supported by the state Government. The Cancer Institute, as the regional cancer centre, is responsible for training personnel and monitoring this programme. The major focus is on health education, professional orientation and extended case-finding in primary health care. There are no organized screening programmes as yet. Low-cost approaches to cervical (Gajalakshmi et al., 1996b), breast and oral cancer detection are being evaluated for their feasibility, performance and efficacy.

Survival analysis

Subjects

The cancer sites considered for the survival analysis, their data quality indices and details of exclusions from the study are shown in Table 2. A total of 12 758 cancer cases among selected sites, registered in Madras during the period 1984–89, formed the basis for this study. The proportion of cases with histological verification varied from 31.3% (for

Table 1. Annual average cancer incidence per 100 000 person-years in Chennai (Madras), India, 1988–92

Site	MALES			FEMALES		
	Number	Crude rate	ASR	Number	Crude rate	ASR
Lip	28	0.3	0.4	25	0.3	0.5
Tongue	371	3.8	5.8	117	1.3	1.9
Salivary gland	34	0.3	0.5	29	0.3	0.4
Mouth	465	4.7	7.5	495	5.4	8.2
Oropharynx	162	1.6	2.7	32	0.3	0.5
Nasopharynx	67	0.7	0.9	27	0.3	0.3
Hypopharynx	403	4.1	6.5	164	1.8	2.4
Oesophagus	641	6.5	10.5	423	4.6	7.0
Stomach	979	10.0	15.9	433	4.7	7.0
Colon	122	1.2	1.8	84	0.9	1.3
Rectum	245	2.5	3.8	174	1.9	2.8
Liver	161	1.6	2.5	32	0.3	0.5
Gallbladder	35	0.4	0.5	26	0.3	0.5
Pancreas	92	0.9	1.4	43	0.5	0.7
Larynx	309	3.1	5.1	38	0.4	0.6
Lung	789	8.0	12.6	142	1.5	2.4
Bone	101	1.0	1.0	34	0.4	0.4
Connective tissue	87	0.9	1.0	83	0.9	1.0
Melanoma of skin	27	0.3	0.4	16	0.2	0.3
Other skin	107	1.1	1.7	71	0.8	1.1
Breast	17	0.2	0.3	1525	16.6	23.5
Cervix uteri				2540	27.7	38.9
Corpus uteri				127	1.4	2.2
Ovary				390	4.2	5.7
Prostate	179	1.8	3.6			
Testis	60	0.6	0.7			
Penis	196	2.0	3.0			
Bladder	162	1.6	2.8	53	0.6	1.0
Kidney	67	0.7	1.0	44	0.5	0.7
Brain	188	1.9	2.2	84	0.9	1.1
Thyroid	53	0.5	0.8	112	1.2	1.6
Hodgkin's disease	123	1.3	1.3	55	0.6	0.6
Non-Hodgkin lymphoma	287	2.9	3.7	149	1.6	2.0
Multiple myeloma	52	0.5	0.8	24	0.3	0.4
Lymphoid leukaemia	134	1.4	1.4	70	0.8	0.8
Myeloid leukaemia	109	1.1	1.3	74	0.8	1.0
All sites	7695	78.3	118.2	8480	92.4	130.9
All sites except skin	7588	77.2	116.5	8409	91.6	129.8

ASR: Age-standardized incidence rate (world population)

pancreas) to 94.1% (for lymphatic leukaemia). Those registered as DCO cases ranged from 1.8% to 10.3% for different sites. These were excluded from the final survival analysis. Cases with no information on follow-up were also excluded. The proportion of cases included in the final survival analysis thus ranged from 76.4% (for pancreas) to 95.5% (for cervix), making a total of 11 246 (88.2%) of the original cases.

Follow-up methods

The methodology for long-term follow-up of cancer patients at the Madras Metropolitan Tumour Registry has been described in detail (Gajalakshmi & Shanta, 1995). Active methods are the main ones used. Cases registered as DCOs are immediately excluded from the analysis, as they have already been subjected to trace-back procedures at the time

Site	ICD 9	No. of cases registered	Data quality indices		Cases excluded from analysis		Cases included for survival analysis	
			% DCO	% HV	DCO	Others	No.	%
Lip	140	46	2.2	65.2	1	6	39	84.8
Tongue	141	505	2.4	68.9	11	62	432	85.5
Oral cavity	143-5	1100	1.8	61.8	20	149	931	84.6
Oropharynx	146	170	1.8	72.9	3	22	145	85.3
Hypopharynx	148	598	2.0	75.9	12	50	536	89.6
Oesophagus	150	1074	5.9	64.3	63	42	969	90.2
Stomach	151	1579	10.3	50.9	162	104	1313	83.2
Pancreas	157	144	6.9	31.3	10	24	110	76.4
Larynx	161	387	6.5	70.0	25	16	346	89.4
Lung	162	775	9.2	50.3	71	48	656	84.6
Breast	174	1632	4.3	73.0	70	216	1346	82.5
Cervix	180	3445	2.1	83.4	71	85	3289	95.5
Urinary bladder	188	201	5.5	76.6	11	34	156	77.6
Hodgkin's disease	201	229	5.2	92.6	12	0	217	94.8
Non-Hodgkin lymphoma	200,202	417	7.4	83.9	31	24	362	86.8
Lymphatic leukaemia	204	202	3.5	94.1	7	5	190	94.1
Myeloid leukaemia	205	200	6.0	89.5	12	11	177	88.5
All leukaemia	204-8	456	8.6	87.9	39	18	399	87.5

Table 2. Cases of cancer registered and data quality indices, Chennai (Madras), India, 1984–89

DCO : Death certificate only; HV : Histological verification

of registration, without success. All other registered incident cases are then checked for matching with the mortality information collected from the Vital Statistics Division and hospital death registers.

Unmatched cases are divided into those registered exclusively from private institutions, and others. No contact in any form (telephone/postal enquiry, house visit) is made with people registered at private institutions, as part of the policy of cancer registration from these hospitals. These cases are traced back to their original case records, or population health registers are scrutinized to elicit any follow-up information that may exist. Cases registered from Government and voluntary institutions are followed up by means of house visits and postal/telephone enquiries. Cases which do not yield follow-up information by any of these methods are excluded from the analysis. Since 1992, we have matched our incident cases with all deaths occurring in Madras, regardless of the stated cause of death on the death certificate. This has greatly contributed to the completeness of follow-up information, especially for cases registered from private institutions.

The closing date for follow-up for the present study was 31 December 1993. Table 3 shows the level of completeness of follow-up achieved for individual cancer sites. The proportion of people whose vital status (i.e. alive/dead) was known at the closing date ranged between 72% (lymphatic leukaemia) and 92.3% (lip). Cases lost to follow-up before the closing date, ranging between 8% and 28% for different sites, had partial follow-up information for a period ranging between one and five years from diagnosis.

Analytical methodology (see Chapters 2, 3 and 5)

The index date for calculation of survival time was the incidence date. The survival time for each case was the time between the index date and the date of death, *or* date of loss to follow-up, *or* 31 December 1993. Cumulative observed and relative survival probabilities were calculated using Hakulinen's method (Hakulinen, 1982; Hakulinen *et al.*, 1994). The expected survival for a group of people in the general population similar to the patient population with respect to age, sex and calendar period of observation were calculated using the abridged life tables of the urban Indian population (Registrar General of India, 1995). In order to facilitate comparison with results from other countries, the age-standardized relative survival (ASRS) was calculated for all age groups and for the age group 0-74 years by directly standardizing site-specific relative survival to the site-specific age distributions of the estimated global incidence of major cancers in 1985.

Results

Table 4 shows the site-specific observed and relative survival at one year, three years and five years for both sexes combined, and at five years for males and females. The five-year relative survival was less than 10% for cancers of the oesophagus, stomach, pancreas and lung. It was 49.5% for female breast cancer and 60.0% for cervical cancer. The lowest survival was observed for pancreatic cancer (5%) and the highest for cervical cancer (60.0%). A higher five-year survival rate was observed in females for cancers of the tongue, oral cavity, oropharynx, hypopharynx, stomach, larynx and lung, as well as for malignant lymphomas and leukaemia.

Site-specific and age-specific number of cases, five-year relative survival and ASRS for all ages and ASRS for the age group 0-74 years are shown in Table 5. Survival from most cancers was highest in age groups below 45 years. Decreasing survival with advancing age was evident for breast and cervical cancers.

Table 6 shows the five-year observed survival by clinical extent of disease for head and neck, breast and cervical cancers. An inverse relationship between clinical extent of disease and survival was observed (Figs. 3-7).

Discussion

The Madras Metropolitan Tumour Registry has a well established cancer information system with effective methods of case-finding, which has now stabilized. The registry has the lowest number of DCNs of the older registries in India, so there is reason to believe that completeness of cancer registration in Madras is adequate. This has been made possible by active case-finding from multiple sources and the rigorous quality control measures adopted by the registry.

The proportion of cases with histological verification of cancer diagnosis is comparable with other Indian registries and other developing countries. Exclusion of DCO cases from the study was minimal for sites with a good prognosis (1-5%) and a little higher for sites with a poor prognosis (6-

10%). Cases with no follow-up in our series are mostly cases registered from private hospitals, since in those cases we refrain from active follow-up by agreement with the hospitals. These exclusions may have introduced some bias into our survival estimates, although a comparison of factors such as age, sex, year of diagnosis and clinical extent of disease in cases excluded from private institutions and those included in the analysis did not reveal any substantial differences. Given the small number of cases excluded on this count, the overall bias in survival estimate is likely to be minimal. If any bias has occurred at all, we assume that it would lead to an overall underestimation of survival rates, because the patients who seek the services of private hospitals usually belong to affluent socioeconomic categories and their survival experience is likely to be better than the average.

The completeness of follow-up is vital for the validity of survival estimates (Table 3). Vital status was known in 72-92% of cancer cases in different sites. It is noteworthy that, in 50% of the cases lost to follow-up, it was known that the person remained alive for a period ranging from two to five years from diagnosis. Therefore, the number of cases that were truly lost to follow-up with little follow-up information ranged between 3% and 17%. Measures to minimize these losses of information have already been tested for feasibility in the Madras Metropolitan Tumour Registry. From 1992 onwards, we have routinely scrutinized all death certificates received from the Vital Statistics Division (not merely those mentioning 'cancer' or 'tumour'), which has improved the collection of mortality data. It is estimated from our postal and house visits that in 9-12% of cases death occurs outside the city and is not recorded by the Madras Vital Statistics Division, owing to the lack of record linkage.

Hence, for all practical purposes, the survival estimates arising from this data can be considered to be unbiased by selection and to reflect an average outcome from the region, thanks to the completeness of registration and satisfactory follow-up. The median survival for different cancer sites is indicative of the aggressiveness of their natural histories, even after treatment.

Health services in Madras are well developed. Services are provided free of charge in Government and voluntary hospitals for those belonging to poorer socioeconomic groups. The lack of compliance with treatment, which varies from 10% to 30% for various cancer sites, is probably mainly due to attitudes and beliefs and only partly due to lack of availability of drugs or lack of access to

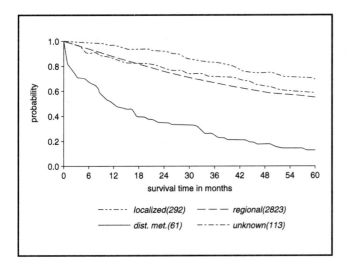

Figure 3. Survival from cervical cancer by clinical extent of disease in Madras, India

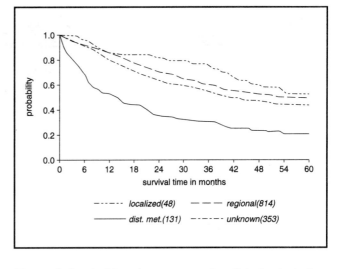

Figure 4. Survival from breast cancer by clinical extent of disease in Madras, India

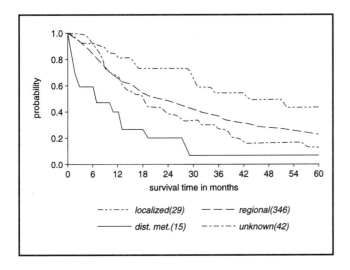

Figure 5. Survival from tongue cancer by clinical extent of disease in Madras, India

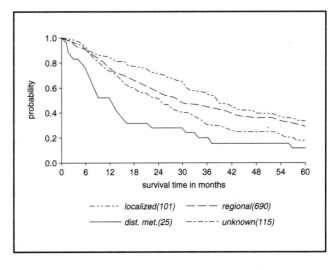

Figure 6. Survival from oral cavity cancer by clinical extent of disease in Madras, India

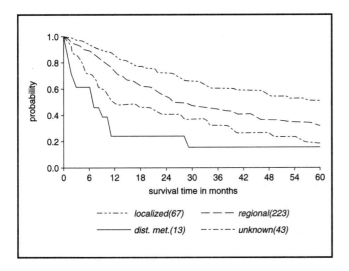

Figure 7. Survival from laryngeal cancer by clinical extent of disease in Madras, India

Table 3. Details of outcome of follow-up of cases in Chennai (Madras), India, 1984–89

ICD-9	Site	No. of cases	Vital status known at closing date (%)	% with partial follow-up information			Median follow-up (in months)
				≤1 yr	2–4 yrs	≥5 yrs	
140	Lip	39	92.3	2.6	5.1	–	30
141	Tongue	432	85.4	6.5	7.6	0.5	16
143–5	Oral cavity	931	81.0	7.1	10.6	1.3	20
146	Oropharynx	145	80.0	11.7	7.6	0.7	18
148	Hypopharynx	536	82.1	16.2	1.1	0.6	11
150	Oesophagus	969	87.8	11.4	0.7	0.1	9
151	Stomach	1313	87.6	11.5	0.8	0.1	8
157	Pancreas	110	86.4	11.8	1.8	–	5
161	Larynx	346	83.8	13.3	2.0	0.9	20
162	Lung	656	85.7	11.4	2.1	0.8	5
174	Breast, female	1346	87.0	5.5	6.2	1.3	34
180	Cervix	3289	83.7	12.2	3.3	0.8	47
188	Bladder	156	89.1	9.6	1.3	–	16
201	Hodgkin's disease	217	90.8	5.1	3.2	0.9	26
200, 202	Non-Hodgkin lymphoma	362	78.5	12.4	7.7	1.4	9
204	Lymphatic leukaemia	190	72.0	17.4	7.4	3.2	8
205	Myeloid leukaemia	177	85.9	8.5	5.6	–	9
204–8	All leukaemia	399	79.7	12.5	6.3	1.5	8

services. This implies that major improvements in cancer survival can be achieved in Madras by early detection and improved compliance with therapy, which can be promoted by means of information and education campaigns to improve the population's awareness of risk factors, symptoms and the facilities available for prevention, early diagnosis and treatment.

Madras has one of the highest reported incidence rates of uterine cervical cancer (Parkin et al., 1997). Though the risk is gradually decreasing, it still remains high, justifying urgent measures to reduce both incidence and mortality. The difficulties of implementing an organized cervical cytology programme have been well described (Sankaranarayanan & Pisani, 1997). Alternative strategies, such as unaided visual inspection to detect early cervical lesions (downstaging), have been shown to be unsatisfactory (Nene et al., 1996; Wesley et al., 1997). There is enough public health observational evidence to prove the usefulness of information and education programmes, using both the mass media and interpersonal approaches, in early detection and improving survival from cervical cancer (Pontén et al., 1995; Jayant et al., 1995, 1996). Our experience in a rural district in Tamil Nadu also confirms the value of increasing public awareness (Gajalakshmi et al., 1996b).

Survival from cervical cancer in Madras is the highest reported in India (Nandakumar et al., 1995a; Jayant et al., 1996; Sankaranarayanan et al., 1995) and is at the higher end of the survival range in other developing countries (Sankaranarayanan et al., 1996). We believe that the reasonably good results achieved in respect of cervical cancer in Madras are due to the possibility of access to good diagnostic and treatment services, in spite of the fact that more than four-fifths of the cancers are already at nonlocalized stages at the time of presentation. Planned educational and case-finding activities should further improve the situation.

Survival from breast cancer is higher than that reported from Bangalore (Nandakumar et al., 1995b) and is at the lower end of the survival range from developing countries and US rates for the period 1967–73 (Sankaranarayanan et al., 1996). Ensuring early diagnosis by targeting risk categories and providing state-of-the-art measures for diagnosis and treatment is likely to improve the outcome in our situation (Gajalakshmi et al., 1997).

The low survival rate in the case of head and neck cancers proves the need for primary prevention as well as early detection measures. Collectively, head and neck cancers are responsible for about 16% of the total cancer burden in Madras. The efficacy of interpersonal communication and

Table 4. Observed and relative survival by site and sex, Chennai (Madras), India, 1984–89

| Site | ICD 9 | Number included | All ages and both sexes combined | | | | | | % Survival rate at 5 years of follow-up | | | | | |
| | | | Observed survival (OS) | | | Relative survival (RS) | | | Male | | | Female | | |
			1 yr	3 yr	5 yr	1 yr	3 yr	5 yr	Number	OS	RS	Number	OS	RS
Lip	140	39	68.5	51.6	40.1	70.3	56.0	46.1	22	41.0	49.9	17	39.2	42.0
Tongue	141	432	66.8	35.6	22.7	68.4	38.3	25.8	341	21.2	24.2	91	29.3	32.2
Oral cavity	143–5	931	76.0	43.7	28.8	78.0	47.2	32.8	447	27.2	31.7	484	30.2	33.8
Oropharynx	146	145	74.6	39.4	18.2	76.6	42.8	20.9	119	16.5	19.2	26	27.2	30.3
Hypopharynx	148	536	58.6	28.4	15.5	59.9	30.6	17.5	380	13.8	16.0	156	20.0	21.3
Oesophagus	150	969	49.1	11.3	5.6	50.4	12.2	6.5	553	5.8	6.8	416	5.4	6.1
Stomach	151	1313	44.9	15.2	6.9	45.9	16.4	7.8	918	6.1	7.1	395	8.4	9.2
Pancreas	157	110	32.2	13.2	4.4	32.8	14.2	5.0	76	6.4	7.2	34	0.0	0.0
Larynx	161	346	70.7	45.6	33.9	72.6	49.5	39.0	304	32.6	37.8	42	43.3	47.3
Lung	162	656	40.3	10.6	6.6	41.4	11.5	7.5	589	6.3	7.2	67	9.2	10.2
Breast	174	1346	82.3	57.2	45.9	83.5	59.7	49.5				1346	45.9	49.5
Cervix	180	3289	87.9	67.4	56.3	89.0	70.0	60.0				3289	56.3	60.0
Bladder	188	156	68.6	33.2	19.1	71.0	36.9	22.8	121	20.7	25.2	35	13.2	15.0
Hodgkin's lymphoma	201	217	67.5	44.7	38.8	68.0	45.7	40.2	160	36.9	38.4	57	44.3	45.7
Non-Hodgkin lymphoma	200,202	362	57.2	31.9	19.4	58.0	33.4	21.1	257	17.5	19.1	105	24.1	25.8
Lymphatic leukaemia	204	190	58.5	34.8	24.5	59.0	35.6	25.4	126	23.0	24.0	64	27.3	28.0
Myeloid leukaemia	205	177	52.1	25.5	16.0	52.8	26.5	17.0	100	15.3	16.3	77	16.5	17.6
All leukaemia	204-8	399	54.5	30.2	20.5	55.1	31.1	21.6	244	19.1	20.2	155	22.4	23.5

mass-media approaches in reducing the long-term prevalence of *pan* tobacco chewing and *bidi* smoking has been well documented in different regions of India (Gupta *et al.*, 1992; Anantha *et al.*, 1995; Sankaranarayanan, 1995). The lack of impact of the Cuban national oral cancer screening programme, in which dentists conduct a visual examination of the oral cavity, is presumably due to low coverage of at-risk groups and poor compliance with referral and treatment (Fernandez Garrote *et al.*, 1995). The efficacy of oral visual inspection in preventing and reducing mortality from oral cancer is currently being evaluated in a randomized intervention trial in India (Mathew *et al.*, 1997). We believe that there is enough evidence to support an education programme to promote primary prevention and case-finding for head and neck cancer in Madras.

The poor survival observed for cancers of the lung, pancreas, stomach and oesophagus reinforce the need to reduce their incidence by means of primary prevention. The poor outcome of treatment in these cancers is well documented. The declining incidence of and mortality from lung cancer among males in some developed countries has been attributed to primary prevention measures (Coleman *et al.*, 1993).

The poor survival observed in the case of lymphoreticular malignancies indicates the need for investment in specialized care centres for diagnosis and treatment, which is currently the only available measure to reduce mortality from these cancers.

The difficulty of obtaining reliable information on clinical extent of disease/stage in population-based cancer registries is well known. However, this information is important for evaluating early detection and survival. We adopted the criteria used in the manual by the National Cancer Registry Programme (National Cancer Registry Programme, 1987). The required information was available in approximately 75–90% of the registered cases. An inverse relationship between clinical extent of disease/stage and survival was seen in all sites. A clear downward trend in survival in cases of advanced cancer of the cervix uteri (Fig. 3), breast (Fig. 4), tongue (Fig. 5), oral cavity (Fig. 6) and larynx (Fig. 7) has been observed, although a certain amount of misclassification cannot be ruled out.

Site	ICD 9	Number of cases by age group						% Relative survival (RS) at 5 years						RS	ASRS%	
		≤34	35–44	45–54	55–64	65–74	75+	≤34	35–44	45–54	55–64	65–74	75+	All ages	0–74	
Lip	140	3	4	7	16	7	2	67.4	101.4	44.6	31.9	59.0	0.0	46.1	39.7	49.7
Tongue	141	18	50	130	143	78	13	21.0	20.8	32.7	25.0	20.2	28.7	25.8	25.5	24.7
Oral cavity	143–5	28	114	269	295	159	66	39.1	47.0	34.0	28.6	29.5	22.7	32.8	31.5	33.7
Oropharynx	146	6	15	43	45	27	9	60.6	21.5	10.2	31.3	5.6	48.9	20.9	27.1	21.6
Hypopharynx	148	37	69	176	145	80	29	22.8	32.0	12.7	15.6	19.3	19.2	17.5	18.9	18.8
Oesophagus	150	39	113	271	297	194	55	9.5	8.0	4.8	6.3	8.4	3.6	6.5	6.0	6.9
Stomach	151	79	176	359	412	233	54	10.2	9.6	9.1	6.4	6.0	8.6	7.8	7.8	7.5
Pancreas	157	12	16	33	31	14	4	24.2	9.1	4.7	5.1	0.0	0.0	5.0	2.8	4.4
Larynx	161	17	45	86	102	80	16	77.9	40.6	39.3	29.3	46.9	11.8	39.0	33.5	39.9
Lung	162	13	81	199	221	108	34	10.9	18.5	7.0	4.8	8.6	0.0	7.5	5.4	7.9
Breast	174	113	357	403	302	123	48	63.6	55.4	50.5	40.1	42.7	19.3	49.5	42.5	48.4
Cervix	180	214	789	1180	791	266	49	77.3	71.9	64.4	47.0	24.7	14.0	60.0	51.5	56.7
Bladder	188	7	16	29	47	41	16	50.8	16.5	21.6	26.9	20.3	0.0	22.8	13.8	23.5
Hodgkin's lymphoma	201	134	25	38	10	8	2	53.3	15.6	17.2	11.2	42.4	0.0	40.2	33.3	35.9
Non-Hodgkin lymphoma	200,202	166	40	53	55	35	13	29.8	31.2	15.9	3.5	9.3	13.0	21.1	16.7	17.7
Lymphatic leukaemia	204	170	3	3	3	10	1	26.8	0.0	0.0	0.0	28.1	0.0	25.4	13.6	16.9
Myeloid leukaemia	205	73	40	27	22	8	7	15.0	20.5	30.9	12.0	0.0	0.0	17.0	11.9	14.7
All leukaemia	204–8	263	46	32	29	21	8	23.3	21.2	25.8	8.9	19.4	0.0	21.6	16.6	20.6

Table 5. Site-specific and age-specific number of cases, five-year relative survival and ASRS, Chennai (Madras), India, 1984–89

ASRS: Age-standardized relative survival

Implications

Notwithstanding the difficulty of organizing and running a population-based cancer information system and studying population-based cancer survival, we feel that both these exercises are of tremendous importance for cancer control and well worth the effort. With the ever-growing database that would accrue for continuing survival studies, active methods of follow-up alone may not be cost-effective. Such studies give an insight into the need to strengthen passive health information systems. This has led to efforts to utilize the information already available in an optimal way. Such studies provide us with a scientific background for the direction that we should take if we wish to achieve a targeted reduction in our cancer burden by rational investment in cancer control.

Our situation calls for investment in early detection of epithelial cancers amenable for treatment, especially the easily accessible sites (e.g. cervix uteri, oral cavity and breast), in primary prevention of those not controllable by available therapy (lung cancer) and in improving drug affordability and supportive care for lymphoid and haematopoietic malignancies. Although the lack of reliable certification of deaths in India will require action in the long term, investment in population-based cancer registries to study incidence and survival seems to be an acceptable and currently feasible solution.

Acknowledgements

We gratefully acknowledge the contribution of a number of colleagues in the cooperating hospitals and institutions in the Government and private sectors and the Vital Statistics Division of Madras Corporation, without whose cooperation this study would not have been possible. We are grateful to the Indian Council of Medical Research, New Delhi, for its financial support for the registry. We are grateful to the Finnish Cancer Society, Helsinki and the International Agency for Research on Cancer (IARC), Lyon for their support for our study of cancer survival. We are grateful to the International Union Against Cancer (UICC), Geneva, and IARC for the award of an International Cancer Research Technology Transfer (ICRETT) fellowship and a special training fellowship, respectively, to Mr. R. Swaminathan, which enabled the data to be

Table 6. Five-year observed survival (%) by clinical extent of disease, Chennai (Madras), India, 1984–89 (number of cases)

Site	Localized	Regional	Distant metastasis	Unknown
Lip	50.0 (8)	32.0 (25)	0.0 (2)	100.0 (4)
Tongue	44.3 (29)	23.0 (346)	6.7 (15)	13.5 (42)
Oral cavity	34.4 (101)	30.3 (690)	12.0 (25)	18.4 (115)
Larynx	51.2 (67)	32.6 (223)	15.4 (13)	16.0 (43)
Breast	53.5 (48)	50.3 (814)	21.2 (131)	44.1 (353)
Cervix	70.4 (292)	55.8 (2823)	12.8 (61)	59.4 (113)

analysed at the Unit of Descriptive Epidemiology, IARC and facilitated the transfer of technology in the field of cancer survival analysis.

References

Anantha, A., Nandakumar, A., Viswanath, N., Venkatesh, T., Pallad, Y.G., Manjunath, P., Kumar, D.R., Murthy, S.G.S., Shivashankariah, S. & Dayananda, C.S. (1995) Efficacy of an anti-tobacco community education program in India. *Cancer Causes Control*, 6, 119–129

Coleman, M.P., Estève, J., Damiecki, P., Arslan, A. & Renard, H. (1993) *Trends in Cancer Incidence and Mortality* (IARC Scientific Publications No. 121). Lyon, International Agency for Research on Cancer

Fernandez Garrote, L., Sankaranarayanan, R., Lence Anta, J.J., Rodriguez Salva, A. & Parkin, D.M. (1995) An evaluation of the oral cancer control program in Cuba. *Epidemiology*, 6, 428–431

Gajalakshmi, C.K. & Shanta, V. (1991) Risk factors for female breast cancer. A hospital based case-control study in Madras, India. *Acta Oncologica*, 30, 569–574

Gajalakshmi, C.K. & Shanta, V. (1995) Methodology for long-term follow-up of cancer cases in a developing environment. *Indian J. Cancer*, 32, 160–168

Gajalakshmi, C.K. & Shanta, V. (1996a) Lifestyle and risk of stomach cancer: A hospital based case control study from Madras, India. *Int. J. Epidemiol.*, 25, 1146–1153

Gajalakshmi, C.K. & Shanta, V. (1996b) Diet and risk of stomach cancer: A case-control study in Madras, India. *Cancer Prevention International*, 2, 97–109

Gajalakshmi, C.K., Ravichandran, K. & Shanta, V. (1996a) Tobacco related cancers in Madras, India. *Eur. J. Cancer Prev.*, 5, 63–68

Gajalakshmi, C.K., Krishnamurthy, S., Ananth, R. & Shanta, V. (1996b) Cervical cancer screening in Tamil Nadu, India : a feasibility study of training the village health nurses. *Cancer Causes Control*, 7, 520–524

Gajalakshmi, C.K., Shanta, V., Swaminathan, R., Sankaranarayanan, R. & Black, R.J. (1997) A population based survival study from female breast cancer in Madras, India. *Br. J. Cancer*, 75, 771–775

Gupta, P.C., Mehta, F.S., Pindborg, J.J., Bhonsle, R.B., Murti, P.R., Daftary, D.K. & Aghi, M.B. (1992) Primary prevention trial of oral cancer in India: a 10-year follow-up study. *J. Oral Pathol. Med.*, 21, 433–439

Hakulinen, T. (1982) Cancer survival corrected for heterogeneity in patient withdrawal. *Biometrics*, 38, 933–942

Hakulinen, T., Gibberd, R., Abeywickrama, K.H. & Soderman, B. (1994) *A Computer Program Package for Cancer Survival Studies, Version 2.0.* Tampere, Finnish Cancer Registry/University of Newcastle, Australia

Jayant, K., Rao, R.S., Nene, B.M. & Dale, P.S. (1995) Improved stage at diagnosis of cervical cancer with increased cancer awareness in a rural Indian population. *Int. J. Cancer*, 63, 161–163

Jayant, K., Rao, R.S., Nene, B.M., Dale, P.S. & Nandakumar, A. (1996) Improved survival in cervical cancer cases in a rural population. *Br. J. Cancer*, 74, 285–287

Mathew, B., Sankaranarayanan, R., Sunilkumar, K., Kuruvila, B., Pisani, P. & Krishnan Nair, M. (1997) Reproducibility and validity of oral visual inspection by trained health workers in the detection of oral cancer and precancer. *Br. J. Cancer*, 76, 390–394

Muir, C., Waterhouse, J., Mack, T., Powell, J. & Whelan, S eds. (1987) *Cancer Incidence in Five Continents,* Volume V (IARC Scientific Publications No. 88). Lyon, International Agency for Research on Cancer

Nagarajan, B. (1996) Risk factors in stomach cancer. In: *Proceedings of the Biennial Conference of the Indian Society of Oncology*. Lucknow, Indian Society of Oncology

Nandakumar, A., Anantha, N. & Venugopal, T.C. (1995a) Incidence, mortality and survival in cancer of the cervix in Bangalore, India. *Br. J. Cancer*, **71**, 1348–1352

Nandakumar, A., Anantha, N., Venugopal, T.C., Sankaranarayanan, R., Thimmasetty, K. & Dhar, M. (1995b) Survival in breast cancer: a population-based study in Bangalore, India. *Int. J. Cancer*, **60**, 593–596

National Cancer Registry Programme (1983) *Annual Report - 1982*. New Delhi, Indian Council of Medical Research

National Cancer Registry Programme (1987) *Code Manual For Population Based Cancer Registry*. New Delhi, Indian Council of Medical Research

Nene, B.M., Deshpande, S., Jayant, K., Budukh, A.M., Dale, P.S., Deshpande, D.A., Chiwate, A.S., Malvi, S.G., Deokar, S., Parkin, D.M. & Sankaranarayanan, R. (1996) Early detection of cervical cancer by visual inspection: a population-based study in rural India. *Int. J. Cancer*, **68**, 770–773

Parkin, D.M., Muir, C.S., Whelan, S.L., Gao, Y.-T., Ferlay, J. & Powell, J., eds. (1992) *Cancer Incidence in Five Continents, Volume VI* (IARC Scientific Publications No. 120). Lyon, International Agency for Research on Cancer

Parkin, D.M., Chen, V.W., Ferlay, J., Galceran, J., Storm, H.H. & Whelan, S.L. (1994) *Comparability and Quality Control in Cancer Registration* (IARC Technical Report No. 19). Lyon, International Agency for Research on Cancer, pp. 61–65

Parkin, D.M., Whelan, S.L., Ferlay, J., Raymond L. & Young J., eds. (1997) *Cancer Incidence in Five Continents, Volume VII* (IARC Scientific Publications No. 143). Lyon, International Agency for Research on Cancer

Pontén, J., Adami, H.O., Bergström, R., Dillner, J., Friberg, J., Gustafsson, L., Miller, A.B., Parkin, D.M., Sparén, P. & Trichopoulos, D. (1995) Strategies for global control of cervical cancer. *Int. J. Cancer*, **60**, 1–26

Registrar General of India. (1995) *SRS Based Abridged Life Tables 1988-92. Occasional Paper No. 4 of 1995*. New Delhi, Office of the Registrar General

Sankaranarayanan, R. (1995) A review of behavioural intervention studies of tobacco use in India. In: Slama, K. ed., *Tobacco and Health*. New York, Plenum Press, pp. 261–266.

Sankaranarayanan, R. & Pisani, P. (1997) Prevention measures in the third world: are they practical? In: Franco, E. & Monsonego, J., eds., *New Developments in Cervical Cancer Screening and Prevention*. Oxford, Blackwell Science Publishers, pp. 70–83

Sankaranarayanan, R., Krishnan Nair, M., Jayaprakash, P.G., Stanley, G., Varghese, C., Ramadas, V., Padmakumary, G. & Padmanabhan, T.K. (1995) Cervical cancer in Kerala: a hospital registry-based study on survival and prognostic factors. *Br. J. Cancer*, **72**, 1039–1042

Sankaranarayanan, R., Swaminathan, R. & Black, R.J. (for Study Group on Cancer Survival in Developing Countries) (1996) Global variations in cancer survival. *Cancer*, **78**, 2461–2464

Shanta, V. & Krishnamurthi, S. (1963) Further study in aetiology of carcinoma of the upper alimentary tract. *Br. J. Cancer*, **17**, 8–23

Shanta, V., Gajalakshmi, C.K. & Swaminathan, R. (1993) *Cancer Incidence and Mortality in Madras: 1982-1991 — A Ten Year Report*. Madras, Madras Metropolitan Tumour Registry

Shanta, V., Gajalakshmi, C.K., Swaminathan, R., Ravichandran, K. & Vasanthi, L. (1994) Cancer registration in Madras Metropolitan Tumour Registry. *Eur. J. Cancer*, **30**, 974–978

Wesley, R., Sankaranarayanan, R., Mathew, B., Chandralekha, A., Aysha, A., Sreedevi Amma, N. & Krishnan Nair, M. (1997) Evaluation of visual inspection as a screening test for cervical cancer. *Br. J. Cancer*, **75**, 436–440

WHO (1976) *International Classification of Diseases for Oncology, First Edition*. Geneva, World Health Organization

WHO (1978) *International Classification of Diseases, Ninth Revision*. Geneva, World Health Organization

Chapter 13

Cancer survival in Rizal, Philippines

D. Esteban, C. Ngelangel, L. Lacaya, E. Robles, M. Monson

Department of Health-Rizal Cancer Registry
Rizal Medical Centre, Pasig, 1600 Metro Manila, Philippines

Introduction

The Republic of the Philippines consists of more than 7000 islands with a total land area of 300 000 km². Rizal province is located adjacent to Metropolitan Manila on Luzon, the second largest island, between latitudes 14°18′N and 14°50′N, and between longitudes 121°7′W and 121°29′W (Fig. 1).

The area covered by the registry comprises 26 municipalities, 14 of which are in Rizal province and 12 in Metropolitan Manila. It encompasses a land area of 1624 km² — 0.54% of the total size of the country. Gently rolling hills and a few rugged ridges which comprise the southern foothills of the Sierra Madre mountain range define the area's eastern topography, while the western part is mostly flat. Within the metropolitan municipal area are located industrial plants of diverse specialization, from food processing to pharmaceutical and chemical industries, from textile manufacturing to the separation of metals from their ores and other metallurgical operations. Of the 14 municipalities of Rizal province, 11 are 'urbanizing' and three are rural.

The population covered by the registry was 5.3 million in 1995, with a male–female ratio of 1:1.06. The population is predominantly young: 33.6% of the population are under 15 years of age and 2.5% over 65. Three-quarters of the population live in the urban catchment areas of the registry.

No information on population-based survival from cancer in the Philippines is available to date. Here we present the results of an analysis of survival of cancer patients diagnosed in the year 1987 from Rizal province, together with background information on cancer registration, health services and follow-up methods used.

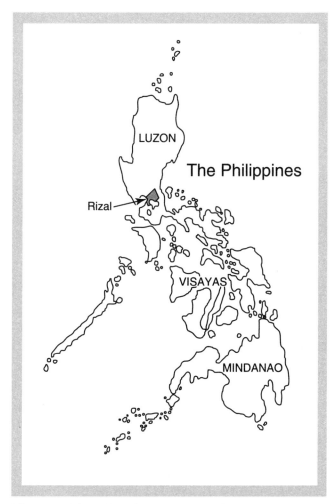

Figure 1. Map showing location of Rizal registry area, Philippines

Cancer registration in Rizal province

The first population-based cancer registry in the Philippines was established in 1974 as one of the activities of the Community Cancer Control Program of the province of Rizal, which at that time comprised 26 municipalities (12 of its municipalities were incorporated into Metropolitan Manila in 1975). From 1974 to 1979, the registry collected data passively, relying on notifications from Government and private physicians and hospitals. Since data collection by passive means was not satisfactory, active registration was started in 1980, with trained registry research assistants abstracting data from hospitals and death certificates.

The registry staff visit the hospitals (N=99) and clinics in the geographical area covered by the registry and enter information about resident cases on the registry abstract form. Death certificate notifications (DCNs) mentioning cancer are

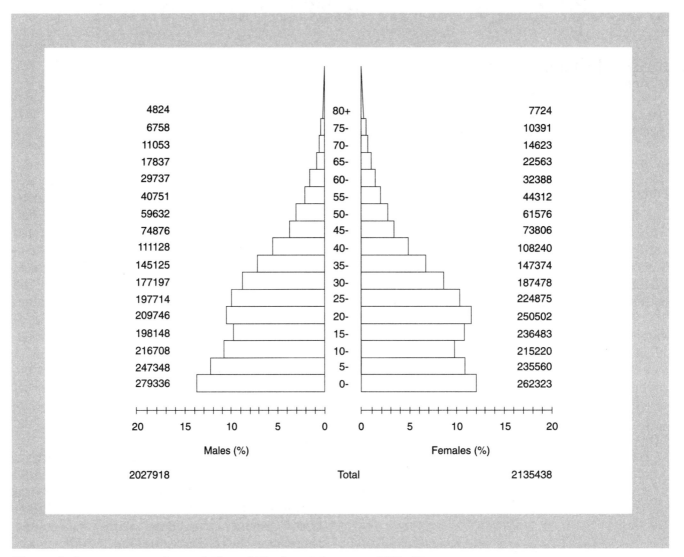

4824	80+	7724
6758	75-	10391
11053	70-	14623
17837	65-	22563
29737	60-	32388
40751	55-	44312
59632	50-	61576
74876	45-	73806
111128	40-	108240
145125	35-	147374
177197	30-	187478
197714	25-	224875
209746	20-	250502
198148	15-	236483
216708	10-	215220
247348	5-	235560
279336	0-	262323

Males (%) Females (%)

2027918   Total   2135438

Figure 2. Average annual population of Rizal registry area, 1983–87

gathered from the municipalities on a special abstract form. These abstracts are checked for completeness and consistency.

To avoid duplication, the abstracts are matched with the file of all previous registrations. Deaths of persons not previously registered are traced back to hospitals, physicians and the person's home address. If no further information is found, these cases are registered as 'death certificate only' (DCO). The proportion of cases with histological verification and the percentage registered as DCO are regularly monitored as indicators of the quality of cancer registration.

After elimination of duplicates, the data are coded and entered into the computer. The *International Classification of Diseases for Oncology*, First Edition (ICD-O) is used to code primary sites and histology (WHO, 1976). *International Classification of Diseases, Ninth Revision* (ICD-9) codes are used for reporting purposes (WHO, 1978).

Detailed descriptions of cancer registration in

Rizal have been published (Laudico *et al.*, 1989, 1993). Incidence data from this registry were published in Volumes V and VI (Muir *et al.*, 1987; Parkin *et al.*, 1992) of *Cancer Incidence in Five Continents*. Cancer incidence data for the periods 1980–82 and 1983–87 were also published in joint technical reports on cancer in the Philippines (Laudico *et al.*, 1989, 1993).

Cancer incidence in Rizal

Table 1 provides the numbers, crude and age-standardized incidence rates for cancers in Rizal province for the period 1983–87 (Parkin *et al.*, 1992). The overall crude and age-standardized incidence rates per 100 000 were 77.0 and 178.4 among males and 87.7 and 174.0 among females, respectively.

The leading cancer sites among males are lung (24.8%), followed by liver (12.5%), prostate (6.1%), stomach (5.5%) and colon (4.2%). The predominant cancers among females are breast (24.1%), uterine cervix (12.3%), lung (6.5%), thyroid (5.6%) and ovary (5.1%). A pattern of increasing incidence of breast, lung and colorectal cancers has recently become evident.

Health care services

The crude mortality rate for Rizal province and Metropolitan Manila in 1985 was 5.9 and 6.3 per 1 000, respectively, while the infant mortality rate was 42.1 and 38.7 per 1000, respectively (Ludovice *et al.*, 1988). The registry catchment area has the most developed health care infrastructure in the Philippines, ensuring access to primary health care services for all the population of the region. Services are provided at subsidized cost in Government facilities. However, there is as yet no health insurance scheme for reimbursement of health care costs for most people, either in Government or in private hospitals or clinics.

There are two comprehensive cancer treatment facilities in Manila. One belongs to the Philippine General Hospital, affiliated to the University of the Philippines; it comes directly under the authority of the Office of the President and has been in operation since the 1950s. The other is located at St. Luke's Medical Centre, a private hospital in Quezon City. There are 99 hospitals, 32 clinics of the Department of Health for outpatient consultations, and scores of private-practice clinics in Metropolitan Manila; there are eight hospitals with radiotherapy facilities. There are now three major Government hospitals (two in Manila, one in Quezon City) with cancer diagnostic facilities (pathology, cytology, haematology, radiological and nonradiological imaging, tumour markers) and therapy facilities (surgery, radiotherapy, chemotherapy, immunotherapy). Imaging and immunocytochemistry services are available in two centres.

A framework for the Philippine Cancer Control Programme was developed in 1987 by the Department of Health. An Advisory Council of the Programme was set up by the Department of Health to advise on policies, priorities and activities in cancer control. The Programme conducts control activities specifically for lung, cervical and breast cancers, which began in 1991. In a knowledge/attitudes/practice (KAP) study in the pilot areas of the Programme in 1989 (Tiglao *et al*, 1990), more than 66.7% of the sample population did not recognize the magnitude of the cancer problem, 33.3% did not know specific procedures to detect cancer or existing treatments for cancer and where they could be obtained, 74.7% perceived the

availability and accessibility of treatment as very difficult, and only 15.4% believed that treatment could be effective. Rizal province was one of the pilot areas of the Programme.

There was no organized early-detection programme in the region during the registration period. Intensive cancer awareness campaigns have been carried out annually since 1975. Currently, a randomized intervention trial in collaboration with the International Agency for Research on Cancer (IARC), France, is under way in the region to evaluate the role of physical examination of the breast in the control of breast cancer. Given the preventable nature of cervical cancer, plans are being developed for a cervical cancer screening programme under the Department of Health's Women and Safe Motherhood Project.

Survival analysis

Subjects
The cancer sites chosen for the survival analysis were lung, breast, cervix, liver, stomach, prostate, colon, rectum and oral cavity, and leukaemia. The number of cases registered, proportion of cases with histological verification, proportion of DCO registrations and number of cases included in the survival analysis for these cancers are shown in Table 2. A total of 1929 cases in these sites were registered in the year 1987. Of these, 330 (17.1%) were DCO registrations; the percentage of DCO cases by site ranged from 3.4% to 42.1%, with the highest proportions in sites with poor survival. These cases, along with a further 199 (with no follow-up information or age/sex unknown or incompatibility in sex, site and histology combination) were excluded from the analysis. The exclusions for individual sites varied between 9.8% to 52.5%. This left 1400 (72.6% of the incident cases) eligible for survival analysis.

Follow-up methods
Both active and passive methods were used to follow up subjects. Seven field assistants were trained to abstract pertinent cancer information from hospital records. They were also trained in the preparation and administration of the follow-up questionnaire. They interviewed patients and/or informants to determine the patient's status (alive and well, alive with disease, migrated, died, unknown) and the date the patient was last known to be alive. The registry records of the study population were reviewed and the patient's status as well as the date of last contact

Table 1. Annual average cancer incidence per 100 000 person-years in Rizal, Philippines, 1983–87

Site	MALES			FEMALES		
	Number	Crude rate	ASR	Number	Crude rate	ASR
Lip	8	0.1	0.3	9	0.1	0.3
Tongue	64	0.8	2.0	62	0.7	1.7
Salivary gland	23	0.3	0.7	29	0.3	0.6
Mouth	75	0.9	2.5	121	1.4	3.5
Oropharynx	20	0.2	0.6	25	0.3	0.7
Nasopharynx	262	3.3	6.3	127	1.5	3.0
Hypopharynx	10	0.1	0.3	6	0.1	0.1
Oesophagus	71	0.9	2.3	50	0.6	1.5
Stomach	342	4.3	11.1	267	3.1	7.4
Colon	257	3.2	7.8	238	2.8	6.6
Rectum	240	3.0	7.3	188	2.2	5.0
Liver	771	9.6	20.7	316	3.7	8.3
Gallbladder	40	0.5	1.3	43	0.5	1.3
Pancreas	127	1.6	4.1	103	1.2	3.1
Larynx	123	1.5	4.0	35	0.4	1.0
Lung	1530	19.1	48.8	487	5.7	13.4
Bone	78	1.0	1.5	63	0.7	1.1
Connective tissue	81	1.0	1.6	68	0.8	1.5
Melanoma of skin	21	0.3	0.6	14	0.2	0.3
Other skin	67	0.8	2.1	55	0.6	1.5
Breast	16	0.2	0.5	1794	21.1	40.9
Cervix uteri				913	10.8	20.1
Corpus uteri				214	2.5	5.5
Ovary				379	4.5	8.2
Prostate	377	4.7	15.2			
Testis	43	0.5	0.7			
Penis	25	0.3	0.6			
Bladder	115	1.4	3.7	46	0.5	1.4
Kidney	93	1.2	2.4	64	0.8	1.5
Brain	119	1.5	2.2	71	0.8	1.1
Thyroid	87	1.1	2.1	415	4.9	7.7
Hodgkin's disease	34	0.4	0.7	24	0.3	0.4
Non-Hodgkin lymphoma	157	2.0	3.9	101	1.2	2.2
Multiple myeloma	27	0.3	0.9	18	0.2	0.5
Lymphoid leukaemia	134	1.7	1.5	93	1.1	1.3
Myeloid leukaemia	121	1.5	2.3	115	1.4	2.0
All sites	6176	77.0	178.4	7443	87.7	174.0
All sites except skin	6109	76.1	176.3	7388	87.0	172.6

ASR: Age-standardized incidence rate (world population)

or date of death (if applicable) were noted. The incident cases of 1987 were also matched with death certificates from the 26 municipalities and the four cities of Metropolitan Manila for the period 1 January 1987 to 31 December 1993 and the date, cause and place of death were noted. Unmatched cases were then matched with the various case-finding lists from the various hospital data sources, to determine whether the patient had consulted other hospitals in the catchment area. Every case which matched the case-finding lists was then followed up at the hospital concerned to confirm the identity of the patient and to gather additional pertinent information, such as diagnosis, tumour stage, treatment, date and status at last contact. Cases were also followed up by contacting the person's attending physician or the

Site	ICD 9	No. of cases registered	Data quality indices		Cases excluded from analysis		Cases included for survival analysis	
			% DCO	% HV	DCO	Others	No.	%
Oral cavity	143-5	44	6.8	88.6	3	3	38	86.4
Stomach	151	118	26.3	60.2	31	11	76	64.4
Colon	153	108	11.1	82.4	12	10	86	79.6
Rectum	154	88	3.4	90.9	3	6	79	89.8
Colorectum	153-4	196	7.7	86.2	15	16	165	84.2
Liver	155	240	42.1	25.0	101	25	114	47.5
Lung	162	430	17.7	65.8	76	24	330	76.7
Breast	174	417	8.6	88.2	36	51	330	79.1
Cervix	180	227	4.4	89.4	10	36	181	79.7
Prostate	185	81	9.9	82.7	8	15	58	71.6
Lymphatic leukaemia	204	51	0.0	100.0	0	5	46	90.2
Myeloid leukaemia	205	55	0.0	100.0	0	9	46	83.6
All leukaemia	204-8	176	28.4	68.8	50	18	108	61.4

Table 2. Cancer cases registered and data quality indices, Rizal, Philippines, 1987

DCO: Death certificate only; HV: Histological verification

hospital where the person was first diagnosed to determine his/her current status and the date of last contact. Additional information on staging (tumour size, lymph node involvement, direct extension, or distant metastasis) and treatment or outcome of treatment was also recorded, where possible: unfortunately, this information was not available for most of the cases. For patients who were lost to follow-up after their discharge from the hospital, the date of discharge was recorded as the date of last contact. People who could not be followed up in the hospital or via their attending physicians because records were no longer available were followed up at their place of residence to determine their current status. Patients with incomplete addresses were followed up through their local health centres or rural health units.

This process revealed the following: a definite vital status (alive/dead) of the cases was known at the closing date for 976 (69.7%) of the cases studied, while the rest (30.3%) were lost to follow-up before the closing date. Among those lost to follow-up, 119 (8.4%) were known to be alive for less than one year, 113 (8.2%) between one and four years and 192 (13.7%) for over five years.

Analytical methodology (see Chapters 2, 3 and 5)
The index date for calculation of survival time was the incidence date. The survival time for each case was the time between the index date and the date of death *or* date of loss to follow-up *or* 31 December 1993. Cumulative observed and relative survival rates were

calculated using Hakulinen's method (Hakulinen, 1982; Hakulinen *et al.*, 1994). The expected survival rates for a group of people in the general population similar to the patient population with respect to age, sex and calendar period of observation were calculated using the model life tables for developing countries for the Far Eastern Region (UN, 1982). Age-standardized relative survival (ASRS) was calculated for all ages and for the age group 0–74 years by directly standardizing the site-specific and age-specific relative survival to the site-specific age distributions of the estimated global incidence of major cancers in 1985 for comparison with other countries.

Results

The cumulative one-year, three-year and five-year site-specific observed and relative survival rates for both sexes combined and site-specific five-year survival rates for males and females are shown in Table 3. The lowest five-year relative survival was for lung cancer (7.2%) and the highest was for breast cancer (45.6%). A five-year survival in excess of 40% was observed for only three cancer sites: oral cavity, colon and breast. For all other sites it was less than 33%.

The site-specific and age-specific number of cases and five-year relative survival, ASRS for all ages and ASRS for the 0–74 age group are shown in Table 4. Owing to the small number of cases in each age category, no distinct impact of age on relative survival could be detected for most cancer sites. Survival was generally better in the younger age groups with the

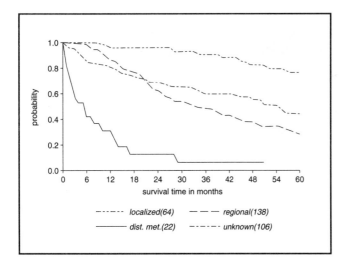

Figure 3. Survival from breast cancer by clinical extent of disease in Rizal, Philippines

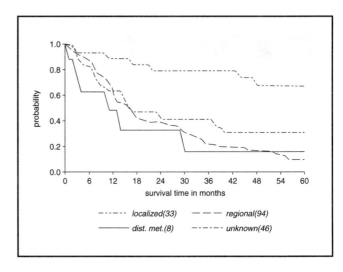

Figure 4. Survival from cervical cancer by clinical extent of disease in Rizal, Philippines

exception of breast cancer, where the lowest survival was encountered in the under-35 age group compared with other age groups.

The observed survival rates by clinical extent of disease for breast and cervical cancers are depicted in Figs. 3 and 4, respectively. Survival rates were higher for people with early clinical disease compared with those with advanced lesions. For breast cancer, the figures were 77.2% for localized disease, 29.2% for regional disease and 6.4% for distant metastatic disease; the corresponding figures for cervical cancer were 67.8%, 11.2% and 16.2%, respectively.

Discussion

Our study is based on a fairly small dataset. Difficulties in the use of active methods to supplement the passive follow-up system meant that our efforts were restricted to cases registered in 1987. Moreover, we wished to explore the possibility of conducting survival studies in our setting and to develop methods to improve follow-up. This is the first population-based cancer survival study in the Philippines and, in spite of the rather limited data obtained, the results on the outcome of cancer care in our region are informative.

A large proportion of cases were excluded from the study for various reasons. The fact that many of these were DCO cases will probably have resulted in an overestimation of survival rates. But a careful look at the results obtained for cancer sites such as oral cavity, breast, cervix and leukaemias shows a survival that is generally poor. From a review of the sporadic reports in hospital-based case series for various sites, these results can probably be attributed to advanced stage of cancer at diagnosis, incomplete treatment and inadequate supportive care because of economic constraints. A

majority of cancers of the oral cavity were categorized as stages III and IV. Surgery was the main method of treatment and the resection rate was estimated to be only 1% for liver cancer (Eufemio *et al.*, 1973), 46% for stomach cancer (Samson *et al.*, 1985) and 57–91% in colorectal cancers (Ceniza *et al.*, 1986). Adenocarcinoma of the lung was predominant among females and squamous-cell carcinoma among males. However, there were few differences in survival between the sexes.

The age-adjusted relative survival rates for breast and cervical cancer in our region are at the lower end of the range observed in other developing countries, and lower than the survival figures observed in the USA 25 years ago (Sankaranarayanan *et al.*, 1996). The five-year relative survival from cervical cancer is poorer than for breast cancer. Given the difficulty of obtaining stage-related information in a routine cancer registration process, particularly in developing countries, the results for these two cancers indicate that a fairly reasonable categorization of the clinical extent of disease has been achieved, although a certain amount of misclassification cannot be ruled out. The probable determinants for late diagnosis of breast cancer among Filipino women were economic factors, lack of awareness of cancer and fear of being diagnosed with cancer (Ngelangel & Lyndon, 1992; Ngelangel *et al.*, 1993). A report on survival based on a large hospital case series revealed a three-year survival rate of 50% from cervical cancer (Sotto, 1987). The low survival in leukaemia is probably due to inadequacies in treatment and general supportive care.

Implications

This survival study has established that, with some additional effort, it was possible to augment the

			All ages and both sexes combined						**% Survival rate at 5 years of follow-up**					
Site	**ICD 9**	**Number included**	**Observed survival (OS)**			**Relative survival (RS)**			**Male**			**Female**		
			1 yr	**3 yr**	**5 yr**	**1 yr**	**3 yr**	**5 yr**	**Number**	**OS**	**RS**	**Number**	**OS**	**RS**
Oral cavity	143-5	38	57.5	33.9	33.9	59.8	38.5	42.5	14	20.4	26.8	24	38.2	46.9
Stomach	151	76	25.7	11.5	9.9	26.7	13.0	12.0	41	14.4	18.3	35	4.3	4.9
Colon	153	86	57.4	38.0	33.7	59.7	42.4	40.5	42	38.9	46.8	44	28.9	34.8
Rectum	154	79	59.9	31.2	20.2	61.7	34.4	23.9	49	17.4	21.1	30	23.1	26.3
Colorectum	153-4	165	58.4	35.1	27.5	60.4	38.8	32.9	91	28.6	34.6	74	26.5	31.2
Liver	155	114	19.9	14.1	12.5	20.5	15.5	14.7	82	11.3	13.3	32	16.3	19.0
Lung	162	330	27.0	9.9	5.9	28.0	11.1	7.2	267	5.7	7.0	63	6.7	7.9
Breast	174	330	82.4	57.2	41.4	83.9	60.5	45.6				330	41.4	45.6
Cervix	180	181	68.5	36.5	26.5	69.6	38.3	29.0				181	26.5	29.0
Prostate	185	58	66.0	29.3	15.6	70.2	35.3	21.3	58	15.6	21.3			
Lymphatic leukaemia	204	46	41.1	28.5	23.7	41.4	28.9	24.4	26	33.0	33.4	20	16.0	16.7
Myeloid leukaemia	205	46	24.0	10.7	10.7	24.5	11.2	11.6	23	5.4	5.9	23	16.2	17.3
All leukaemia	204-8	108	31.2	17.9	16.3	31.6	18.6	17.3	56	17.7	18.8	52	15.3	16.3

Table 3. Observed and relative survival by site and sex, Rizal, Philippines, 1987

routine cancer registration follow-up system to provide a dataset suitable for survival analysis. In the absence of a reliable mortality registration system in our setting and in many other developing countries, information on incidence and survival are important for evaluating the outcome of primary and secondary prevention. The results of this study imply that much still needs to be done to educate the public about cancer and implement all aspects of cancer prevention. The results are perhaps explained by: (1) the lack of favourable knowledge, attitudes, and practices regarding cancer among the target population, which means that many cancer patients seek treatment only when the disease is already far advanced; (2) the lack of resources to organize and implement primary and secondary preventive measures properly; (3) the lack of resources for adequate cancer treatment; and (4) the natural course of the disease itself.

More focused studies are required to collect information on prognostic variables and treatment in order to define approaches to early detection and treatment in more detail and to review whether the full potential of existing health services is being realized. In 1996, the Asian Development Bank, in cooperation with the Philippines Department of Health, initiated the Philippine Adult Health Project. The project report (Havas & Ngelangel, 1996) concludes that there are considerable shortcomings in available data, medical education, national policy issues, treatment guidelines and practices, and quality control of testing and screening services. Changes in programmes, medical education, public policies, additional financial resources, collaboration with nongovernmental organizations, cooperation and compliance by the public, political and administrative support from the Government, and technical assistance from abroad will be necessary. A single strategy will not suffice by itself. The goal of the Philippine Cancer Control Programme is to improve the survival of cancer patients over the coming years, by implementing its various prevention and education programmes.

Acknowledgements

Thanks are due to the Philippine Cancer Control Programme for financial support for this study through the Department of Health Non-Communicable Disease Control Services Division, Manila and to the International Agency for Research on Cancer (IARC), Lyon, France for scientific collaboration.

References

Ceniza, N., Rafols, R.N., Kanglaon, R., Estrada, E., Delalaon, V. & Borja, C. (1986) Colorectal carcinoma: Cebu (Velez) General Hospital experience. *Cebu Inst. Med. J.*, 1, 11–18

Eufemio, G.G., Laudico, A.V., Bulan, M.B., Banes, H.N.M., Domingo, E.O. & Garcia, C.R. (1973) Local experience

Table 4. Site-specific and age-specific number of cases, five-year relative survival and ASRS, Rizal, Philippines, 1987

Site	ICD 9	Number of cases by age group						% Relative survival (RS) at 5 years						RS	ASRS%	
		≤34	35–44	45–54	55–64	65–74	75+	≤34	35–44	45–54	55–64	65–74	75+	All ages	0–74	
Oral cavity	143–5	4	1	3	8	16	6	71.6	101.0	0.0	23.7	56.3	44.4	42.5	41.8	41.2
Stomach	151	5	10	9	20	19	13	20.4	10.3	21.7	14.7	8.5	0.0	12.0	9.6	13.9
Colon	153	13	9	11	21	16	16	38.5	30.8	43.4	67.1	26.0	39.6	40.5	41.1	42.1
Rectum	154	8	9	11	24	22	5	0.0	22.0	15.4	49.6	27.0	0.0	23.9	17.4	29.4
Colorectum	153–4	21	18	22	45	38	21	20.2	27.0	32.0	58.4	26.9	28.2	32.9	33.1	36.5
Liver	155	17	16	25	23	21	12	11.1	38.3	7.2	8.0	10.0	19.1	14.7	14.1	12.9
Lung	162	7	32	69	98	95	29	0.0	11.0	3.0	8.3	9.5	0.0	7.2	5.2	7.7
Breast	174	34	84	95	58	47	12	24.5	44.4	51.9	37.6	52.5	68.2	45.6	49.3	44.5
Cervix	180	19	42	54	39	24	3	32.1	42.4	29.7	17.8	18.5	0.0	29.0	24.6	28.0
Prostate	185	0	0	6	12	22	18	–	–	0.0	33.6	40.5	10.6	21.3	18.7	34.9
Lymphatic leukaemia	204	38	2	4	0	0	2	27.3	50.0	0.0	–	–	0.0	24.4	14.5	18.0
Myeloid leukaemia	205	27	5	2	6	2	4	15.0	0.0	33.4	18.4	0.0	0.0	11.6	11.1	13.7
All leukaemia	204–8	73	8	7	6	6	8	21.5	0.0	0.0	18.4	20.9	0.0	17.3	12.9	15.9

ASRS: Age-standardized relative survival

in the treatment of liver cancer by hepatic artery cannulation and infusion of chemotherapeutic agents. *Phil. J. Surg. Spec.*, **28**, 208–225

Hakulinen, T. (1982) Cancer survival corrected for heterogeneity in patient withdrawal. *Biometrics*, **38**, 933–942

Hakulinen, T., Gibberd, R., Abeywickrama, K.H. & Soderman, B. (1994) *A Computer Program Package for Cancer Survival Studies, Version 2.0*. Tampere, Finnish Cancer Registry/University of Newcastle, Australia

Havas, S. & Ngelangel, C.A. (1996) Assessment of the cancer control efforts in the Philippines. *Phil. J. Int. Med.*, **34**, 115–118

Laudico, A.V., Esteban, D. & Parkin, D.M. (1989) *Cancer in the Philippines* (IARC Technical Report No. 5). Lyon, International Agency for Research on Cancer

Laudico, A.V., Esteban, D., Ngelangel, C.A., Reyes, L.M., Parkin, D.M. & Olivier, S. (1993) *Cancer in the Philippines*. Manila, Philippines Cancer Society

Ludovice, Z.A., Faraon, A.O., Andaya, J.A., Gregorio, S.P., Aquino, I.S. & Guerrero, E.T. (1988) *Philippine Health Statistics 1985*. Manila, Health Intelligence Service, Department of Health

Muir, C., Waterhouse, J., Mack, T., Powell, J. & Whelan, S., eds. (1987) *Cancer Incidence in Five Continents*, Volume V (IARC Scientific Publications No. 88). Lyon, International Agency for Research on Cancer

Ngelangel, C.A. & Lyndon, L. (1992) Breast cancer in the Philippines: determinants of stage at diagnosis. *Phil. J. Int. Med.*, **30**, 231–247

Ngelangel, C.A., Cordero, C.P. & Lacaya, L. (1993) Woman & child health care knowledge, beliefs & practices among Filipino women randomly selected from the 1989 telephone directory of Metro Manila. *Phil. J. Int. Med.*, **31**, 89–101

Parkin, D.M., Muir, C.S., Whelan, S.L., Gao, Y.-T., Ferlay, J. & Powell, J., eds. (1992) *Cancer Incidence in Five Continents*, Volume VI (IARC Scientific Publications No. 120). Lyon, International Agency for Research on Cancer

Samson, P.S., Lopana, J.L. & Gener, R.M. (1985) What awaits the Filipino patient with gastric cancer? The predictive value of hypersensitivity skin test. *Phil. J. Surg. Spec.*, **40**, 70–79

Sankaranarayanan, R., Swaminathan, R. & Black, R.J. (for Study Group on Cancer Survival in Developing Countries) (1996) Global variations in cancer survival. *Cancer*, **78**, 2461–2464

Sotto, L.S.J. (1987) Carcinoma of the cervix. In: Sotto, L.S.J. & Manalo, A.M. eds., *Gynecologic Oncology for the Clinician*, Manila, pp. 53–109

Tiglao, T.V., Tempongco, T.V. & Baltazar, J.C. (1990) *Knowledge, Attitudes, Beliefs and Practices on Cancer in Selected Philippine Provinces*. Manila, Department of Health-Philippine Cancer Control Program

UN (1982) *Model Life Tables for Developing Countries* (Population Studies No. 77). New York, United Nations Department of International Economic and Social Affairs

WHO (1976) *International Classification of Diseases for Oncology*, First Edition. Geneva, World Health Organization

WHO (1978) *International Classification of Diseases, Ninth Revision*. Geneva, World Health Organization

Chapter 14

Cancer survival in Chiang Mai, Thailand

Nimit Martin, Songphol Srisukho, Orathai Kunpradist, Maitree Suttajit

Maharaj Nakorn Chiang Mai Hospital
Faculty of Medicine, Chiang Mai University
Chiang Mai, Thailand

Introduction

Thailand is divided into 76 provinces grouped within four geographical regions: north, north-east, south and central. The northern region is predominantly mountainous with much cooler temperatures than the rest of the country and is the home of several minority tribes, both indigenous and immigrant. Chiang Mai province is one of the 17 provinces of this northern region and has a population of 1.7 million (as at 1 January 1990) living in an area of 20 107 km^2. It is situated in the upper part of the northern region, about 310 m above sea level and at latitude 16°N and longitude 99°E (Fig. 1). The annual average number of wet days is around 120, with an average

annual rainfall of around 125 cm. More than two-thirds of the province is covered with mountains and forests.

Chiang Mai province consists of one municipality and 22 health districts. The population is predominantly rural, and less than one-tenth of the population live in the municipal area of Chiang Mai city. The province has an agrarian economy, dependent on the cultivation of rice, peanuts, soya beans, litchis, strawberries and tobacco. The main industries are tobacco-leaf drying, rice-milling and food and beverage manufacture.

The first population-based cancer registry in Thailand was established in the province in 1986, and data on patients diagnosed with cancer in the province are collected actively. The registry has established a database of incident cases of cancer in the province since 1983 by retrospective data collection. Incidence data from the registry for the periods 1983–87 and 1988–92 were included in Volumes VI and VII of *Cancer Incidence in Five Continents* (Parkin *et al.*, 1992, 1997). The registry has evolved methods to follow up all the registered patients. In this chapter, we describe the survival experience of incident cancer patients in Chiang Mai.

Chiang Mai population-based cancer registry

The first hospital-based cancer registry in the country was established at the University Hospital of Chiang Mai in 1963 to collect hospital-based data on cancer. Population-based cancer registration in the province began in 1986, with the aim of studying the pattern of cancer incidence retrospectively since 1983. This project was supported by the China Medical Board and the Faculty of Medicine, University of Chiang Mai. The registry now covers the entire population of the province (1.7 million), the age structure of which is shown in Fig. 2. Twenty-four per cent of the population are aged under 14, and six per cent are aged 65 years or over.

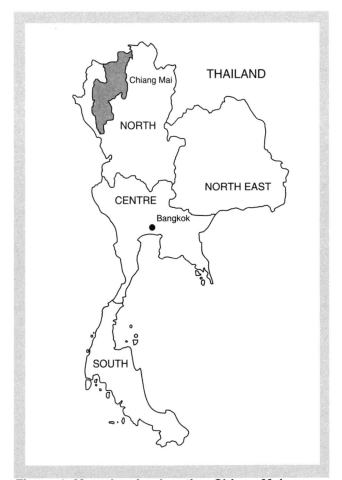

Figure 1. Map showing location Chiang Mai province, Thailand

The registry follows the methods described by IARC for cancer registration and quality control (Jensen *et al.*, 1991; Parkin *et al.*, 1994). Its collaboration with IARC has helped to improve and stabilize cancer registration in our province. Case-finding is predominantly active. The registry staff regularly visit the University Hospital, six other Government hospitals, 20 community hospitals, eight private hospitals and a number of private pathology laboratories and clinics to collect information on cancer patients. The data are abstracted on a standard form for further processing. Copies of death certificates are collected from the offices of the Chiang Mai Public Health Service. All certified cancer deaths are reviewed and matched with the incident case records of the registry. The cases for which no matching records are found are traced back to the data sources in order to obtain relevant data. The cases which cannot be traced back to records in the data sources are registered as 'death certificate only' (DCO).

The classification system of the *International Classification of Diseases for Oncology,* First Edition (ICD-O) (WHO, 1976) is used to code the primary site and histology of the cancers. These codes are then converted to *International Classification of Diseases, Ninth Revision* (ICD-9) codes (WHO, 1978), using the CONVERT programme (Ferlay, 1994) for reporting of incidence and survival data.

The registry is supervised by the cancer committee of the Faculty of Medicine, University of Chiang Mai. A physician from the cancer committee is responsible for the day-to-day operation of the registry and for monitoring and verification of data collection. The registry staff comprises seven nurses and a clerk.

Incidence data for the period 1988-91 were included in IARC Technical Report No. 16, *Cancer in Thailand 1988–91* (Vatanasapt *et al.*, 1993) and later published in the international literature (Vatanasapt *et al.*, 1995). The most recently published data are for the period 1988–92 (Parkin *et al.*, 1997).

Cancer services in Chiang Mai province

Cancer diagnostic services (clinical consultations and radiological and pathological investigations) are available at most public and private hospitals in the province. However, diagnostic and cancer-related therapeutic facilities are available within the same institution only at the University Hospital (Maharaj Nakorn Chiang Mai Hospital).

Cancer surgery services are provided at several locations: the University Hospital, five Government hospitals, two community hospitals and eight private hospitals. The radiotherapy equipment available at the University Hospital includes one superficial-voltage X-ray therapy machine, two cobalt machines, three linear accelerators and one remote after-loading device for brachytherapy. There are five radiotherapy consultants responsible for planning and supervising therapy. Cancer chemotherapy services are provided at the University Hospital, two Government and six private hospitals. The services provided are mostly free, or at least subsidized, at the University and Government facilities. Most hospitals in the province provide palliative care.

Early detection activities

There are no organized screening programmes or officially promulgated cancer control programmes in the province. However, the cancer unit of the University Hospital has assumed the leading role in the provision of cancer care in the region. There are sporadic health education campaigns about common cancers in the region. Mammography and Pap smear services are available on demand in selected hospitals and clinics.

Cancer patterns in Chiang Mai

Table 1 gives the age-standardized incidence rates of major cancers in Chiang Mai for the period 1988–92 (Parkin *et al.*, 1997). Cancer is more common in females, with an age-standardized rate of 155.6 per 100 000, compared with 148.4 among males. Lung cancer accounts for almost one-quarter of all male cases and one-fifth of female cases, and is the most common cancer in both sexes. The incidence of this cancer is much higher in Chiang Mai, in both sexes, than elsewhere in Thailand. The incidence rate among females in Chiang Mai is one of the highest reported anywhere in the world. Adenocarcinomas accounted for half the cancers in both sexes registered with a specified histology; two-thirds of female lung cancers were adenocarcinomas. The male-to-female ratio of lung cancer incidence in Chiang Mai in the period 1988–92 was 1.1:1. In a case–control study involving 115 people with lung cancer in Chiang Mai, smoking cigarettes and indigenous cigars was associated with a nonsignificant increased risk of lung cancer, while chewing *miang* (fermented wild-tea leaves) was associated with elevated risk of lung cancer in women (Simarak *et al.*, 1977).

Liver cancer is the second most common cancer among males (14% of all cases) and the fourth most

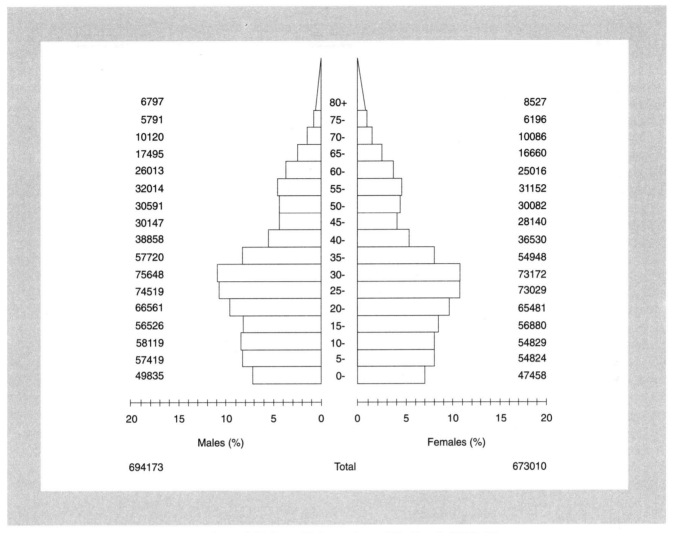

Figure 2. Average annual population of Chiang Mai province, Thailand, 1988–92

common among females in Chiang Mai. Among the histologically verified cancers (35%), hepatocellular carcinoma accounted for 48% of liver cancers and cholangiocarcinoma for 45%. In a case-control study of residents of north-east Thailand, chronic infection with hepatitis B was associated with a relative risk of 15.2 (Srivatanakul *et al.*, 1991). Although an early correlation study found that estimated mortality from liver cancer in two municipal areas in Thailand was apparently related to exposure to aflatoxin-contaminated foodstuffs (Shank *et al.*, 1972a) and aflatoxin has been detected in a variety of market foodstuffs in Thailand (Shank *et al.*, 1972b), a recent study involving direct measurement of aflatoxin–albumin adducts in sera from humans suggest that intake is rather low. This is consistent with the low prevalence of G-to-T mutations at codon 249 of the *p53* gene in Thai patients with hepatocellular carcinoma (Wild *et al.*, 1992). It seems unlikely that aflatoxin exposure is a major risk factor for hepatocellular carcinoma in Thailand.

Uterine cervical cancer is the second most common malignant neoplasm among women, accounting for one-sixth of all female cases. A case–control study in Bangkok reported an increased risk associated with early onset of sexual intercourse and number of sexual partners (Wangsuphachart *et al.*, 1987). The high fertility of women in rural areas of Thailand in the past is also likely to be an important determinant of cervical cancer risk. This again would explain the current low incidence of breast cancer. The habit of betel quid chewing is common in the villages, particularly among women, and this has been shown to be a risk factor for mouth cancer in both sexes (Simarak *et al.*, 1977; Vatanasapt *et al.*, 1991).

Survival analysis

Subjects

During the period 1983–92, the registry identified 17 226 incident cases of cancer in the province. The distribution of these cases, with the proportion of

Table 1. Annual average cancer incidence per 100 000 person-years in Chiang Mai, Thailand, 1988–92

Site	MALES			FEMALES		
	Number	Crude rate	ASR	Number	Crude rate	ASR
Lip	7	0.2	0.2	15	0.4	0.4
Tongue	59	1.7	2.0	37	1.1	1.2
Salivary gland	12	0.3	0.4	16	0.5	0.5
Mouth	77	2.2	2.5	66	2.0	2.0
Oropharynx	50	1.4	1.6	29	0.9	0.9
Nasopharynx	88	2.5	2.6	48	1.4	1.5
Hypopharynx	74	2.1	2.4	18	0.5	0.6
Oesophagus	70	2.0	2.3	46	1.4	1.5
Stomach	245	7.1	7.5	154	4.6	4.9
Colon	139	4.0	4.2	122	3.6	3.7
Rectum	101	2.9	3.1	92	2.7	2.8
Liver	659	19.0	20.1	303	9.0	9.7
Gallbladder	104	3.0	3.3	92	2.7	3.0
Pancreas	85	2.4	2.7	74	2.2	2.4
Larynx	158	4.6	5.3	55	1.6	1.8
Lung	1140	32.8	36.0	941	28.0	30.3
Bone	23	0.7	0.6	18	0.5	0.6
Connective tissue	17	0.5	0.5	20	0.6	0.7
Melanoma of skin	21	0.6	0.6	15	0.4	0.5
Other skin	132	3.8	4.2	98	2.9	3.0
Breast	2	0.1	0.1	477	14.2	14.6
Cervix uteri				864	25.7	25.6
Corpus uteri				110	3.3	3.5
Ovary				152	4.5	4.4
Prostate	122	3.5	4.1			
Testis	22	0.6	0.5			
Penis	78	2.2	2.4			
Bladder	168	4.8	5.3	78	2.3	2.5
Kidney	50	1.4	1.6	48	1.4	1.5
Brain	66	1.9	2.0	55	1.6	1.8
Thyroid	37	1.1	1.1	88	2.6	2.5
Hodgkin's disease	43	1.2	1.2	15	0.4	0.4
Non-Hodgkin lymphoma	131	3.8	3.8	84	2.5	2.6
Multiple myeloma	14	0.4	0.4	10	0.3	0.3
Lymphoid leukaemia	34	1.0	1.2	22	0.7	0.7
Myeloid leukaemia	93	2.7	2.6	88	2.6	2.7
All sites	4791	138.0	148.4	5006	148.8	155.6
All sites except skin	4659	134.2	144.2	4908	145.9	152.6

ASR: Age-standardized incidence rate (world population)

histologically verified cases and those registered as DCO by site, are shown in Table 2. A histological verification of diagnosis was available in 68.8% of cases. The proportion varied from site to site: it was below 50% in liver, pancreas and brain cancers and ranged between 50% and 80% in cancers of the oesophagus, stomach, colon, gallbladder, lung and bone. It was higher for other sites.

A total of 1723 subjects (10%) were registered on a DCO basis. For more than two-thirds of these cases, the primary site was unknown. They were excluded from the final analysis.

For 915 cases (5.3%), no follow-up information was available after registration. Even active methods were not successful in tracing them back. These cases, and six more with invalid cancer data, were

Table 2. Cancer cases registered and data quality indices, Chiang Mai, Thailand, 1983–92								
Site	ICD 9	No. of cases registered	Data quality indices		Cases excluded from analysis		Cases included for survival analysis	
			% DCO	% HV	DCO	Others	No.	%
Lip	140	37	2.7	94.6	1	1	35	94.6
Tongue	141	173	0.6	94.8	1	0	172	99.4
Salivary gland	142	41	0.0	92.7	0	0	41	100.0
Oral cavity	143-5	275	1.1	90.2	3	33	239	86.9
Oropharynx	146	139	0.0	95.0	0	14	125	89.9
Nasopharynx	147	258	1.9	90.7	5	31	222	86.0
Hypopharynx	148	182	0.0	93.4	0	18	164	90.1
Oesophagus	150	241	2.1	58.5	5	18	218	90.5
Stomach	151	747	3.2	74.3	24	68	655	87.7
Colon	153	447	4.0	70.5	18	37	392	87.7
Rectum	154	369	1.6	84.3	6	18	345	93.5
Colorectum	153-4	816	2.9	76.7	24	55	737	90.3
Liver	155	1619	7.0	40.1	114	56	1449	89.5
Gallbladder	156	339	2.7	53.4	9	23	307	90.6
Pancreas	157	241	1.2	43.6	3	22	216	89.6
Larynx	161	383	1.0	86.4	4	37	342	89.3
Lung	162	3489	3.9	59.9	135	159	3195	91.6
Bone	170	61	11.5	54.1	7	9	45	73.8
Connective tissue	171	78	1.3	94.9	1	10	67	85.9
Skin melanoma	172	67	0.0	100.0	0	1	66	98.5
Other skin	173	410	1.0	98.8	4	4	402	98.0
Breast	174	791	1.6	94.3	13	14	764	96.6
Cervix	180	1574	0.7	97.4	11	8	1555	98.8
Corpus uteri	182	165	9.1	84.2	15	13	137	83.0
Ovary	183	292	0.7	89.4	2	30	260	89.0
Vagina	184	75	1.3	96.0	1	6	68	90.7
Prostate	185	183	1.1	87.4	2	24	157	85.8
Testis	186	43	0.0	86.0	0	8	35	81.4
Penis	187	143	0.0	92.3	0	22	121	84.6
Bladder	188	425	0.5	89.9	2	30	393	92.5
Kidney	189	142	2.8	82.4	4	24	114	80.3
Brain & nervous system	191-2	212	13.2	45.8	28	18	166	78.3
Thyroid	193	211	0.9	85.3	2	33	176	83.4
Hodgkin's disease	201	95	0.0	100.0	0	10	85	89.5
Non-Hodgkin lymphoma	200,202	381	0.0	100.0	0	48	333	87.4
Multiple myeloma	203	42	0.0	100.0	0	2	40	95.2
Lymphatic leukaemia	204	98	0.0	100.0	0	10	88	89.8
Myeloid leukaemia	205	277	0.0	100.0	0	25	252	91.0
All leukaemia	204-8	480	0.0	100.0	0	39	441	91.9
Primary site uncertain	195-9	1791	70.4	22.2	1260	2	529	29.5
All sites	140-208	17226	10.0	68.8	1723	2644	14582	84.7

DCO : Death certificate only; HV : Histological verification excluded from the final analysis. Thus 14 582 cases (84.7% of registered cases) were eligible for the survival analysis.

Follow-up methods

Follow-up data about registered cancer patients were obtained by a mixture of passive and active methods. The first method used was matching with death certificates. For the remaining cases thought to be alive, follow-up information was obtained by repeated scrutiny of hospital case records, postal enquiries and, if these measures failed to establish a patient's vital status, home visits. For more than half the cases, information on vital status was obtained by reply-paid postal enquiries.

The closing date for follow-up was 30 June 1994. The details of the outcome of follow-up by site are shown in Table 3. The vital status of the person (alive/dead) was known in 77.2% of cases, and the rest were lost to follow-up prior to the closing date: 1.4% in less than one year, 11.3% between one and five years and 10.1% more than five years from the date of diagnosis of cancer.

Analytical methodology (see Chapters 2, 3 and 5)

The duration of survival for each case was calculated from the date of diagnosis to the date of death *or* the date of loss to follow-up *or* 30 June 1994. Cumulative observed and relative survival probabilities were calculated using Hakulinen's method (Hakulinen, 1982; Hakulinen *et al.*, 1994). The expected survival of the patient population was calculated using the life tables for the whole of Thailand (National Statistical Office, 1994). For comparison of survival rates with other reported experiences, site-specific and age-specific relative survival rates were directly standardized to the site-specific age distributions of the estimated global incidence of major cancers in the world in 1985.

Results

The observed and relative survival at one, three and five years from diagnosis for both sexes combined is shown in Table 4 for various cancer sites. The same table shows observed and relative survival at five years for males and females for different cancer sites. Five-year relative survival was over 50% for cancers of the lip, skin (non-melanoma), female breast, cervix, corpus uteri, vagina and vulva, testis, penis and thyroid. The highest survival rate (92.7%) was observed for non-melanoma skin cancer. Five-year survival was less than 10% for cancers of the oesophagus, stomach, liver, gallbladder, pancreas

and lung. The lowest survival (0.5%) was observed for liver cancer. Survival ranged from 10% to 20% for tumours of the oral cavity, larynx, kidney and central nervous system and leukaemias. The survival rates varied from 20% to 50% for cancers of the tongue, pharynx, colorectum, bone, connective tissue, skin (melanoma), ovary, prostate and bladder and in Hodgkin's disease and non-Hodgkin lymphoma.

No major differences in survival were observed in either sex for major cancers such as lung and liver. A higher survival among females was seen for cancer sites including the tongue, oral cavity, oropharynx, nasopharynx, oesophagus, larynx, connective tissue, kidney and brain, and for Hodgkin's disease. The five-year age-specific relative survival, age-standardized relative survival (ASRS) for all ages and for the age group 0–74 years by site are shown in Table 5. There is a general trend of declining survival with old age for most cancer sites.

Table 6 shows five-year observed survival in relation to clinical extent of disease for cancers of the lip, tongue, oral cavity, larynx, colon, rectum, breast and uterine cervix. Figs. 3–10 depict the observed survival by clinical extent of disease until five years from the date of diagnosis of these cancers. The survival was around 90% for localized cancers of breast and uterine cervix, and 74.3% for localized cancers of colon. More than half the patients with regional disease in colon, breast and cervical cancers survived for five years.

Discussion

In our situation, factors relating to the completeness of cancer registration, exclusions and completeness of follow-up are likely to influence the survival results. Active case-finding from multiple sources and the data quality indicators (the proportion of histologically verified cases and the low proportion of DCO registrations) indicate that cancer registration is fairly complete.

If the cases without follow-up information happen to represent a sample of all cases, the bias introduced is likely to be minimal. If, on the other hand, these patients have poor natural histories and health behaviours (which is likely to be the case), the results obtained may overestimate the true survival. However, we believe that this overestimation is minor. The completeness of follow-up is also fairly adequate. In 87% of cases included, either their vital status (alive/dead) was known at the closing date or they were known to have been alive for more than five years from diagnosis.

Site	Number included	Vital status (alive/dead) known (%)	% lost to follow-up		
			<1 year	1–5 years	>5 years
Lip	35	51.4	0.0	25.7	22.9
Tongue	172	77.3	0.6	12.8	9.3
Salivary gland	41	51.2	0.0	29.3	19.5
Oral cavity	239	87.0	0.8	5.9	6.3
Oropharynx	125	78.4	3.2	10.4	8.0
Nasopharynx	222	75.7	2.3	11.7	10.3
Hypopharynx	164	85.9	4.1	8.7	1.3
Oesophagus	218	96.8	0.5	2.7	0.0
Stomach	655	91.3	1.8	3.2	3.7
Colon	392	64.8	3.8	20.9	10.5
Rectum	345	76.2	2.6	12.2	9.0
Colorectum	737	70.1	3.3	16.8	9.8
Liver	1449	97.8	0.8	1.3	0.1
Gallbladder	307	93.5	1.6	3.6	1.3
Pancreas	216	92.1	2.8	4.2	0.9
Larynx	342	84.2	0.6	7.3	7.9
Lung	3195	95.3	1.4	2.8	0.5
Bone	45	64.4	4.4	20.0	11.2
Connective tissue	67	71.6	3.0	9.0	16.4
Skin melanoma	66	63.6	1.5	15.2	19.7
Other skin	402	30.8	0.2	32.8	36.1
Breast	764	41.6	0.0	32.2	26.2
Cervix	1555	36.9	0.1	28.5	34.5
Corpus uteri	137	34.6	3.6	32.1	16.7
Ovary	260	66.9	2.7	14.6	15.8
Vagina	68	57.4	1.5	25.0	16.1
Prostate	157	69.4	2.5	17.2	10.9
Testis	35	57.1	2.9	17.1	22.9
Penis	121	58.7	2.5	19.8	19.0
Bladder	393	69.5	1.3	16.0	13.2
Kidney	114	86.8	1.0	6.1	6.1
Brain & nervous system	166	84.3	3.1	6.0	6.6
Thyroid	176	56.8	4.5	21.6	17.1
Hodgkin's disease	85	74.1	4.7	12.9	8.3
Non-Hodgkin lymphoma	333	77.5	1.8	10.8	6.9
Multiple myeloma	40	85.0	5.0	2.5	7.5
Lymphatic leukaemia	88	90.9	0.0	2.3	6.8
Myeloid leukaemia	252	89.3	1.2	5.6	3.9
All leukaemia	441	90.9	0.7	4.3	4.1
Primary site uncertain	529	94.1	1.9	3.6	0.4
All sites	14582	77.2	1.4	11.3	10.1

Table 3. Outcome of follow-up in Chiang Mai, Thailand, 1983–92

In our study, very low survival was experienced by patients with head and neck cancer (except those with lip cancer). Most of the head and neck cancers are associated with tobacco and alcohol consumption, and the symptoms of the disease most often appear only after the tumour has grown and spread to the surrounding tissues and lymph glands. The information available on clinical extent of disease at presentation indicates that more than 80% of the patients presented with regional extension of

Table 4. Observed and relative survival by site and sex, Chiang Mai, Thailand, 1983–92

Site	ICD 9	Number included	Observed survival (OS)			Relative survival (RS)			Male			Female		
			1 yr	3 yr	5 yr	1 yr	3 yr	5 yr	Number	OS	RS	Number	OS	RS
Lip	140	35	68.6	57.0	53.4	73.1	68.5	71.3	13	67.0	88.9	22	45.4	60.8
Tongue	141	172	49.4	28.9	27.4	52.3	34.1	35.9	106	19.3	26.8	66	39.8	48.3
Salivary gland	142	41	82.9	60.4	47.8	85.1	65.2	55.0	20	35.7	42.1	21	59.3	66.4
Oral cavity	143–5	239	38.1	20.2	14.8	40.3	23.9	19.4	141	11.1	15.5	98	20.4	24.9
Oropharynx	146	125	47.5	23.3	16.9	50.8	28.4	23.3	84	15.6	22.4	41	19.2	24.7
Nasopharynx	147	222	61.3	33.0	27.2	62.1	34.5	29.4	148	24.1	26.4	74	33.5	35.1
Hypopharynx	148	164	45.2	24.8	15.5	48.3	30.2	21.4	135	15.7	22.3	29	14.8	18.0
Oesophagus	150	218	14.4	4.0	2.9	15.1	4.7	3.8	130	1.7	2.2	88	4.8	6.3
Stomach	151	655	27.3	11.9	7.5	28.1	12.9	8.6	411	7.8	9.2	244	7.0	7.7
Colon	153	392	55.2	38.0	33.3	56.8	41.3	38.4	210	33.7	39.6	182	32.5	36.6
Rectum	154	345	58.3	28.8	21.9	59.9	31.3	25.2	185	22.9	26.8	160	21.0	23.6
Colorectum	153–4	737	56.7	33.6	27.6	58.2	36.5	31.8	395	28.6	33.6	342	26.7	30.1
Liver	155	1449	6.8	1.5	0.4	6.9	1.6	0.5	975	0.0	0.0	474	0.8	1.1
Gallbladder	156	307	21.5	5.5	3.5	22.2	6.0	4.1	148	3.9	4.6	159	3.2	3.8
Pancreas	157	216	19.6	5.1	3.2	20.1	5.6	3.7	118	3.8	4.3	98	2.6	3.0
Larynx	161	342	49.8	22.2	16.2	51.9	25.2	20.2	250	14.4	18.5	92	21.0	23.9
Lung	162	3195	17.6	4.4	2.7	18.0	4.7	3.1	1743	2.6	3.0	1452	2.8	3.1
Bone	170	45	57.6	33.7	33.7	58.0	34.8	36.1	29	47.3	48.4	16	12.5	14.3
Connective tissue	171	67	65.1	37.3	35.3	65.9	38.8	37.9	30	27.2	29.8	37	40.9	43.0
Skin melanoma	172	66	72.4	42.0	36.5	75.2	47.2	43.7	42	34.8	43.8	24	39.9	44.3
Other skin	173	402	88.3	77.1	73.9	92.5	88.6	92.7	225	72.4	92.7	177	75.8	92.9
Breast	174	764	88.1	69.2	59.4	89.3	72.0	63.7				764	59.4	63.7
Cervix	180	1555	86.9	70.3	65.0	87.6	72.3	68.2				1555	65.0	68.2
Corpus uteri	182	137	81.4	68.1	64.1	82.5	71.3	69.5				137	64.1	69.5
Ovary	183	260	64.2	47.2	42.6	64.7	48.5	44.9				260	42.6	44.9
Vagina	184	68	82.2	57.9	51.2	84.4	62.6	59.2				68	51.2	59.2
Prostate	185	157	65.2	43.7	28.7	70.2	54.8	42.3	157	28.7	42.3			
Testis	186	35	85.6	51.7	47.9	86.6	53.5	50.7	35	47.9	50.7			
Penis	187	121	75.7	55.1	48.9	77.9	60.3	56.8	121	48.9	56.8			
Bladder	188	393	58.2	38.4	31.0	60.7	43.6	38.3	266	31.6	39.7	127	29.6	35.2
Kidney	189	114	39.4	19.2	14.0	40.1	20.2	15.3	55	10.2	11.4	59	17.4	18.6
Brain & nervous system	191–2	166	39.0	22.1	17.9	39.3	22.7	18.7	83	12.3	13.0	83	23.7	24.6
Thyroid	193	176	60.7	52.1	48.3	61.6	54.6	52.7	59	46.9	52.1	117	48.8	52.9
Hodgkin's disease	201	85	49.3	27.2	27.2	50.2	28.6	29.6	57	20.0	22.0	28	41.2	43.6
Non-Hodgkin lymphoma	200,202	333	45.9	27.2	22.4	46.9	28.9	24.7	217	24.0	26.5	116	18.8	20.5
Multiple myeloma	203	40	52.1	20.4	14.6	53.5	22.3	16.9	26	19.1	22.8	14	7.1	8.0
Lymphatic leukaemia	204	88	37.5	14.7	13.2	37.7	15.0	13.7	53	12.8	13.2	35	13.5	14.1
Myeloid leukaemia	205	252	28.7	14.7	10.1	29.2	15.4	10.9	142	10.3	11.2	110	9.6	10.2
All leukaemia	204–8	441	26.8	12.6	9.7	27.2	13.1	10.4	247	9.5	10.2	194	10.0	10.6

Table 5. Site-specific and age-specific number of cases, five-year relative survival and ASRS, Chiang Mai, Thailand, 1983–92

Site	ICD 9	Number of cases by age group						% Relative survival (RS) at 5 years						RS	ASRS%	
		≤34	35–44	45–54	55–64	65–74	75+	≤34	35–44	45–54	55–64	65–74	75+	All ages	0–74	
Lip	140	2	1	5	9	4	14	101.0	101.0	55.9	59.6	26.5	111.7	71.3	70.9	60.6
Tongue	141	1	8	20	45	50	48	101.2	38.1	41.6	33.2	26.1	48.5	35.9	37.5	34.7
Salivary gland	142	2	7	12	6	8	6	100.9	56.7	58.0	26.7	45.2	94.1	55.0	55.4	45.7
Oral cavity	143–5	12	4	25	73	53	72	35.1	25.1	16.3	23.4	16.1	10.9	19.4	19.2	21.3
Oropharynx	146	11	4	6	28	32	44	73.5	50.6	0.0	13.8	12.6	19.3	23.3	20.7	21.1
Nasopharynx	147	25	37	68	58	29	5	58.1	40.9	27.0	18.6	14.7	33.0	29.4	27.9	26.6
Hypopharynx	148	0	4	8	42	58	52	–	25.6	15.3	22.4	22.7	18.6	21.4	19.0	19.1
Oesophagus	150	1	4	27	60	68	58	0.0	0.0	0.0	2.7	7.7	4.0	3.8	3.5	3.3
Stomach	151	39	57	121	221	152	65	19.3	8.6	5.3	7.4	10.9	6.3	8.6	7.9	8.7
Colon	153	33	44	68	131	65	51	31.8	36.0	56.8	35.3	25.9	42.8	38.4	38.5	35.6
Rectum	154	46	37	57	78	90	37	29.4	35.7	24.6	25.9	14.8	45.8	25.2	32.1	22.6
Colorectum	153–4	79	81	125	209	155	88	30.3	36.6	42.4	31.1	19.2	43.1	31.8	34.9	29.2
Liver	155	108	177	294	459	312	99	2.5	0.0	0.0	0.6	0.6	0.0	0.5	0.5	0.6
Gallbladder	156	4	16	68	97	73	49	0.0	13.8	6.1	2.9	1.7	13.2	4.1	6.7	4.1
Pancreas	157	10	17	37	72	61	19	0.0	7.0	0.0	0.0	4.5	22.2	3.7	9.7	2.5
Larynx	161	3	9	43	97	129	61	33.7	53.0	30.6	25.8	10.2	13.2	20.2	23.0	25.8
Lung	162	71	176	685	1259	756	248	4.8	4.2	3.1	2.8	3.3	3.2	3.1	3.2	3.2
Bone	170	31	2	5	2	2	3	40.2	50.2	20.8	0.0	59.5	0.0	36.1	22.7	31.7
Connective tissue	171	19	13	9	15	10	1	50.6	48.1	34.9	26.9	23.9	0.0	37.9	23.5	32.8
Skin melanoma	172	13	2	8	18	12	13	35.9	50.5	39.3	31.9	39.4	118.2	43.7	39.2	39.2
Other skin	173	27	23	58	98	99	97	89.3	92.9	84.3	86.6	84.0	137.0	92.7	85.7	86.4
Breast	174	80	198	213	164	78	31	69.0	67.7	65.0	54.8	61.9	74.2	63.7	65.0	62.7
Cervix	180	216	449	399	318	139	34	83.6	76.4	66.1	54.2	50.8	78.2	68.2	66.5	64.9
Corpus uteri	182	5	15	48	46	16	7	20.1	94.9	83.2	55.4	64.0	47.6	69.5	63.0	67.1
Ovary	183	60	40	67	63	25	5	62.3	61.0	45.4	31.9	9.6	37.4	44.9	39.0	39.3
Vagina	184	8	10	12	19	8	11	37.8	78.2	60.4	64.4	28.4	52.4	59.2	53.9	54.3
Prostate	185	1	0	4	20	70	62	0.0	–	79.5	39.7	46.1	31.6	42.3	36.3	45.9
Testis	186	15	5	10	4	0	1	71.3	61.1	31.5	27.4	–	0.0	50.7	63.4	63.3
Penis	187	12	8	27	43	17	14	45.1	64.0	52.7	46.3	70.9	128.1	56.8	60.6	56.6
Bladder	188	13	14	42	134	118	72	40.0	26.2	32.0	35.5	36.1	69.3	38.3	49.0	34.6
Kidney	189	11	8	26	40	26	3	45.9	25.2	8.0	21.7	4.9	0.0	15.3	14.1	19.1
Brain & nervous system	191–2	82	23	21	26	9	5	25.9	4.9	0.0	24.0	12.9	30.9	18.7	16.7	13.1
Thyroid	193	27	32	35	42	29	11	79.3	84.5	51.4	36.0	19.4	15.8	52.7	40.4	46.7
Hodgkin's disease	201	24	15	10	22	8	6	48.4	30.1	24.0	13.2	13.7	29.4	29.6	34.4	34.8
Non-Hodgkin lymphoma	200,202	106	33	50	81	38	25	31.3	37.2	17.5	20.3	9.3	27.6	24.7	23.8	22.7
Multiple myeloma	203	3	3	6	15	9	4	67.4	50.8	0.0	9.5	0.0	60.6	16.9	34.7	27.3
Lymphatic leukaemia	204	65	9	3	6	3	2	11.7	22.7	35.0	0.0	36.5	0.0	13.7	14.6	18.1
Myeloid leukaemia	205	92	31	35	49	34	11	15.1	10.0	11.6	8.2	0.0	21.1	10.9	12.7	10.7
All leukaemia	204–8	203	52	49	73	46	18	11.3	13.5	12.6	7.1	3.4	12.5	10.4	10.3	9.8

ASRS: age-standardized relative survival

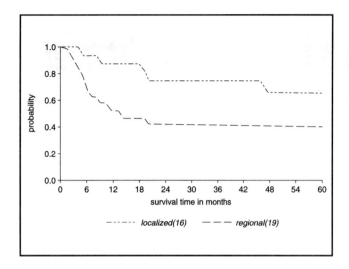

Figure 3. Survival from lip cancer by clinical extent of disease in Chiang Mai, Thailand

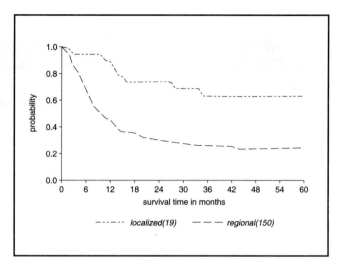

Figure 4. Survival from tongue cancer by clinical extent of disease in Chiang Mai, Thailand

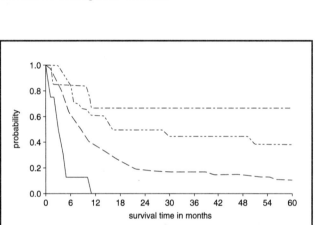

Figure 5. Survival from oral cavity cancer by clinical extent of disease in Chiang Mai, Thailand

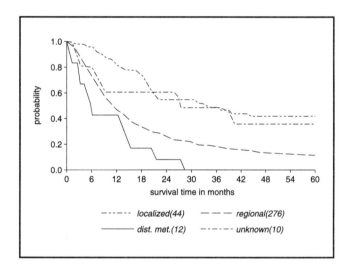

Figure 6. Survival from laryngeal cancer by clinical extent of disease in Chiang Mai, Thailand

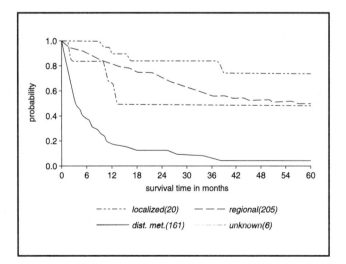

Figure 7. Survival from colon cancer by clinical extent of disease in Chiang Mai, Thailand

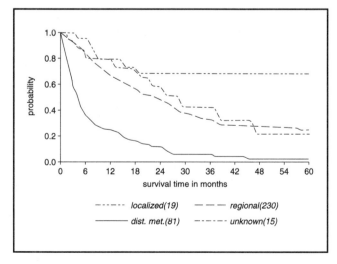

Figure 8. Survival from rectal cancer by clinical extent of disease in Chiang Mai, Thailand

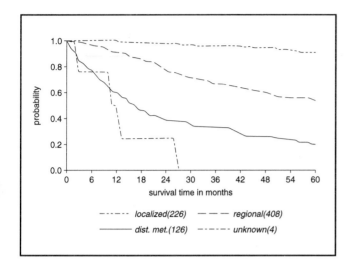

Figure 9. Survival from breast cancer by clinical extent of disease in Chiang Mai, Thailand

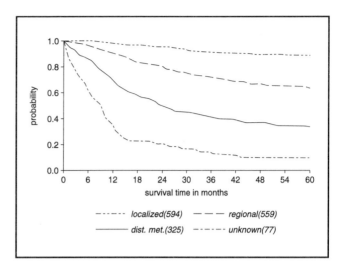

Figure 10. Survival from cervical cancer by clinical extent of disease in Chiang Mai, Thailand

disease at diagnosis. Regional extension implies that the disease has spread to surrounding organs/tissues, or cervical regional lymph nodes, or both. It is an established fact that the control of disease in the regional lymph nodes has always been difficult, even with the most radical therapies. Locoregional persistence (residual disease) or recurrence has always been a major cause of failure in the treatment of head and neck cancers. Distant metastases are not common in most head and neck cancers.

The results obtained in the case of localized oral cavity cancer and both localized and regionally spread laryngeal cancers were exceedingly low. This may be a reflection of stage misclassification. Site misclassification is likely to be relevant for estimated survival from laryngeal cancer. Supraglottic laryngeal cancers generally have a poor prognosis compared with glottic cancers, in view of their higher probability of spreading regionally, both to the regional nodes and to the surrounding tissues, particularly cartilage. It is also likely that some oropharyngeal or laryngopharyngeal cancers were misclassified as laryngeal cancers, and vice versa.

The poor survival observed in cancers of the oesophagus, stomach, liver, pancreas and lung point to the importance of prevention to control these cancers. The harsh fact that there are only a very few long-term survivors of liver cancer indicates the need to invest resources in vaccinating people against hepatitis B infection and educating them about prevention of cholangiocarcinoma by prudent dietary habits and prompt treatment of infection.

Information on clinical extent of disease indicates that most colorectal cancers are diagnosed at an advanced stage, when the disease has spread regionally. This is responsible for the poor overall survival. People with rectal cancer have poorer survival than those with colon cancer. Prognosis in colorectal cancer is related to stage at presentation and the completeness of resection. The higher survival in the case of colon cancer with regional extension (51.2%) compared with that observed in rectal cancer (24.4%) may be due to better surgical resection, possibly with more complete resection of lymph nodes in the case of colon cancer compared with rectal cancer. Comparable survival in localized cases of colon and rectal cancer probably reflects the better surgical management possible in both these situations.

Two-thirds of women with breast cancer survive for five years. This figure compares favourably with the results reported from Khon Kaen, Thailand (Sriamporn *et al.*, 1995), India (Krishnan Nair *et al.*, 1993; Nandakumar *et al.*, 1995a; Gajalakshmi *et al.*, 1997) and some countries in Europe (Berrino *et al.*, 1995). The good prognosis in breast cancer in our setting seems to be related to the comparatively high proportion of patients (30%) who present with localized disease and the availability of fairly high-quality treatment for all cases. There is a specific interest in the diagnosis and management of breast cancer in the cancer unit at the Chiang Mai University Hospital. The high five-year survival (90.9%) observed in localized cancer and the plausible survival (53.8%) observed in patients with regional disease indicate that staging is done fairly accurately within the limitations of the investigative facilities in the province and availability of and access to adequate treatment facilities. Survival across different age groups is comparable.

Table 6. Five-year observed survival (%) by clinical extent of disease for selected sites, Chiang Mai, Thailand, 1983–92

Site	Localized	Regional extension	Distant metastasis	Unknown
Lip	67.3	42.1	-	-
Tongue	62.2	23.4	0.0	0.0
Oral cavity	38.6	11.1	0.0	66.7
Larynx	42.1	11.7	0.0	36.0
Colon	74.3	51.2	4.1	50.0
Rectum	68.4	24.4	1.9	21.1
Breast	90.9	53.8	21.5	0.0
Cervix	89.0	64.5	34.5	10.2

Survival from cervical cancer in our region also compares favourably with results reported from Khon Kaen (Sriamporn *et al.*, 1995), India (Nandakumar *et al.*, 1995b; Sankaranarayanan *et al.*, 1995) and some regions of Europe (Berrino *et al.*, 1995). Once again, clinical extent of disease is an important prognostic factor in cervical cancer. More than one-third of cervical cancer patients (38%) in our province present in localized stages, for which the five-year survival was satisfactorily high at 89%. Another third presented with regional extension of disease, and their five-year survival was 64.5%. Radiotherapy plays a major role in the management of uterine cervical cancer, and the opportunity to provide such treatment adequately in our setting and the presentation of cases at an early stage are thought to be responsible for the high overall survival observed for cervical cancer.

The survival of ovarian cancer patients is less satisfactory when compared with the prospects of survival from cervical and endometrial cancers. Epithelial ovarian cancers are generally diagnosed at an advanced stage when surgical treatment is often not possible, or surgery alone will not effect a complete cure. Both surgical excision and aggressive chemotherapy have a role to play in the case of moderately advanced tumours. Many ovarian tumours in Chiang Mai are diagnosed at a stage where even debulking is not possible.

Low five-year survival was observed from lymphomas and leukaemias in our setting. The poor survival in leukaemias is probably a reflection of general inability to provide consistently aggressive treatment (multidrug remission-induction protocols, high quality supportive care and follow-up treatment) which is important in improving the outcome from these diseases.

The age-standardized relative survival for large bowel, breast, cervix and testicular cancers in our region correspond to the higher range of survival reported for developing countries (Sankaranarayanan *et al.*, 1996). However, the survival experience in our province indicates that there is considerable scope for further improvement in survival by early detection and appropriate treatment in several cancer sites. On the other hand, investment in prevention of liver and lung cancer is very important in order to achieve a measurable reduction in overall cancer incidence and mortality. There is an urgent need for rational reassessment of existing resources for cancer care and its reallocation to preventive, therapeutic and palliative care.

Acknowledgements

The co-operation extended by the collaborating institutions to the cancer registry and to the survival project is gratefully acknowledged. Thanks are due to the International Agency for Research on Cancer (IARC) for training our staff in registration and survival analysis.

References

Berrino, F., Sant, M., Verdecchia, A., Capocaccia, R., Hakulinen, T. & Estève, J., eds. (1995) *Survival of Cancer Patients in Europe: the EUROCARE Study* (IARC Scientific Publications No. 132). Lyon, International Agency for Research on Cancer

Ferlay, J. (1994) *ICD Conversion Programs For Cancer* (IARC Technical Report No. 21). Lyon, International Agency for Research on Cancer

Gajalakshmi, C.K., Shanta, V., Swaminathan, R., Sankaranarayanan, R. & Black, R.J. (1997) A population based survival study from female breast cancer in Madras, India. *Br. J. Cancer*, **75**, 771–775

Hakulinen, T. (1982) Cancer survival corrected for heterogeneity in patient withdrawal. *Biometrics*, **38**, 933–942

Hakulinen, T., Gibberd, R., Abeywickrama, K.H. & Soderman, B. (1994) *A Computer Program Package for Cancer Survival Studies, Version 2.0.* Tampere, Finnish Cancer Registry/University of Newcastle, Australia

Jensen, O.M., Parkin, D.M., MacLennan, R., Muir, C.S. & Skeet, R.G. (1991) *Cancer Registration: Principles and Methods* (IARC Scientific Publications No. 95). Lyon, International Agency for Research on Cancer

Krishnan Nair, M., Sankaranarayanan, R., Sukumaran Nair, K., Sreedevi Amma, N., Varghese, C., Padmakumari, G. & Cherian, T. (1993) Overall survival from breast cancer in Kerala, India, in relation to menstrual, reproductive and clinical factors. *Cancer*, **71**, 1791–1796

Nandakumar, A., Anantha, N., Venugopal, T.C., Sankaranarayanan, R., Thimmasetty, K. & Dhar, M. (1995a) Survival in breast cancer: a population-based study in Bangalore, India. *Int. J. Cancer*, **60**, 593–596

Nandakumar, A., Anantha, N. & Venugopal, T.C. (1995b) Incidence, mortality and survival in cancer of the cervix in Bangalore, India. *Br. J. Cancer*, **71**, 1348–1352

National Statistical Office (1994) *Population and Housing Census, Whole Kingdom, 1990.* Thailand, Office of the Prime Minister

Parkin, D.M., Muir, C.S., Whelan, S.L., Gao, Y.-T., Ferlay, J. & Powell, J., eds. (1992) *Cancer Incidence in Five Continents*, Volume VI (IARC Scientific Publications No. 120). Lyon, International Agency for Research on Cancer

Parkin, D.M., Chen, V.W., Ferlay, J., Galceran, J., Storm, H.H. & Whelan, S.L. (1994) *Comparability and Quality Control in Cancer Registration* (IARC Technical Report No. 19). Lyon, International Agency for Research on Cancer, pp. 61–65

Parkin, D.M., Whelan, S.L., Ferlay, J., Raymond L. & Young J., eds. (1997) *Cancer Incidence in Five Continents*, Volume VII (IARC Scientific Publications No. 143). Lyon, International Agency for Research on Cancer

Sankaranarayanan, R., Krishnan Nair, M., Jayaprakash, P.G., Stanley, G., Varghese, C., Ramadas, V., Padmakumary, G. & Padmanabhan, T.K. (1995) Cervical cancer in Kerala: a hospital registry-based study on survival and prognostic factors. *Br. J. Cancer*, **72**, 1039–1042

Sankaranarayanan, R., Swaminathan, R. & Black, R.J. (for Study Group on Cancer Survival in Developing Countries) (1996) Global variations in cancer survival. *Cancer*, **78**, 2461–2464

Shank, R.C., Bhamarapravati, N., Gordon, J.E. & Wogan, G.N. (1972a) Dietary aflatoxins and human liver cancer. IV. Incidence of primary liver cancer in two municipal populations of Thailand. *Food Cosmet. Toxicol.*, **10**, 171–179

Shank, R.C., Wogan, G.N., Gibson, J.B. & Nondasuta, A. (1972b) Dietary aflatoxins and human liver cancer. II. Aflatoxins in market foods and foodstuffs of Thailand and Hong Kong. *Food Cosmet. Toxicol.*, **10**, 61–69

Simarak, S., de Jong, U.W., Breslow, N., Dahl, C.J., Ruckphaopunt, K., Scheelings, P. & MacLennan, R. (1977) Cancer of the oral cavity, pharynx/larynx and lung in north Thailand: case-control study and analysis of cigarette smoke. *Br. J. Cancer*, **36**, 130–140

Sriamporn, S., Black, R., Sankaranarayanan, R., Kamsa-ad, S., Parkin, D.M. & Vatanasapt, V. (1995) Cancer survival in Khon Kaen province, Thailand. *Int. J. Cancer*, **61**, 296–300

Srivatanakul, P., Parkin, D.M., Jiang, Y.-Z., Khlat, M., Kao-Ian, U.T., Sontipong, S. & Wild, C. (1991) The role of infection by *Opisthorchis viverrini*, hepatitis B virus and aflatoxin exposure in the etiology of liver cancer in Thailand. *Cancer*, **68**, 2411–2417

Vatanasapt, V., Sriamporn, S. & MacLennan, R. (1991) Contrasts in risk factors for cancers of the oral cavity and hypopharynx and larynx in Khon Kaen, Thailand. In: Varma, A.K., ed., *Oral Oncology Volume II. Proceedings of the International Congress on Oral Cancer.* New Delhi, Macmillan India Ltd, pp. 39–42

Vatanasapt, V., Martin, N., Sriplung, H., Chindavijak, K., Sontipong, S., Sriamporn, S., Parkin, D.M. & Ferlay, J. (1993) *Cancer in Thailand 1988–1991* (IARC Technical Report No. 16). Lyon, International Agency for Research on Cancer

Vatanasapt, V., Martin, N., Sriplung, H., Chindavijak, K., Sontipong, S., Sriamporn, S., Parkin, D.M. & Ferlay, J. (1995) Cancer incidence in Thailand 1988–1991. *Cancer Epidemiol. Biomarkers Prev.*, **4**, 475–483

Wangsuphachart, V., Thomas, D.B., Koetswang, A. & Riotton, G. (1987) Risk factors for invasive cervical cancer and reduction of risk by "PAP" smears in Thai women. *Int. J. Epidemiol.*, **16**, 362–366

WHO (1976) *International Classification of Diseases for Oncology,* First Edition. Geneva, World Health Organization

WHO (1978) *International Classification of Diseases, Ninth Revision.* Geneva, World Health Organization

Wild, C.P., Shrestha, S.M., Anwar, W.A. & Montesano, R. (1992) Field studies of aflatoxin exposure, metabolism and induction of genetic alterations in relation to HBV infection and hepatocellular carcinoma in The Gambia and Thailand. *Toxicol Lett.*, **64/65**, 455–461

Chapter 15

Cancer survival in Khon Kaen, Thailand

Vanchai Vatanasapt, Supanee Sriamporn, Supot Kamsa-ard,
Krittika Suwanrungruang, Prasit Pengsaa,
D. Jintakanon Charoensiri, Jitjaroen Chaiyakum, Montien Pesee

Cancer Unit, Faculty of Medicine
Khon Kaen University, Khon Kaen, Thailand 40002

Introduction

Khon Kaen province is situated in the north-eastern region of Thailand (Fig. 1). It covers an area of 13 404 km² and has a population of 1.6 million people (1994). The climate is tropical, with the mean temperature around 28°C. The average annual rainfall is approximately 119 cm. Agriculture, particularly rice cultivation, is the traditional occupation of the people; however, there has been increased industrialization in recent years, especially in agroindustry and industrial establishments such as paper pulp mills and breweries, which pollute the environment.

Oncologists at the Faculty of Medicine of Khon Kaen University initiated a hospital-based cancer

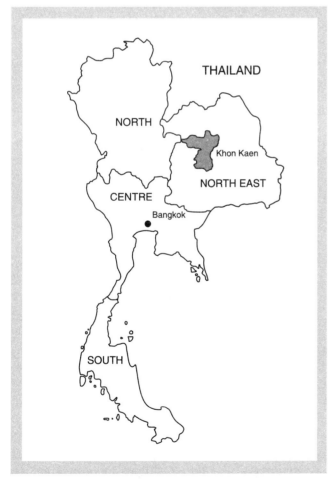

Figure 1. Map showing location of Khon Kaen province, Thailand

registry in 1984 at Srinagarind Hospital. The success of this initiative and the apparent limitations of hospital data for public health purposes prompted the establishment of a population-based cancer registry with the aim of registering all incident cases in Khon Kaen province since 1988. The registry made additional efforts to collect, retrospectively, information on all incident cases of cancer since 1984. Thus a cancer database with information on new cases occurring in this region became available for epidemiological and clinical research, as well as for public health purposes.

The first report of the registry, with results of the first year of operation, was published in 1989 (Vatanasapt *et al.*, 1989). Incidence data from the registry were included for the first time in Volume VI of *Cancer Incidence in Five Continents* (Parkin *et al.*, 1992). Recently, a preliminary analysis of population-based cancer survival from this province was published, one of the first comprehensive analyses of population-based survival on major cancer sites in a developing country population (Sriamporn *et al.*, 1995).

Khon Kaen population-based cancer registry

The Khon Kaen population-based cancer registry is based at the Cancer Unit of the Srinagarind Hospital, Khon Kaen. It is under the administrative control of the Cancer Unit and a registry advisory committee consisting of representatives from each department of the university's faculty of medicine and other major data sources.

The registry staff consist of four nurses, one computer technician, one statistician and two clerks. Technical collaboration with the Unit of Descriptive Epidemiology of the International Agency for Research on Cancer (IARC), France was established at the inception of the population-based cancer registry. This helped us to develop a system of case-finding suited to local conditions.

Cancer registration is carried out using the methodology described in IARC Scientific Publication No. 95, *Cancer Registration: Principles and*

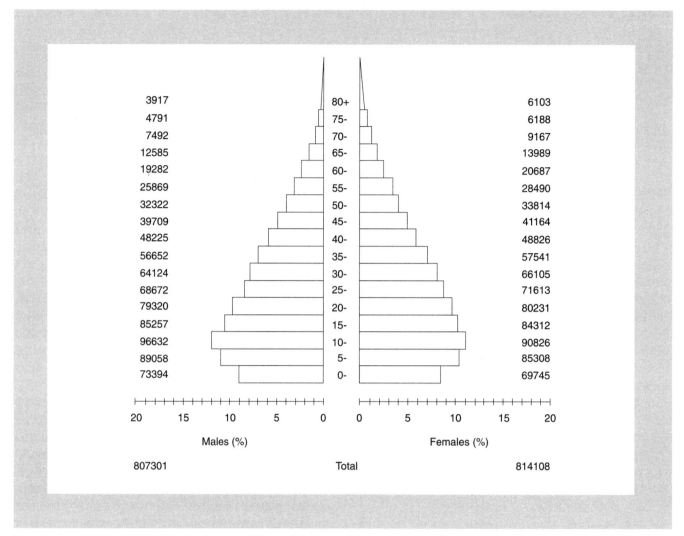

Figure 2. Average annual population of Khon Kaen province, Thailand, 1988–92

Methods (Jensen *et al.*, 1991). Registration is mainly active: regular visits are made by the registry staff to data sources where the records are scrutinized and relevant information abstracted. The major data sources for the registry are Srinagarind Hospital (a university hospital with 800 beds), six other public hospitals, 19 district hospitals and eight private hospitals in the province. Death certificates which mention cancer as a cause of death are obtained from the Office of the Chief Medical Officer by registry staff. All certified cancer deaths are reviewed and matched with the incident case records of the registry. The cases for which no matching records are found are traced back to find further relevant information. The cases which cannot be traced back to their hospital/physician records are categorized as death certificate only (DCO) registrations.

Three staff members of the registry received advanced training in cancer registration, epidemiological methods and biostatistics at IARC and practical training in cancer registries in Denmark and Leeds, United Kingdom. Three physicians from

the Cancer Unit supervise methods of data collection and verify the validity of the collected information. The methods of cancer registration in Khon Kaen have been described in detail (Vatanasapt *et al.*, 1993, 1995).

The registry covers the entire population of the Khon Kaen province. The population age structure (Fig. 2) is typical of a developing country with 31% of the population aged under 15 years and 4% over 65 years.

Completed data abstracts are checked manually and the data are entered into the database files, using CANREG (Coleman & Bieber, 1991). The name, age, sex, address and site of cancer are checked in order to detect duplicates. All cases of multiple primary cancers are verified by the medical staff of the registry. The *International Classification of Diseases for Oncology,* First Edition (ICD-O) is used to code primary site and morphology of the cancers registered (WHO, 1976). These are converted to *International Classification of Diseases, Ninth Revision* (ICD-9) codes for reporting purposes (WHO, 1978).

Incidence data for the period 1988–89 and 1988–92 were included in Volumes VI and VII, respectively, of *Cancer Incidence in Five Continents* (Parkin *et al.*, 1992, 1997). Data for the period 1988-91 were included in IARC Technical Report No. 16 *Cancer In Thailand, 1988–1991* (Vatanasapt *et al.*, 1993) and were later peer-reviewed and published in the international literature (Vatanasapt *et al.*, 1995).

Cancer incidence in Khon Kaen

Table 1 shows the age-standardized incidence rates of major cancers in Khon Kaen (Parkin *et al.*, 1997). Cancer was more common in males, with an age-standardized incidence rate of 190.6 per 100 000, compared with 132.4 among females. Liver cancer, the most frequent cancer in both sexes, accounts for half the male cases and more than one-quarter of female cases. Less than one-quarter of liver cancers are confirmed by biopsy; however, cholangiocarcinoma predominates among those cases which are histologically confirmed, constituting 90% of all liver cancers in Khon Kaen province. In contrast, hepatocellular carcinoma accounts for between one-half and three-quarters of liver cancers in other regions of Thailand (Vatanasapt *et al.*, 1995). It is unlikely that cholangiocarcinomas are overrepresented in the biopsy series, as diagnosis is fairly straightforward with characteristic ultrasonography findings. Cervical cancer is the second most common cancer among females, accounting for 15% of all cases. Lung cancer in males accounts for 8% of all male cases.

The high risk of liver cancer in Khon Kaen province is associated with liver fluke infestation (*Opisthorchis viverrini*) (Parkin *et al.*, 1993). The widespread local habit of consuming raw cyprinoid fish, which is often infected with *Opisthorchis viverrini*, is responsible for the high prevalence of infestation in humans in north-eastern Thailand (Prekusaraj, 1984; Harinasuta & Harinasuta, 1984). The regional incidence of cholangiocarcinoma correlates significantly with the observed pattern of *Opisthorchis viverrini* infestation (Vatanasapt *et al.*, 1990; Srivatanakul *et al.*, 1991), and infestation was associated with a relative risk of 5–6 in case–control studies (Parkin *et al.*, 1991; Haswell Elkins *et al.*, 1994). Interestingly, regular use of betel nut, particularly among females, was also associated with an increased risk of cholangiocarcinoma.

The mechanisms of carcinogenesis by liver fluke infestation are not clear, although factors such as increased cellular proliferation due to *Opisthorchis viverrini* infestation, induction of nitric oxide synthase by resultant inflammation and enhanced activity of certain carcinogen-metabolizing enzymes of the P450 system have been suggested as being possibly responsible for the increased risk.

Lung cancer is the second most common cancer among males, although it is much less common than liver cancer, followed by colon and stomach cancer. Among females, cancer of the uterine cervix accounts for 15% and breast cancer for 7% of all cancers.

Health care services in Khon Kaen

Health care in Khon Kaen province is provided free of charge for people of poor socioeconomic status, and at subsidized cost for others, in the public hospitals of the Ministry of Health. These hospitals are the major providers of primary and specialized health care in the region. The public health care facilities consist of the University Hospital (Srinagarind Hospital), the regional provincial hospital in Khon Kaen (580 beds), two health promotion centres, a military hospital, two other hospitals in the city of Khon Kaen and 20 district hospitals. The ratio of physicians to population in the province is 1:3000.

The Cancer Unit at Srinagarind Hospital provides comprehensive diagnostic and therapeutic services for cancer. Pathology, radiology, imaging, surgery, radiotherapy, chemotherapy, paediatric oncology and palliative care services are available at this institution. There are four pathology laboratories in the province, two public and two private. Diagnostic radiological facilities with varying degrees of sophistication are available in seven public and eight private hospitals and some of the 19 community health centres.

Cancer-related surgical services are available at the University Hospital, the regional provincial hospital and three private hospitals. Radiotherapy services are available only at the University Hospital. The facilities include two cobalt machines (for external radiotherapy); a low dose-rate caesium 137 afterloading device and a high dose-rate cobalt 60 afterloading device for brachytherapy. A linear accelerator and facilities for high dose-rate iridium 192 are being installed. Cancer chemotherapy is usually practised only at the University Hospital, although paediatric oncology services are available at the regional hospital and three private hospitals. Some patients also go to the cities of Bangkok and Chiang Mai for treatment.

Table 1. Annual average cancer incidence per 100 000 person-years, Khon Kaen, Thailand, 1988–92

Site	MALES			FEMALES		
	Number	Crude rate	ASR	Number	Crude rate	ASR
Lip	7	0.2	0.3	59	1.8	2.7
Tongue	22	0.7	1.0	21	0.6	0.8
Salivary gland	6	0.2	0.3	8	0.2	0.3
Mouth	33	1.0	1.7	68	2.1	3.0
Oropharynx	14	0.4	0.7	6	0.2	0.2
Nasopharynx	65	2.0	2.6	23	0.7	0.9
Hypopharynx	11	0.3	0.5	1	0.0	0.0
Oesophagus	34	1.1	1.5	12	0.4	0.5
Stomach	84	2.6	4.1	52	1.6	2.1
Colon	107	3.3	4.9	81	2.5	3.3
Rectum	63	2.0	3.0	48	1.5	1.9
Liver	2119	65.6	97.4	927	28.5	39.0
Gallbladder	41	1.3	1.8	47	1.4	2.1
Pancreas	21	0.7	0.9	16	0.5	0.7
Larynx	22	0.7	1.2	5	0.2	0.2
Lung	355	11.0	17.0	132	4.1	5.3
Bone	29	0.9	1.2	40	1.2	1.7
Connective tissue	26	0.8	0.9	19	0.6	0.7
Melanoma of skin	7	0.2	0.4	14	0.4	0.6
Other skin	77	2.4	3.9	81	2.5	3.4
Breast	0	0	0	236	7.2	8.4
Cervix uteri				517	15.9	18.8
Corpus uteri				54	1.7	2.0
Ovary				126	3.9	4.4
Prostate	48	1.5	2.8			
Testis	18	0.6	0.6			
Penis	45	1.4	1.8			
Bladder	65	2.0	3.2	14	0.4	0.5
Kidney	31	1.0	1.2	19	0.6	0.7
Brain	72	2.2	2.7	67	2.1	2.3
Thyroid	23	0.7	1.0	106	3.3	3.5
Hodgkin's disease	12	0.4	0.4	12	0.4	0.5
Non-Hodgkin lymphoma	69	2.1	2.7	50	1.5	1.8
Multiple myeloma	4	0.1	0.2	3	0.1	0.1
Lymphoid leukaemia	38	1.2	1.2	27	0.8	0.8
Myeloid leukaemia	41	1.3	1.4	43	1.3	1.5
All sites	4207	130.3	190.6	3384	103.9	132.4
All sites except skin	4130	127.9	186.8	3303	101.4	129.0

ASR: Age-standardized incidence rate (world population)

Early detection activities

Though a national cancer control committee has recently been established, there is as yet no official provincial cancer control programme. However, the Cancer Unit at the University Hospital has assumed a leading role in providing cancer preventive and therapeutic services in the province. Opportunistic Pap smear screening is offered in the district hospitals through the gynaecology services. Approximately one-third of the married female population have used Pap smear services at least once. So far, more health-conscious people have been screened, whereas some high-risk groups, such as promiscuous women, have not been the target of screening. Opportunistic mammography is also available at Khon Kaen, and health education about the control of common cancers in the region is also provided. Screening for liver cancer (cholangiocarcinoma), the most common cancer in Khon Kaen, has been attempted, using stool examination for *Opisthorchis viverrini* and ultrasonography.

Survival analysis

Subjects
A total of 11 937 cases were registered during the period 1985–92. The distribution of cases by site is shown in Table 2. Of these, 1569 cases (13.1%) were DCO registrations. The proportion of histologically verified cases varied from 15% to 100% according to site. Only 15% of the liver cancers were histologically verified, whereas in sites like lung and gallbladder just over half the cases had histological confirmation. More than three-quarters of those with cancer in head and neck sites, breast, uterine cervix, ovary and thyroid were histologically verified.

Those registered as DCO cases and 30 patients with no information on age were excluded from the survival analysis (Table 2). This left 10 338 cases for further analysis.

Follow-up methods
Patients were followed up until death *or* date of loss to follow-up *or* 31 December 1995. The methods used by the registry to establish the vital status (i.e. alive/dead) of cancer patients include both passive and active measures. The passive method consists of matching the patients with death certificates mentioning cancer as a cause of death. For the remaining cases, follow-up information was collected by routine scrutiny of hospital case-records, enquiries with treating physicians and general practitioners and reply-paid postal enquiries addressed to patients and to the village headman. Annual follow-up on the anniversary of the date of incidence was attempted for presumed survivors by sending a reply-paid postcard inquiring about the current status of the patient. If no reply was received, a second postcard was sent to the headman of the village requesting the same information. House visits were also performed in a few cases.

Analytical methodology (see Chapters 2, 3 and 5)
The duration of survival for each case was calculated from the date of diagnosis of cancer to date of death *or* the last date of follow-up. Cumulative observed survival and relative survival rates were calculated using Hakulinen's method (Hakulinen, 1982; Hakulinen *et al.*, 1994). The abridged life table for

the whole of Thailand for the period under study was used for calculating expected survival (National Statistical Office, 1994). For comparison of relative survival rates with other reported experiences, site-specific and age-specific relative survival rates were directly standardized to the site-specific age distributions of the estimated global incidence of major cancers in 1985.

Results
The proportion of five-year survivors was 10% or less in people with liver, pancreas and lung cancer (Table 3). The percentage of five-year survivors was 70% or more in cancer sites such as lip, skin (non-melanoma), corpus uteri, and thyroid. The relative survival was generally higher among females, with the exception of cancers of the lip, oesophagus, gallbladder, larynx, lung, skin (melanoma), urinary bladder and all leukaemias. The survival experience from liver cancer was about the same in both sexes.

Table 4 shows the five-year relative survival by age groups and for all ages combined and age-standardized relative survival (ASRS) for all ages and for the age group 0–74 years in different cancer sites. There was a trend of decreasing five-year relative survival with increasing age for cancers such as nasopharynx, colon, cervix and myeloid leukaemia. Increasing survival with increasing age was evident in cancer of the larynx. No trend was explicitly seen among other cancers.

Discussion
It is important to consider data quality, the effect of exclusions and the completeness of follow-up when interpreting and comparing the survival experience. The Khon Kaen registry has eight years' operational experience and, within this short period, registration has been fairly stable. The registry uses multiple sources (*N*=30, approx.) and data are actively searched for and abstracted. On average, two notifications are received for each registered case. The overall proportion of histologically verified cases in the registry is low (47%), but this is due to a high proportion of liver cancers, which tend not to involve biopsy/cytology for diagnosis. For most other sites, the proportion of histologically verified cases exceeds 80%. Similarly, for most major sites, the proportion of cases registered as DCO did not exceed 10%. It is also possible that the diagnostic information in some death certificates is of poor quality, as a proportion of death certificates are not

Table 2. Cancer cases registered and data quality indices, Khon Kaen, Thailand, 1985–92

Site	ICD 9	No. of cases registered	Data quality indices		Cases excluded from analysis		Cases included for survival analysis	
			% DCO	% HV	DCO	Others	No.	%
Lip	140	104	0.0	80.8	0	1	103	99.0
Tongue	141	61	0.0	83.6	0	0	61	100.0
Oral cavity	143-5	147	1.4	83.7	2	0	145	98.6
Oropharynx	146	28	0.0	92.9	0	0	28	100.0
Nasopharynx	147	182	1.1	87.9	2	2	178	97.8
Hypopharynx	148	31	0.0	87.1	0	0	31	100.0
Oesophagus	150	76	5.3	48.7	4	1	71	93.4
Stomach	151	244	8.2	65.6	20	0	224	91.8
Colon	153	296	11.5	50.0	34	0	262	88.5
Rectum	154	179	0.0	72.1	0	0	179	100.0
Colorectum	153-4	475	7.2	58.3	34	0	441	92.8
Liver	155	4272	14.2	14.7	606	12	3654	85.5
Gallbladder	156	146	3.4	56.8	5	0	141	96.6
Pancreas	157	73	2.7	28.8	2	0	71	97.3
Larynx	161	62	3.2	74.2	2	0	60	96.8
Lung	162	688	14.0	50.7	96	3	589	85.6
Bone	170	119	48.7	31.1	58	0	61	51.3
Connective tissue	171	66	0.0	87.9	0	0	66	100.0
Skin melanoma	172	41	0.0	100.0	0	0	41	100.0
Other skin	173	276	2.5	87.7	7	0	269	97.5
Breast	174	417	1.9	87.1	8	0	409	98.1
Cervix	180	869	5.4	75.9	47	2	820	94.4
Corpus uteri	182	79	0.0	77.2	0	0	79	100.0
Ovary	183	264	3.8	78.4	10	1	253	95.8
Prostate	185	75	0.0	84.0	0	0	75	100.0
Testis	186	30	0.0	83.3	0	0	30	100.0
Penis	187	84	0.0	76.2	0	0	84	100.0
Bladder	188	125	0.0	79.2	0	0	125	100.0
Kidney	189	74	5.4	83.8	4	0	70	94.6
Brain & nervous system	191-2	178	18.0	25.3	32	0	146	82.0
Thyroid	193	279	0.0	85.7	0	0	279	100.0
Hodgkin's disease	201	48	0.0	100.0	0	0	48	100.0
Non-Hodgkin lymphoma	200,202	217	0.0	100.0	0	0	217	100.0
Lymphatic leukaemia	204	124	0.0	100.0	0	1	123	99.2
Myeloid leukaemia	205	129	0.0	100.0	0	0	129	100.0
All leukaemia	204-8	382	25.7	74.3	98	1	283	74.1
Primary site uncertain	195-9	1151	40.7	38.0	468	5	678	58.9
All sites	140-208	11937	13.1	47.1	1569	30	10338	86.6

DCO : Death certificate only; HV : Histological verification

Table 3. Observed and relative survival by site and sex, Khon Kaen, Thailand, 1985–92

| Site | ICD 9 | Number included | All ages and both sexes combined | | | | | | % Survival rate at 5 years by sex | | | | | |
| | | | Observed survival (OS) | | | Relative survival (RS) | | | Male | | | Female | | |
			1 yr	3 yr	5 yr	1 yr	3 yr	5 yr	Number	OS	RS	Number	OS	RS
Lip	140	103	85.3	74.7	63.1	88.3	82.2	74.4	8	100.0	110.2	95	59.0	70.1
Tongue	141	61	48.6	27.9	20.1	50.0	30.4	23.2	37	4.5	5.2	24	43.5	49.9
Oral cavity	143-5	145	61.7	40.3	31.7	64.3	45.5	39.3	52	24.6	31.0	93	35.6	43.6
Oropharynx	146	28	39.3	22.4	22.4	40.6	25.0	26.7	17	19.2	22.9	11	30.2	35.8
Nasopharynx	147	178	73.1	38.8	26.8	74.1	40.6	29.1	116	18.8	20.8	62	40.5	42.6
Oesophagus	150	71	41.9	28.0	25.5	43.0	30.3	29.4	49	28.2	33.0	22	19.9	22.5
Stomach	151	224	39.6	17.6	15.3	40.6	19.1	17.5	156	12.7	14.9	68	21.4	23.3
Colon	153	262	59.9	42.6	31.9	61.3	45.8	36.6	141	28.8	33.8	121	34.9	39.0
Rectum	154	179	66.0	38.6	29.1	67.3	41.2	32.7	106	23.5	27.2	73	37.6	40.2
Colorectum	153-4	441	62.4	41.0	30.9	63.7	44.0	35.1	247	26.7	31.1	194	35.7	39.2
Liver	155	3654	22.7	10.4	7.5	23.2	11.1	8.4	2556	7.5	8.5	1098	7.5	8.3
Gallbladder	156	141	36.6	16.5	13.8	37.3	17.6	15.5	70	15.6	17.9	71	11.7	13.0
Pancreas	157	71	20.4	9.3	4.6	20.7	9.8	5.1	46	4.0	4.5	25	4.9	5.1
Larynx	161	60	69.5	49.9	36.4	71.8	55.9	44.5	52	41.4	52.0	8	12.5	13.4
Lung	162	589	26.4	12.5	8.8	27.2	13.6	10.1	439	8.8	10.3	150	8.5	9.5
Bone	170	61	61.1	39.6	34.3	61.7	40.8	36.0	34	33.2	34.9	27	36.5	38.3
Connective tissue	171	66	55.6	32.3	25.9	56.2	33.4	27.5	40	23.3	24.4	26	27.3	29.8
Skin melanoma	172	41	73.2	52.6	44.8	75.1	56.8	51.2	16	46.5	57.4	25	41.5	45.3
Other skin	173	269	89.2	74.3	67.3	93.0	83.8	82.0	129	57.0	73.3	140	77.5	89.7
Breast	174	409	88.0	61.6	44.9	88.8	63.3	47.1				409	44.9	47.1
Cervix	180	820	84.6	64.2	54.5	85.4	66.1	57.5				820	54.5	57.5
Corpus uteri	182	79	87.8	77.7	74.6	88.6	80.2	78.7				79	74.6	78.7
Ovary	183	253	57.5	39.4	34.0	58.0	40.5	35.6				253	34.0	35.6
Prostate	185	75	85.2	47.1	29.5	90.6	57.3	41.1	75	29.5	41.1			
Testis	186	30	60.4	40.1	40.1	60.8	40.9	41.6	30	40.1	41.6			
Penis	187	84	77.3	60.8	60.8	79.1	65.1	67.7	84	60.8	67.7			
Bladder	188	125	75.0	53.3	49.7	76.9	57.6	57.2	107	52.3	61.5	18	37.1	39.0
Kidney	189	70	41.9	21.2	21.2	42.3	21.8	22.4	43	17.1	18.2	27	27.8	29.1
Brain & nervous system	191-2	146	53.9	37.6	32.5	54.3	38.5	34.0	76	26.8	28.2	70	39.6	41.1
Thyroid	193	279	93.0	87.0	82.8	93.9	89.9	88.0	52	64.8	73.0	227	86.4	90.7
Hodgkin's disease	201	48	65.4	39.6	29.4	66.1	40.8	31.1	32	13.9	14.8	16	60.2	62.3
Non-Hodgkin lymphoma	200,202	217	59.5	33.6	26.2	60.3	35.0	28.0	115	23.1	25.0	102	29.5	31.2
Lymphatic leukaemia	204	123	54.6	32.5	27.3	54.8	32.9	27.8	75	28.5	29.1	48	25.1	25.5
Myeloid leukaemia	205	129	38.2	20.3	15.9	38.5	20.7	16.5	71	18.5	19.4	58	12.7	13.0
All leukaemia	204-8	283	44.9	25.1	20.1	45.1	25.5	20.7	166	21.2	22.0	117	18.8	19.2
Primary site uncertain	195-9	678	25.3	12.6	9.2	25.8	13.4	10.3	401	7.3	8.2	277	12.4	13.5

issued by a physician. The possibility also exists that some DCO cases were not actually cancers.

Apart from the DCO cases, only a tiny proportion (0.3%) was excluded from the analysis because no information was available about the patient's age. The proportion of cases excluded from the analysis for any reason was 25% in leukaemia, 15% in liver and lung cancers and around 5% for

Table 4. Site-specific and age-specific number of cases–relative survival and ASRS, Khon Kaen, Thailand, 1985-92

Site	ICD 9	Number of cases by age group						% Relative survival (RS) at 5 years						RS	ASRS%
		≤34	35–44	45–54	55–64	65–74	75+	≤34	35–44	45–54	55–64	65–74	75+	All ages	0–74
Lip	140	3	3	8	27	42	20	101.2	101.6	83.0	90.7	69.1	0.0	74.4	65.4	81.9
Tongue	141	4				17	8	0.0	51.0	12.9	32.2	25.5	0.0	23.2	20.4	25.5
Oral cavity	143–5	5	4	22	34	45	35	100.8	38.2	50.0	34.3	24.4	48.8	39.3	39.1	36.6
Oropharynx	146	1	3	5	11	2	6	100.8	101.9	0.0	11.5	60.0	0.0	26.7	16.2	20.3
Nasopharynx	147	29	21	54	37	28	9	74.2	31.9	24.9	17.8	11.0	0.0	29.1	20.2	25.3
Oesophagus	150	4	8	9	28	12	10	0.0	0.0	29.8	42.4	20.4	45.7	29.4	31.7	26.5
Stomach	151	17	13	56	60	56	22	10.6	11.4	19.3	7.7	25.9	37.1	17.5	23.1	16.7
Colon	153	24	28	56	73	50	31	56.2	45.1	31.3	30.9	18.6	59.0	36.6	41.3	29.1
Rectum	154	16	14	48	53	37	11	30.9	28.2	26.4	37.4	46.1	0.0	32.7	22.1	37.4
Colorectum	153–4	40	42	104	126	87	42	48.0	38.8	28.6	33.7	32.1	46.0	35.1	38.6	33.4
Liver	155	86	351	926	1308	733	250	22.0	12.6	7.5	6.0	10.4	10.4	8.4	10.1	10.0
Gallbladder	156	3	14	29	33	50	12	0.0	17.1	24.2	0.0	15.0	49.2	15.5	21.9	11.1
Pancreas	157	1	18	12	23	12	5	0.0	7.7	0.0	5.5	0.0	0.0	5.1	1.6	2.5
Larynx	161	0	1	9	18	23	9	–	0.0	29.9	38.8	52.9	65.3	44.5	41.7	34.9
Lung	162	19	49	124	171	152	74	22.1	18.4	6.3	8.6	8.4	19.7	10.1	12.6	9.3
Bone	170	33	4	6	5	12	1	38.8	0.0	62.4	21.6	40.5	0.0	36.0	24.9	34.7
Connective tissue	171	31	10	7	7	7	4	31.4	29.2	0.0	25.0	47.6	0.0	27.5	19.9	27.8
Skin melanoma	172	1	4	11	9	13	3	0.0	76.4	42.6	43.4	62.6	48.2	51.2	47.3	47.0
Other skin	173	14	17	43	66	66	63	71.0	102.4	74.9	68.8	75.7	135.7	82.0	76.0	76.1
Breast	174	42	124	122	82	31	8	59.4	47.3	40.1	47.8	48.7	146.5	47.1	47.3	47.0
Cervix	180	82	206	270	158	84	20	76.6	63.0	54.8	53.7	35.0	44.4	57.5	54.0	55.4
Corpus uteri	182	2	13	36	17	8	3	100.8	66.5	93.0	86.4	27.6	63.4	78.7	68.9	70.4
Ovary	183	56	51	73	46	21	6	58.9	27.6	28.2	33.0	28.1	32.9	35.6	33.3	33.6
Prostate	185	0	2	1	10	43	19	–	102.1	0.0	47.4	31.2	67.5	41.1	56.5	34.5
Testis	186	18	7	1	2	2	0	53.3	20.9	0.0	0.0	58.2	–	41.6	36.0	36.8
Penis	187	7	20	25	19	6	7	33.8	94.5	55.5	76.1	119.8	23.6	67.7	56.3	69.2
Urinary bladder	188	11	14	28	31	25	16	57.0	65.9	71.7	46.7	58.8	38.1	57.2	49.7	57.8
Kidney	189	23	10	23	9	4	1	35.8	20.4	18.9	36.7	0.0	0.0	22.4	16.1	21.9
Brain & nervous system	191–2	75	16	11	26	12	6	36.5	41.5	31.2	19.3	55.4	0.0	34.0	28.3	35.5
Thyroid	193	81	52	69	38	27	12	100.9	99.2	85.7	62.6	79.2	20.9	88.0	68.6	80.7
Hodgkin's disease	201	15	7	10	10	5	1	29.5	22.6	39.8	12.2	61.1	0.0	31.1	28.4	30.5
Non-Hodgkin lymphoma	200,202	80	25	42	31	27	12	34.4	34.3	14.9	28.0	23.5	23.6	28.0	26.6	27.4
Lymphatic leukaemia	204	103	8	4	5	3	0	29.0	20.4	0.0	43.4	0.0	–	27.8	17.7	21.9
Myeloid leukaemia	205	55	30	16	19	6	3	22.1	17.0	14.6	13.6	0.0	0.0	16.5	12.7	15.8
All leukaemia	204–8	175	42	22	28	12	4	25.1	16.7	11.2	17.9	0.0	0.0	20.7	14.0	17.4
Primary site uncertain	195–9	46	61	177	236	111	47	39.6	11.8	7.0	5.3	11.6	0.0	10.3	9.1	11.4

– No cases

ASRS: Age-standardized relative survival

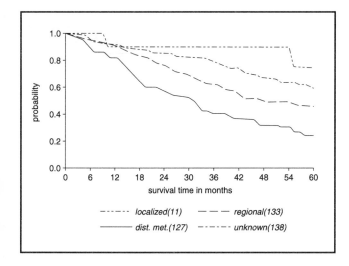

Figure 3. Survival from breast cancer by clinical extent of disease in Khon Kaen, Thailand

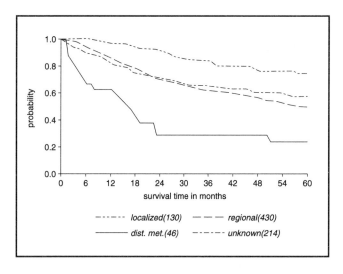

Figure 4. Survival from cervical cancer by clinical extent of disease in Khon Kaen, Thailand

most other major cancer sites. An effort to obtain follow-up information was made for all the cases. The person's vital status at the closing date was known in 62% of cases. The rest were lost to follow-up at various times prior to the closing date: 19% were known to be alive for a period of less than one year from the date of diagnosis of cancer, 11% between one and five years and 8% for more than five years.

The five-year relative survival of patients with cancers of the mouth and pharynx (excluding lip cancer) was 40% or less. The proportion of patients surviving from cancers such as tongue, oropharynx and nasopharynx was less than 30% at five years. Information on the clinical extent of disease at presentation for these cancer sites was unknown in the majority of cases, but presumably most cancers presented at an advanced stage. In nasopharyngeal cancer, there was a clear trend of decreasing survival with increasing age. The few cases in different age groups for other sites of head and neck cancer do not allow interpretation of the effect of age on prognosis. Three-quarters of patients aged under 35 survived five years, compared with none among those aged 75+ years, except in the case of oral cavity cancer.

The relative survival rates of patients with cancers of the stomach, liver, gallbladder, pancreas and lung were less than 20%. The failure of treatment in the above sites means that emphasis needs to be placed on preventive action to control these invariably fatal malignancies. Survival from liver cancer, especially cholangiocarcinoma, was better in the periphery than in the central group (Vatanasapt *et al.*, 1996). About 30% of males and around 40% of females with colorectal cancer survive for five years. It is likely that this poor survival rate is a reflection of advanced disease at the time of presentation.

The five-year relative survival in breast cancer was 47%. This is much lower than the survival experience of breast cancer patients in developed countries, where improved awareness and the availability of mammography have resulted in the diagnosis of many breast cancers at early stages. There have also been a number of therapeutic advances in the management of breast cancer, particularly adjuvant chemotherapy and hormone therapy for those with stage II and stage III cancers. A combination of these factors is thought to be responsible for the improving survival rates in breast cancer over the last two decades in developed countries. Information on clinical extent of disease of breast cancers in Khon Kaen is available for two-thirds of registered cases. Localized cancers constituted less than 5% of the cases for which information on clinical extent was available. This is likely to be the major factor in the comparatively low survival of breast cancer patients in Khon Kaen. Three-quarters of patients (75%) with localized cancer and just under half of the patients (46%) with regional disease survived five years (Fig. 3). The poor overall survival observed in Khon Kaen may be partly a reflection of lack of compliance or difficulty in ensuring multimodality therapy in moderately advanced breast cancer.

Cervical cancer is mainly managed with radiotherapy. Early cancers (stage I and a proportion of stage II A) are treated with intracavitary radiotherapy. Stage II B and stage III cancers are treated with a combination of external radiotherapy and intracavitary therapy. Stage IV cancers are treated with palliative intent, mostly with external radiation only, though occasionally intracavitary treatment is attempted. Almost 20% of the cases of cervical cancer for which information on clinical stage is available (74%) presented at localized stages. This figure is higher than that observed for breast cancer. The five-year observed survival rates for cervical cancer with localized (75%) and regional (50%) disease (Fig. 4) were comparable with the corresponding rates for breast cancer. Radiotherapy facilities are well developed in Khon Kaen, and this may explain the reasonable prognosis observed with cervical cancer.

Five-year age-adjusted relative survival for colorectal, breast and cervical cancers was lower than the survival observed in the USA during the period 1967–73 (Sankaranarayanan et al., 1996) and that reported from Europe during the period 1978–85 (Berrino et al., 1995). They were in the lower range of survival reported from other developing countries.

The high five-year survival observed in cases of localized disease indicates that, if patients are diagnosed in early stages, the existing treatment facilities are capable of achieving improved survival. The figures observed for the early stages of breast and cervical cancers may still be lower than those seen in developed countries, which may be partly explained by stage misclassification, due both to limited investigative facilities and to the nonstandardized criteria for determination of clinical extent of disease.

Survival from cancer of the ovary was poor. Prognosis in ovarian cancer is determined by histology, stage at presentation and treatment. Chemotherapy has a major role in the management of nonlocalized ovarian cancer. Recent improvements in survival in ovarian cancer in developed countries are attributed to diagnosis at an early stage (mostly by ultrasonography) and advances in adjuvant chemotherapy. The poor survival from ovarian cancer in Khon Kaen is likely to be a reflection of both advanced disease and lack of some treatment modalities, particularly chemotherapy.

Patients with thyroid cancer have a very good prognosis, which is well established. Better prognosis was seen among people under 45 years of age: the predominant follicular carcinoma, due in part to iodine deficiency, indicated worse survival than papillary cases. These findings should alert the clinician to follow and manage nodular goitre cases more carefully (Vatanasapt et al., 1991, 1992). Advanced disease and old age at presentation in this young population are likely to be responsible for the poor survival in prostate cancer. Subjects with brain tumours also have a poor prognosis.

The low five-year survival rates for testicular cancer, lymphoma and leukaemia suggest

difficulties in providing adequate chemotherapy-based treatment for these tumours. Over the last two decades, the outcome from these cancers has greatly improved in developed countries, thanks to a better understanding of the natural history of the disease, advances in chemotherapy and supportive care.

Implications

The results obtained by analysis of survival data are valuable in the local context for the direction of cancer control efforts. It is very clear that major reductions in cancer morbidity and mortality cannot be achieved in Khon Kaen unless the high incidence of liver cancer is reduced. All liver cancers have a very poor prognosis whatever treatment is used, with very few long-term survivors. However, there are increasing prospects for prevention of both cholangiocarcinoma and hepatocellular carcinoma, given the current state of knowledge about the causation of these tumours. Investment in educating the public about liver fluke infestation, motivating people to avoid eating raw, pickled, smoked or undercooked fish and treatment of established infestation with praziquantel are important for controlling cholangiocarcinoma. For hepatocellular carcinoma, promoting hepatitis B vaccination as part of extended immunization programmes is a priority. There is an urgent need for the resources currently used for the early detection and treatment of this incurable tumour to be diverted to prevention.

Early detection by raising professional and public awareness is a priority area for cancers such as colon/rectum, breast and cervix. Development of and strict adherence to consensus management protocols for sites such as breast, ovary, testis, lymphomas and leukaemias are likely to improve prognosis in these cancers, although it should be realized that some of these are comparatively uncommon cancers. Fine-needle aspiration of thyroid nodules or goitres is recommended in order to detect thyroid cancer early and plan definitive treatment, especially when the person is young.

Tobacco control activities are important for prevention of head and neck and lung cancers, given their low survival rates.

In the absence of reliable mortality data, the survival rates observed by this study provide a valid baseline for the evaluation of further progress in early detection, treatment and improved access by the population to the available cancer care facilities. The rationale for investment in cancer control can be clearly seen from the cancer survival experience in Khon Kaen.

Acknowledgements

The authors gratefully acknowledge the cooperation of health care authorities and providers, without which cancer registration and this study on cancer survival would not have been possible. Our thanks are due to S. Horasith and P. Usantia for their data collection efforts. The assistance provided by the International Agency for Research on Cancer (IARC), Lyon, France, in cancer registration and augmentation of patient follow-up, through a collaborative research agreement, is gratefully acknowledged. The authors wish to thank the International Union Against Cancer (UICC), Geneva, Switzerland, for the award of an International Cancer Research Technology Transfer (ICRETT) fellowship to Mrs. S. Sriamporn, which enabled her to undertake a detailed analysis of our survival data at IARC's Unit of Descriptive Epidemiology.

References

Berrino, F., Sant, M., Verdecchia, A., Capocaccia, R., Hakulinen, T. & Estève, J., eds. (1995) *Survival of Cancer Patients in Europe: the EUROCARE Study* (IARC Scientific Publications No. 132). Lyon, International Agency for Research on Cancer

Coleman, M.P., Estève, J., Damiecki, P., Arslan, A. & Renard, H. (1993) *Trends in Cancer Incidence and Mortality* (IARC Scientific Publications No. 121). Lyon, International Agency for Research on Cancer

Hakulinen, T. (1982) Cancer survival corrected for heterogeneity in patient withdrawal. *Biometrics*, **38**, 933–942

Hakulinen, T., Gibberd, R., Abeywickrama, K.H. & Soderman, B. (1994) *A Computer Program Package for Cancer Survival Studies, Version 2.0.* Tampere, Finnish Cancer Registry/University of Newcastle, Australia

Harinasuta, C. & Harinasuta, T. (1984) Opisthorchis viverrini: life cycle, intermediate hosts, transmission to man and geographical distribution in Thailand. *Drug Res.*, **34**, 1164–1167

Haswell Elkins, M.R., Mairiang, E., Mairiang, P., Chaiyakum, J., Chamadol, N., Loapaiboon, V., Sithithaworn, P. & Elkins, D.B. (1994) Cross-sectional study of *Opisthorchis viverrini* infection and cholangiocarcinoma in communities within a high-risk area in northeast Thailand. *Int. J. Cancer*, **59**, 505–509

Jensen, O.M., Parkin, D.M., MacLennan, R., Muir, C.S. & Skeet, R.G. (1991) *Cancer Registration: Principles and Methods* (IARC Scientific Publications No. 95). Lyon, International Agency for Research on Cancer

National Statistical Office (1994) *Population and Housing Census, Whole Kingdom, 1990.* Thailand, Office of the Prime Minister

Parkin, D.M., Srivatanakul, P., Khlat, M., Chenvidhya, D., Chotiwan, P., Insiripong S., L'Abbe K.A. & Wild, C.P. (1991) Liver cancer in Thailand. A case-control study of cholangiocarcinoma. *Int. J. Cancer,* **48**, 323–328

Parkin, D.M., Muir, C.S., Whelan, S.L., Gao, Y.-T., Ferlay, J. & Powell, J., eds. (1992) *Cancer Incidence in Five Continents,* Volume VI (IARC Scientific Publications No. 120). Lyon, International Agency for Research on Cancer

Parkin, D.M., Oshima, H., Srivatanakul, P. & Vatanasapt, V. (1993) Cholangiocarcinoma: epidemiology, mechanisms of carcinogenesis and prevention. *Cancer Epidemiol. Biomarkers Prev.,* **2**, 537–544

Parkin, D.M., Whelan, S.L., Ferlay, J., Raymond L. & Young J., eds. (1997) *Cancer Incidence in Five Continents,* Volume VII (IARC Scientific Publications No. 143). Lyon, International Agency for Research on Cancer

Prekusaraj, S. (1984) Public health aspects of opisthorchiasis in Thailand. *Drug Res.,* **34**, 1119–1120

Sankaranarayanan, R., Swaminathan, R. & Black, R.J. (for Study Group on Cancer Survival in Developing Countries) (1996) Global variations in cancer survival. *Cancer,* **78**, 2461–2464

Sriamporn, S., Black, R., Sankaranarayanan, R., Kamsa-ad, S., Parkin, D.M. & Vatanasapt, V. (1995) Cancer survival in Khon Kaen province, Thailand. *Int. J. Cancer,* **61**, 296–300

Srivatanakul, P., Parkin, D.M., Jiang, Y.-Z., Khlat, M., Kao-Ian, U.T., Sontipong, S & Wild, C. (1991) The role of infection by *Opisthorchis viverrini*, hepatitis B virus and aflatoxin exposure in the etiology of liver cancer in Thailand. *Cancer,* **68**, 2411–2417

Vatanasapt, V., Titapant, V., Tangvoraphonkchai, V. & Pengsaa, P. (1989) *Cancer Incidence in Khon Kaen, Thailand 1985–88.* Khon Kaen, University of Khon Kaen

Vatanasapt, V., Tangvoraphonkchai, V., Titapant, V., Pipitgool, V., Viriyapap, D. & Sriamporn, S. (1990) A high incidence of liver cancer in Khon Kaen province, Thailand. *S.E. Asian J. Trop. Med. Publ. Hlth.,* **21**, 382–387

Vatanasapt, V., Taksaphan, P., Chowchuen, B., Komthong, R., Pesee, M., Sriamporn, S., Boonrowdchu, D. & Comesuk, K. (1991) Thyroid cancer: results of treatment and complications. *Thai. J. Surgery,* **12**, 63–68

Vatanasapt, V., Taksaphan, P., Komthong, R., Chowchuen, B., Sriamporn, S., Boonrowdchu, D. & Teerasan, P. (1992) The epidemiology of thyroid cancer in Northeast Thailand. *Asian J. Surgery*, **15**, 84–89

Vatanasapt, V., Martin, N., Sriplung, H., Chindavijak, K., Sontipong, S., Sriamporn, S., Parkin, D.M. & Ferlay, J.

(1993) *Cancer in Thailand, 1988–1991* (IARC Technical Report No. 16). Lyon, International Agency for Research on Cancer

Vatanasapt, V., Martin, N., Sriplung, H., Chindavijak, K., Sontipong, S., Sriamporn, S., Parkin, D.M. & Ferlay, J. (1995) Cancer incidence in Thailand 1988-1991. *Cancer Epidemiol. Biomarkers Prev.*, **4**, 475–483

Vatanasapt, V., Bhudhisawasdi, V., Mairiang, P., Sukeepais-arncharoen, W., Chaiyakam, J. & Songsivilai, S. (1996) *Liver Cancer in Thailand: Research and Development Leading to Liver Cancer Control Programme.* Bangkok, Thailand Research Fund, pp. 149–151

WHO (1976) *International Classification of Diseases for Oncology,* First Edition. Geneva, World Health Organization

WHO (1978) *International Classification of Diseases, Ninth Revision.* Geneva, World Health Organization

An overview of cancer survival in developing countries

R. Sankaranarayanan[1], R. J. Black[1], R. Swaminathan[2], D.M. Parkin[1]

[1]International Agency for Research on Cancer
Lyon,
France

[2]Cancer Institute (WIA)
Chennai (Madras) 600036
India

Population-based cancer survival data from developing countries

This book describes cancer survival for 10 populations in five countries (China, Cuba, India, Philippines and Thailand). This is the first time that the results of a standardized analysis of population-based survival data from developing countries have been presented and discussed. The reasons for the paucity of information about cancer survival from developing countries are readily understandable. Cancer registries are a recent phenomenon in some developing countries, and do not exist at all in many others. The initial emphasis for many registries in developing countries is to provide valid estimates of cancer incidence patterns and trends in the regions they cover by concentrating resources on collecting information on the identification details, date of incidence, primary site, morphology and method of diagnosis. Since passive data reporting is not feasible in many developing countries, the registries use active methods of data collection, in which their staff visit a number of potential reporting sources in their region and collect cancer information. This process is often challenging and time-consuming. Once the basic registration process has become established, some registries are able to focus on related functions, such as routine collection of follow-up data on incident cases.

Obtaining adequate information about the vital status of registered cancer patients is as challenging as case-finding. In general, active measures to obtain follow-up information must be pursued if reliable cancer survival analysis is contemplated in developing-country settings. The 10 cancer registries in the present study have used a variety of methods to achieve this. They are presented in detail in each of the registry chapters, and are summarized in Table 1. Death registration in

developing countries is often incomplete — not all deaths are registered, and the recorded cause of death may be inaccurate, or missing. Thus any follow-up effort that relies only on matching the incident cancer database with death certificates mentioning 'cancer' as the cause of death will be grossly inadequate. Some registries (e.g. Madras, India) have tried to overcome this limitation by matching incident cancer cases with the entire mortality database, irrespective of the cause of death mentioned in the certificates.

Cancer hospitals in many countries have unified medical records systems which allow repeated review of records to trace any hospital deaths or details of clinical follow-up. Hospital cancer registries, where they are present, generally have quite extensive information on the follow-up of registered cases (provided that this takes place in the same institution).

Reply-paid postal enquiries are useful for establishing vital status in certain settings. The registries in Thailand and India use this method extensively for follow-up. Enquiries addressed to consulting physicians are also occasionally useful. If all the above methods failed to establish the patients' vital status at the closing date of the study, many registries resort to house visits performed by registry staff, trained social workers or health workers from the local health or municipal offices.

Variations in cancer survival

The results of the analysis, summarized in Tables 2–4 and 6–7, reveal wide variations in survival from many cancer sites between the developing-country populations studied. The variations were less marked for cancer sites such as hypopharynx, oesophagus, stomach, liver, gallbladder, lung and bone tumours.

Table 1. Follow-up methods used by cancer registries in developing countries

Method of follow-up	Qidong, China	Shanghai, China	Cuba	Bangalore, India	Barshi, India	Mumbai (Bombay), India	Chennai (Madras), India	Rizal, Philippines	Chiang Mai, Thailand	Khon Kaen, Thailand
Matching with death certificates mentioning cancer	+	+	+	+	+	+	+	+	+	+
Matching with all death certificates irrespective of cause of death	+	+	+				+			
Scrutiny of hospital case records	+	+	+	+	+	+	+	+	+	+
Postal enquiries		+		+	+	+	+		+	+
Telephone enquiries				+		+	+			
Enquiries to physicians, local health/municipal offices	+	+						+	+	+
House visits	+	+		+	+	+	+	+	+	+
Matching with population register			+							

Within the range of age-standardized relative survival (ASRS) estimates, Shanghai, in China, reported the highest figures for all cancer sites except the hypopharynx, oesophagus, liver, bone, cervix, vagina, prostate, brain, thyroid and leukaemia (Table 4). Khon Kaen, in Thailand, reported the highest survival for cancers of the oesophagus, bone, melanoma, brain and thyroid, while Chiang Mai, in Thailand, reported the highest figures for cancers of the uterine cervix, vagina, skin, hypopharynx, and prostate. Cuba reported the highest survival for leukaemia, and Rizal (Philippines) the highest for liver cancer.

Interpretation of cancer survival rates is not straightforward. A number of factors should be taken into account, including the accuracy and completeness of cancer registration, the completeness of follow-up, host factors such as sex and age, tumour-related factors, including stage at diagnosis, and possible effects of treatment (see Chapter 4).

Variations by sex and age

The five-year relative survival rates for 13 selected cancer sites (oral cavity, oesophagus, stomach, colorectum, liver, larynx, lung, breast, cervix, ovary,

Hodgkin's disease, non-Hodgkin's lymphoma and leukaemia) from the participating registries are presented graphically in Appendix 1 of this chapter.

Table 2 shows five-year relative survival by site and sex for the 10 registries. Generally, a higher survival among females was observed for cancers of the tongue, salivary gland, oral cavity, nasopharynx and kidney, and to a lesser extent, for cancers of the oropharynx, oesophagus, colon, rectum, lung, melanoma, brain, thyroid and lymphoma. Lower survival among females was observed for urinary bladder cancers in all registries and for stomach, pancreas and larynx in some. Sex differences in cancer survival have been a matter of intense discussion (Wiebelt & Hakulinen, 1991). It seems likely that the observed female advantage in survival from most cancers in developed countries is the result of more favourable distributions of prognostic factors, particularly stage.

The five-year relative survival rates were generally higher for young adults than for older age groups in respect of most cancer sites in most registries, although this was less evident for colorectal and breast cancer (Table 3). The declining relative survival with increasing age was most marked for cervical cancer in all registries.

Table 2. Five-year relative survival (%) by site and sex in developing countries

Site	ICD-9	Qidong M	Qidong F	Shanghai M	Shanghai F	Cuba M	Cuba F	Bangalore M	Bangalore F	Barshi F	Bombay F	Madras M	Madras F	Rizal M	Rizal F	Chiang Mai M	Chiang Mai F	Khon Kaen M	Khon Kaen F
Lip	140			83.4	89.7							49.9	42.0			88.9	60.8	110.2	70.1
Tongue	141			44.7	50.5	21.8	35.1					24.2	32.2			26.8	48.3	5.2	49.9
Salivary gland	142			56.8	71.9											42.1	66.4		
Oral cavity	143–5			53.2	50.9	45.8	56.9					31.7	33.8	26.8	46.9	15.5	24.9	31.0	43.6
Oropharynx	146			47.1	67.9	36.3	23.6					19.2	30.3			22.4	24.7	22.9	35.8
Nasopharynx	147	24.9	34.8	49.7	62.2											26.4	35.1	20.8	42.6
Hypopharynx	148			25.7	14.2							16.0	21.3			22.3	18.0		
Oesophagus	150	4.2	4.0	10.5	12.7							6.8	6.1			2.2	6.3	33.0	22.5
Stomach	151	15.1	13.0	24.8	22.3							7.1	9.2	18.3	4.9	9.2	7.7	14.9	23.3
Small intestine	152	6.7	17.9	26.2	38.1														
Colon	153	29.8	32.8	43.1	44.0	34.2	41.0							46.8	34.8	39.6	36.6	33.8	39.0
Rectum	154	26.9	23.1	41.3	44.3	40.7	42.6							21.1	26.3	26.8	23.6	27.2	40.2
Colorectum	153–4	27.6	25.3	42.3	44.1	36.9	41.6							34.6	31.2	33.6	30.1	31.1	39.2
Liver	155	1.8	2.7	4.3	4.8									13.3	19.0	0.0	1.1	8.5	8.3
Gallbladder	156			10.8	8.7											4.6	3.8	17.9	13.0
Pancreas	157	5.8	5.1	6.9	5.1							7.2	0.0			4.3	3.0	4.5	5.1
Larynx	161			53.3	42.7							37.8	47.3			18.5	23.9	52.0	13.4
Lung	162	3.4	4.1	12.1	11.3	10.0	12.6					7.2	10.2	7.0	7.9	3.0	3.1	10.3	9.5
Bone	170			19.3	19.6											48.4	14.3	34.9	38.3
Connective tissue	171			61.4	60.1											29.8	43.0	24.4	29.8
Skin melanoma	172			42.5	48.9											43.8	44.3	57.4	45.3
Other skin	173			74.6	70.7											92.7	92.9	73.3	89.7
Breast	174		55.7		72.0		60.8		45.1		55.1		49.5		45.6		63.7		47.1
Cervix	180		33.6		51.9		55.9		40.4	33.3	50.7		60.0		29.0		68.2		57.5
Corpus uteri	182				76.8		60.9										69.5		78.7
Ovary	183				44.2		43.3										44.9		35.6
Vagina	184				47.1												59.2		
Prostate	185			40.1		45.1								21.3		42.3		41.1	
Testis	186			65.8												50.7		41.6	
Penis	187			67.9												56.8		67.7	
Bladder	188	43.7	21.3	64.1	51.2							25.2	15.0			39.7	35.2	61.5	39.0
Kidney	189			46.5	49.4											11.4	18.6	18.2	29.1
Brain & nervous system	191–2	8.5	7.9	29.8	40.8											13.0	24.6	28.2	41.1
Thyroid	193			71.7	82.8											52.1	52.9	73.0	90.7
Hodgkin's disease	201			51.0	44.4	54.0	56.2	57.2	61.0			38.4	45.7			22.0	43.6	14.8	62.3
Non-Hodgkin lymphoma	200,202			31.8	35.9	35.6	39.0	32.4	38.7			19.1	25.8			26.5	20.5	25.0	31.2
Multiple myeloma	203	1.4	3.3	26.4	18.6	16.7	19.8	30.2	16.3							22.8	8.0		
Lymphatic leukaemia	204			18.3	20.3	29.1	33.4	31.8	28.3			24.0	28.0	33.4	16.7	13.2	14.1	29.1	25.5
Myeloid leukaemia	205	15.8	3.8	16.9	17.8	15.8	6.0	14.9	29.0			16.3	17.6	5.9	17.3	11.2	10.2	19.4	13.0
All leukaemia	204–8	6.1	3.2	15.1	15.8	22.3	20.0	21.4	26.4			20.2	23.5	18.8	16.3	10.2	10.6	22.0	19.2
Primary site uncertain	195–9			11.8	10.4											3.9	4.0	8.2	13.5

Table 3. Five-year relative survival (%) by age group and selected sites

Registry	Oral cavity						Larynx					
	0–34	35–44	45–54	55–64	65–74	75–99	0–34	35–44	45–54	55–64	65–74	75–99
Shanghai	88.1	70.6	80.8	62.1	35.7	13.6	75.4	80.6	71.0	54.6	50.2	31.6
Cuba	52.9	36.1	41.9	38.7	47.0	91.6						
Madras	39.1	47.0	34.0	28.6	29.5	22.7	77.9	40.6	39.3	29.3	46.9	11.8
Rizal	71.6	101.0	0.0	23.7	56.3	44.4						
Chiang Mai	35.1	25.1	16.3	23.4	16.1	10.9	33.7	53.0	30.6	25.8	10.2	13.2
Khon Kaen	100.8	38.2	50.0	34.3	24.4	48.8	–	0.0	29.9	38.8	52.9	65.3

Registry	Colon						Rectum					
	0–34	35–44	45–54	55–64	65–74	75–99	0–34	35–44	45–54	55–64	65–74	75–99
Qidong	44.1	48.0	29.2	35.7	30.3	16.0	19.3	34.8	35.5	29.8	23.8	6.4
Shanghai	39.3	45.9	53.7	45.4	42.0	32.9	37.9	45.4	55.7	47.4	40.7	21.3
Cuba	39.1	42.9	30.9	35.6	35.8	54.3	36.0	33.0	34.0	43.8	41.5	50.1
Rizal	38.5	30.8	43.4	67.1	26.0	39.6	0.0	22.0	15.4	49.6	27.0	0.0
Chiang Mai	31.8	36.0	56.8	35.3	25.9	42.8	29.4	35.7	24.6	25.9	14.8	45.8
Khon Kaen	56.2	45.1	31.3	30.9	18.6	59.0	30.9	28.2	26.4	37.4	46.1	0.0

Registry	Breast						Cervix					
	0–34	35–44	45–54	55–64	65–74	75–99	0–34	35–44	45–54	55–64	65–74	75–99
Qidong	59.8	60.8	62.1	47.0	51.8	23.2	50.3	42.2	47.4	41.6	28.0	6.9
Shanghai	70.5	74.9	76.9	69.9	70.0	58.0	66.9	76.6	59.5	59.8	46.1	36.9
Cuba	53.7	62.1	57.9	55.7	58.7	104.0	66.0	60.8	53.4	54.1	40.2	47.7
Bangalore	49.5	50.1	44.3	44.1	36.3	25.6	46.1	46.1	41.6	35.7	31.0	27.8
Barshi							31.8	39.4	34.5	24.7	28.5	84.7
Bombay	59.5	56.1	53.7	53.7	55.8	49.6	66.5	57.4	42.3	46.3	44.5	20.9
Madras	63.6	55.4	50.5	40.1	42.7	19.3	77.3	71.9	64.4	47.0	24.7	14.0
Rizal	24.5	44.4	51.9	37.6	52.5	68.2	32.1	42.4	29.7	17.8	18.5	0.0
Chiang Mai	69.0	67.7	65.0	54.8	61.9	74.2	83.6	76.4	66.1	54.2	50.8	78.2
Khon Kaen	59.4	47.3	40.1	47.8	48.7	146.5	76.6	63.0	54.8	53.7	35.0	44.4

Registry	Ovary						Hodgkin's disease					
	0–34	35–44	45–54	55–64	65–74	75–99	0–34	35–44	45–54	55–64	65–74	75–99
Shanghai	66.5	57.4	42.7	38.0	32.4	25.3	71.4	55.9	30.5	31.7	29.7	0.0
Cuba	60.3	46.8	42.0	26.2	41.4	92.5	63.8	65.5	61.0	29.1	6.3	46.8
Bangalore												
Madras							53.3	15.6	17.2	11.2	42.4	0.0
Chiang Mai	62.3	61.0	45.4	31.9	9.6	37.4	48.4	30.1	24.0	13.2	13.7	29.4
Khon Kaen	58.9	27.6	28.2	33.0	28.1	32.9	29.5	22.6	39.8	12.2	61.1	0.0

Inter-registry comparison of results

The aim of this section is to compare results for developing-country cancer registries on a site-by-site basis, between the registries themselves and also between developing and developed countries in general. To this end, published survival data from the USA and Europe were compared with the results of the present study.

For whites in the USA, two datasets were used:

(1) Data from the 'End Results Program', including survival of cancer patients from the state of Connecticut, one-fifth of cancer patients in California and patients registered at the Charity Hospital in New Orleans and the University of Iowa Hospital for the period 1950–73 (Axtell et al., 1976);

(2) Survival reported from the 'Surveillance End Results Epidemiology' (SEER) programme in the USA for the white population (Ries et al., 1990; Kosary et al., 1995) for the periods 1974–86 and 1986–91.

Table 4. Comparison of age-standardized relative survival rates (0–74 years) from selected cancers in the USA, Europe and developing countries

Site	US White 1967–73	US White 1974–86	US White 1986–91	Europe 1978–85	China Qidong 1982–91	China Shanghai 1988–91	Cuba 1988–89	India Bangalore 1982–89	India Barshi 1988–92	India Bombay 1982–86	India Madras 1984–89	Philippines Rizal 1987	Thailand Chiang Mai 1983–92	Thailand Khon Kaen 1985–92	DC[a] range 1982–92[b]
Lip						80.4	93.4				49.7		60.6	81.9	49.7 – 93.4
Tongue				42.3		51.0	25.0				24.7		34.7	25.5	24.7 – 51.0
Oral cavity				49.3		64.0	42.4				33.7	41.2	21.3	36.6	21.3 – 64.0
Oropharynx				34.7		67.9	29.9				21.6		21.1	20.3	20.3 – 67.9
Nasopharynx				40.2	25.2	51.6							26.6	25.3	25.2 – 51.6
Hypopharynx				20.5		14.6					18.8		19.1		14.6 – 19.1
Oral & Pharynx	–	54.5[c]	55.0	37.1											
Oesophagus	5.9	9.4	12.7	5.8	4.6	14.8					6.9		3.3	26.5	3.3 – 26.5
Stomach	12.6	16.8	19.5	23.0	17.2	28.2					7.5	13.9	8.7	16.7	7.5 – 28.2
Colon	46.9	55.2	62.5	45.4	34.1	45.4	35.7					42.1	35.6	29.1	29.1 – 45.4
Rectum	45.1	53.9	61.8	40.9	28.5	45.7	39.7					29.4	22.6	37.4	22.6 – 45.7
Colorectum	46.0	54.8	62.3	43.1	29.6	45.5	37.2					36.5	29.2	33.4	29.2 – 45.5
Liver	10.1	6.5[c]	10.3		2.1	5.1						12.9	0.6	10.0	0.6 – 12.9
Gallbladder						12.6							4.1	11.1	4.1 – 12.6
Pancreas	2.8	4.2	5.6	6.4	6.0	7.2					4.4		2.5	2.5	2.5 – 7.2
Larynx	64.2	70.2	69.6	58.2		60.9					39.9		25.8	34.9	25.8 – 60.9
Lung	9.7	14.6	15.7	9.9	3.9	13.8	10.2				7.9	7.7	3.2	9.3	3.2 – 13.8
Bone				42.9		21.9							31.7	34.7	21.9 – 34.7
Connective tissue						62.4							32.8	27.8	27.8 – 62.4
Skin melanoma	66.7	81.5	87.2			46.8							39.2	47.0	39.2 – 47.0
Other skin						74.8							86.4	76.1	74.8 – 86.4

Table 4. (Contd) Comparison of age-standardized relative survival rates (0–74 years) from selected cancers in the USA, Europe and developing countries

Site	US White			Europe	China		Cuba	India				Philippines	Thailand		DC[a]
					Qidong	Shanghai		Bangalore	Barshi	Bombay	Madras	Rizal	Chiang Mai	Khon Kaen	range
	1967–73	1974–86	1986–91	1978–85	1982–91	1988–91	1988–89	1982–89	1988–92	1982–86	1984–89	1987	1983–92	1985–92	1982–92[b]
Breast (female)	65.0	76.1	83.6	68.7	55.7	72.7	57.9	44.1		55.1	48.4	44.5	62.7	47.0	44.1 – 72.7
Cervix	58.7	68.2	70.1	61.5	42.0	61.9	54.3	39.9	32.0	49.5	56.7	28.0	64.9	55.4	28.0 – 64.9
Corpus uteri	80.0	88.8	88.2	76.2		76.7	58.7						67.1	70.4	58.7 – 76.7
Ovary	36.7	45.1	53.2	38.4		45.0	41.1						39.3	33.6	33.6 – 45.0
Vagina				62.5		48.9							54.3		48.9 – 54.3
Prostate	61.9	75.3	88.9			42.3	35.9					34.9	45.9	34.5	34.5 – 45.9
Testis	68.6	92.1	95.3	85.2		70.8							63.3	36.8	36.8 – 70.8
Penis				71.5		72.4							56.6	69.2	56.6 – 72.4
Bladder	67.8	81.1	86.1		42.8	66.1					23.5		34.6	57.8	23.5 – 66.1
Kidney	45.1	56.4	64.0	49.5		49.2							19.1	21.9	19.1 – 49.2
Brain				15.2	8.2	34.5							13.1	35.5	8.2 – 35.5
Thyroid						74.3							46.7	80.7	46.7 – 80.7
Hodgkin's disease	61.5	77.3	79.6	71.3		55.2	54.8	59.0			35.9		34.8	30.5	30.5 – 59.0
NHL[d]	32.2	55.7	54.2			35.5	37.4	32.8			17.7		22.7	27.4	17.7 – 37.4
Multiple myeloma	14.3	29.2	38.5		2.7	37.3	12.2	31.5							2.7 – 37.3
Leukaemia	22.5	39.9	48.1	35.4	4.7	16.9	21.3	22.6			20.6	15.9	9.8	17.4	4.7 – 22.6
Primary uncertain						13.0							4.2	11.4	4.2 – 13.0

[a] Developing countries

[b] Period varies for individual registries

[c] Data for 1981–86

[d] NHL: non-Hodgkin lymphoma

In the USA, the National Cancer Act of 1971 mandated the collection, analysis and dissemination of data useful in the prevention, diagnosis and treatment of cancer. This led to the establishment of the SEER programme, which succeeded earlier programmes (the End Results Program and the Third National Cancer Survey) of the US National Cancer Institute. The SEER programme collects cancer data on a routine basis from designated population-based cancer registries in various areas of the USA, covering 9.5% of the US population (states of Connecticut, Hawaii, Iowa, New Mexico, Utah, ten counties of Georgia, metropolitan areas of Atlanta, Detroit, San Francisco (Oakland), Seattle (Puget Sound area), and American Indians of Arizona).

The 'European Cancer Registry-based Study of Survival and Care of Cancer Patients' (EUROCARE) has the objective of estimating, comparing and interpreting the survival of cancer patients in different European populations. A description of survival rates of cancer patients diagnosed during the period 1978–85 from 30 population-based cancer registries in 11 European countries (Denmark, Estonia, Finland, France, Germany, Italy, Netherlands, Poland, Spain, Switzerland and United Kingdom) was published in 1995 (Berrino *et al.,* 1995). A pooled dataset from this study, for the period 1978–85, was used to represent European populations for comparative purposes.

Data for US whites and European populations were age-standardized to the 'world' patient population, as described in Chapter 3.

The comparison of age-standardized relative survival rates for selected cancers in the developing countries, Europe and USA is shown in Table 4. The proportion of patients within different clinical-extent-of-disease categories at the time of presentation for selected cancer sites in eight developing-country cancer registries and for the US-SEER programme (1986–91) is shown in Table 5. Relative and observed survival in relation to clinical extent of disease for these selected cancer sites in these cancer registries is shown in Tables 6 and 7. Comparative data for Europe are not available.

Oral cavity and pharyngeal cancers

For all the subsites within the oral cavity and pharynx, age-standardized relative survival in the developing-country regions (except Shanghai) was lower than in Europe, although comparatively high survival was reported from Shanghai for all subsites except hypopharynx. Information on clinical extent of disease was available from Cuba, Chiang Mai and Madras for tongue and oral cavity cancers. In Cuba, one-third of patients presented with localized disease, compared with one-tenth of patients in the other two regions. The high proportion of localized cancers and the comparatively high survival from oral cavity cancer in Cuba may be due to the ongoing oral cancer screening programme in that country (Fernandez Garrote *et al.,* 1995). The survival rates for localized and regionally spread oral cavity cancer in the three developing-country registries with stage-specific data were lower than in the USA (Table 6). The results for oral cancer presenting with distant metastases were based on very few cases. No evidence of improvement in survival from oral cavity and pharyngeal cancer has been seen in the USA over the period 1973–89 (Miller *et al.,* 1993).

Surgical resection and radiation therapy are the mainstays of treatment for these cancers. For most small primary cancers without regional spread (stages I and II), wide surgical excision or radiotherapy alone can result in local tumour control and long-term survival. While local tumour control is better with surgery, radiotherapy offers more acceptable cosmetic and functional results. For more extensive primary tumours or regional metastatic disease, a combination of surgery and radiotherapy is generally used. However, long-term survival prospects are poor, even for moderately advanced oral and pharyngeal cancer. Data from many clinical trials indicate that chemotherapy does not result in better survival prospects from this cancer than those achieved using surgery and radiotherapy.

Surgery and radiotherapy facilities are widely available in the health services of the developing countries represented in this study. Early detection linked with these services can lead to considerable gains in survival outcome from these cancers in these regions, even if co-morbidity is a major limiting factor in achieving improved survival.

There is some evidence that screening for oral cancer results in the detection of a high proportion of early-stage cancers (Fernandez Garrote *et al.,* 1995; Mathew *et al.,* 1999). Whether screening for oral cancer will result in increased survival and reduced mortality remains to be established (Sankaranarayanan, 1997; Mathew *et al.,* 1997). The vast potential for prevention of oral cancer by tobacco control and dietary changes should not be overlooked in overall control measures. A reduced incidence of oral precancerous lesions has been reported in a primary prevention trial (Gupta *et al.,* 1986, 1992).

Oesophagus

Age-standardized relative survival in Qidong, Madras and Chiang Mai registries was lower than in the USA for 1988–91, and comparable with that reported from Europe in 1978–85 and the USA in 1967–73. Survival in Shanghai is similar to that in the USA, while the reasons for the apparently high survival in Khon Kaen are not clear. We speculate that they may be related to misclassification at diagnosis, in view of the high proportion of clinically diagnosed cases.

There has been some improvement in short-term survival (one-year and two-year survival) in the USA, which has been attributed to improvements in diagnosis, staging, availability of parenteral nutrition and increasing use of combinations of chemotherapy and radiation in the treatment of unresectable oesophageal cancer (Miller et al., 1993). Almost half the histologically verified oesophageal cancers in the US SEER white patients are adenocarcinomas, compared with one-quarter to one-third in European registries, and less than one-fifth in the developing-country registries (Parkin et al., 1997). Adenocarcinomas mainly occur in the lower third of the oesophagus. These cancers are more suitable for surgical therapy, which offers the best chance for long-term survival in oesophageal cancer. Hence lower-third tumours have a better prognosis than other cancers located in the middle or upper third of the oesophagus. These facts should be considered when interpreting the results. Radiotherapy can also result in long-term control of selected small localized cancers; it relieves dysphagia from advanced cancers for a varying period of time (3–9 months) in the vast majority of patients.

By the time the symptoms of swallowing difficulty appear, the disease is usually too advanced to be amenable to radical surgery or radiotherapy. Early detection procedures (e.g. barium swallow followed by gastro-oesophageal endoscopy or brush cytology using disposable endoscopy brushes) involve sophisticated and costly equipment and are not readily accepted for use in routine field conditions. Thus, there are no suitable screening or diagnostic tests available to detect this cancer at an early stage, and there are no specific symptoms leading to clinical suspicion of early oesophageal cancer. Hence the potential of early detection and treatment to improve outcomes is quite limited. Alcohol, tobacco and dietary factors are the major risk factors for oesophageal cancers, and primary prevention remains the main approach for reducing mortality from this cancer.

Stomach

The five-year survival rates reported from Qidong and Khon Kaen registries are comparable with those in the USA and Europe: those from Madras, Rizal, and Chiang Mai are lower. The survival reported from Shanghai is higher than the US and European results: this may be related to the early detection efforts in Shanghai (see Chapter 7). Short-term and long-term survival rates in the USA have increased only very slightly during the period 1973–89 (Miller et al., 1993). In spite of the continuing worldwide decline in incidence, it is still the second most common cancer globally and the most common cancer in many developing countries (Parkin et al., 1993). Symptoms of the disease are nonspecific, and hence most of these cancers are quite advanced by the time they are detected clinically.

Screening for stomach cancer, though probably effective in reducing mortality from the disease, is largely confined to Japan, since the resources required for double-contrast radiography and follow-up gastroscopy are expensive (Pisani & Parkin, 1996). Survival from gastric cancer in Japan is relatively good: four-year cumulative survival increased from 55.8%, 31.4% 24.2% and 27.4% in 1976 in teaching hospitals, large, medium and small hospitals, respectively, to 59.6%, 47.5%, 41.2% and 39.3% respectively in 1986, in the data reported from the population-based Osaka cancer registry (Tanaka et al., 1994). This is partly due to a much more favourable stage distribution as a consequence of the screening programme, but survival within stage in Japan is also higher than elsewhere: five-year survival rates were 94%, 56%, 30% and 9%, respectively, for stage I-to-stage IV stomach cancers in Japan during the period 1963–66; these improved to 96%, 81%, 61% and 14% during the period 1979-90 (Taira et al., 1993). The improvement in stage-specific survival in Japan has been brought about by progress in surgical techniques, particularly systematic lymph node dissection.

The intestinal type of gastric cancer mostly occurs in the pyloric antrum, while the diffuse type generally involves the upper and middle part of the stomach, and these often present at an advanced stage, since the tumours in the proximal region of the stomach are technically difficult to find with endoscopy and contrast radiography. Pyloric cancers have the best prognosis, and those of the fundus have the worst prognosis. The widely documented decline in gastric cancer is mostly restricted to the intestinal type (Correa & Chen, 1994), and consequently the proportion of cancers which are of the diffuse type is on the increase in many countries.

A decline in overall gastric cancer survival may even occur in future, owing to the increasing proportions of proximal, diffuse-type tumours.

The potential for reduced mortality and improved survival through early detection is limited primarily by the cost of photofluorographic screening and follow-up by gastroscopy of around 10% of screened subjects. Primary prevention seems to be a more realistic long-term control strategy for developing countries. Dietary factors and infection with *Helicobacter pylori* seem to be important in the causation of the intestinal type of stomach cancer. Large gains in the control of stomach cancer are likely with the better understanding of the role of these factors, particularly in developing countries.

Colon

In all developing-country registries, age-standardized relative survival was lower than in the USA. Survival in Shanghai was comparable with that in Europe and in the USA in the period 1967–73. The distribution of cases by stage in Cuba was similar to that in the USA, but the proportion of localized cancers in Chiang Mai was much lower (Table 5). However, the stage-specific relative survival rates from Chiang Mai were similar to those in the USA, and the lower overall relative survival seems to be due to the low proportion of localized cancers (5% vs. 36% in the USA). In Cuba, however, survival was lower within each stage category (Table 6).

Survival from colon cancer has increased for both sexes in the USA, and this has been attributed to earlier diagnosis, improvements in diagnostic tests and refinement of surgical techniques (Miller *et al.*, 1993). The increased use of sigmoidoscopy and faecal occult blood tests, with the resulting high frequency of colonoscopy, appears to have played a role in reducing mortality from colorectal cancer in the USA (Chu *et al.*, 1994).

The most important aspects of treatment of colon cancer are adequacy of surgery and appropriate multimodality treatment for patients who are at high risk of recurrence. A significant overall survival benefit with routine adjuvant chemotherapy with 5-fluorouracil and levamisole in moderately advanced colon cancer is now evident (Moertel *et al.*, 1990; Krook *et al.*, 1991). The role of adjuvant radiotherapy in resected colon cancer is not as well defined as it is for rectal cancer. It is likely that the current advances in adjuvant therapy will have an impact on survival in future years.

Major gains in survival could be achieved in developing countries by early detection and adequate treatment. Though colon cancer is not a common cancer in many developing-country populations, its incidence is likely to increase with the social and dietary changes associated with socioeconomic development. Tumours occurring in the caecum and ascending colon are diagnosed in more advanced stages than cancers in the rectosigmoid and descending colon, partly due to the fact that early detection procedures such as sigmoidoscopy and air contrast barium enema are more successful in identifying early left-sided tumours. Thus right-sided tumours have a poor prognosis compared with left-sided colon cancers. These are relatively more common in developing countries, since it is tumours of the left colon (rectosigmoid region) that show a particular increase in incidence with increasing affluence and have become proportionately more important in developed countries. This may account for some of the differences in survival when colon cancer is considered as a whole.

Rectum

Age-standardized relative survival from rectal cancer in all registries included in this study was lower than that in the USA in the periods 1986–91 and 1974–86. With the exception of Shanghai, the survival rates were also lower than the US rates in 1967–73 and European rates in 1978–85. The proportion of localized rectal cancer in Cuba was similar to that in the US SEER study, but the proportion in Chiang Mai was much lower (Table 5). However, the stage-specific survival rates reported from Chiang Mai and Cuba were lower than those in the USA. Some of this may be due to stage misclassification, as well as to differences in the availability and effectiveness of treatment.

The increases in survival observed in the USA during 1973–89 have been attributed to early diagnosis, improved surgical techniques and the recent increased use of radiotherapy (Miller *et al.*, 1993). As in colon cancer, surgery is the mainstay of treatment. Surgical techniques have been advanced and refined over the years to allow preservation of the anal sphincter in an increasing proportion of patients. Adjuvant radiotherapy benefits those patients who remain at high risk for locoregional failure despite complete surgery, when the tumour invades through the muscle wall and involves lymph nodes. Adjuvant chemotherapy based on 5-fluorouracil and adjuvant radiotherapy have been shown to reduce overall recurrence rates and prolong patient survival in the case of moderately advanced rectal cancer. As in colon cancer, significant gains in survival could be achieved in developing countries

Table 5. Proportion (%) of cases by clinical extent of disease for selected sites

Registry	Lip No.	L	R	D	U	Tongue No.	L	R	D	U	Oral cavity No.	L	R	D	U
Cuba						233	35	33	3	29	384	37	19	1	43
Madras	39	21	64	5	10	432	7	80	3	10	931	11	74	3	12
Chiang Mai	35	46	54	0	0	172	11	87	1	1	239	8	86	3	3
US-SEER, White[a,b]											11 004	38	42	8	12

Registry	Colon No.	L	R	D	U	Rectum No.	L	R	D	U	Colon and rectum No.	L	R	D	U
Cuba	1092	31	23	8	38	708	41	24	6	29	1800	35	23	7	35
Chiang Mai	392	5	52	41	2	345	6	67	23	4	737	5	59	33	3
US-SEER, White[a]	38 122	36	39	20	5	15 707	42	34	16	8	53 829	38	37	19	6

Registry	Larynx No.	L	R	D	U	Breast No.	L	R	D	U	Cervix No.	L	R	D	U
Cuba						2375	38	30	5	27	1531	44	25	2	29
Bangalore						1361	32	46	8	14	2155	16	70	5	9
Barshi											247	19	64	2	15
Bombay						2872	33	45	13	9	2354	34	51	10	5
Madras	346	19	65	4	12	1346	4	60	10	26	3289	9	86	2	3
Rizal						330	19	42	7	32	181	18	52	5	25
Chiang Mai	342	13	81	3	3	764	30	53	16	1	1555	38	36	21	5
Khon Kaen						409	3	32	31	34	820	16	52	6	26
US-SEER, White[a]	4640	51	32	11	6	66 261	59	32	6	3	5007	54	31	8	7

[a] 1986–91

[b] oral cavity and pharynx combined

L: Localized; R: Regional; D: Distant metastasis; U: Unstaged

by early detection and provision of adequate treatment. It should be noted that rectal cancer is more common than colon cancer in most Asian countries (Parkin *et al.*, 1997).

Liver

Age-standardized relative survival from liver cancer was uniformly poor in all registries. This essentially preventable cancer is a major problem in many developing countries. Although surgery can achieve long-term survival in patients with localized liver cancer, such cases are rare, and surgical management is limited by concomitant cirrhosis in many patients. Thus, early detection and treatment seem to have very little to contribute to the overall reduction in mortality from liver cancer.

Though screening with alpha-fetoprotein and ultrasonography resulted in early detection of liver cancer in an intervention trial in Qidong, China, the five-year survival rates were similar in both the intervention and the control groups (Chen *et al.*, unpublished; *see Chapter 6*).

While hepatocellular carcinomas are the most common liver cancer in many regions of the world, cholangiocarcinoma accounts for most (approx. 90%) of liver cancers in Khon Kaen, Thailand (*see Chapter 15*) and a little less than half the liver cancers in Chiang Mai (*see Chapter 14*). Cholangiocarcinomas account for about one-fifth of histologically confirmed liver cancers in the US SEER whites and rather less in the European registries (Parkin *et al.*, 1997). Though these are totally different cancers, both have the same grave prognosis.

Epidemiological and laboratory investigations have yielded possible preventive strategies for both types of liver cancers. The role of hepatitis viruses (IARC, 1994a), liver flukes (IARC, 1994b) and aflatoxins (IARC, 1993) in the causation of liver cancers has been well established. Vaccination against hepatitis B infection is the most important preventive measure currently available for the control of liver cancer. Recently, there has been observational evidence of decreasing incidence of liver cancer among children in Taiwan as a consequence of the nationwide hepatitis B vaccination programme introduced in 1984 (Chang *et al.*, 1997). Control of liver fluke infection has a major potential to control liver cancer in Thailand.

Pancreas

Survival from pancreatic cancer was low in all registries (Table 4). This cancer is difficult to diagnose at an early stage, owing to the absence of specific symptoms and early signs. Though resection of all or part of the pancreas with adjacent tissues can achieve long-term survival, tumours are seldom diagnosed early enough to allow this procedure. The most frequently recognized symptoms (e.g. jaundice, pain and weight loss) signify advanced disease, by which time more than four-fifths of pancreatic cancers will have encroached on to other organs. The results of radiotherapy are also disappointing, owing to the bioaggressiveness of the tumour and the radiosensitivity of the surrounding tissues.

There are no specific screening or diagnostic tests to detect this cancer at an early stage. Smoking, alcohol consumption and dietary factors have been implicated as risk factors. Tobacco control and balanced nutrition seem to be the only viable current measures to prevent pancreatic cancer.

Larynx

Age-standardized relative survival reported from all registries in this study was lower than that reported from the USA for all the three periods beginning 1973 (Ries *et al.*, 1990; Miller *et al.*, 1993; Kosary *et al.*, 1995). The low survival in the developing-country registries seems to be due to advanced stage at presentation (Table 5). As with many other cancer sites, survival in Shanghai is similar to that in Europe. The stage-specific survival rates reported from the Madras and Chiang Mai cancer registries are considerably lower than those reported from the USA (Table 6). Stage and site misclassification and inadequacies in treatment (particularly in regional disease where a combination of surgery and radiotherapy is increasingly used) may account for these differences. Advanced laryngeal cancers involve infiltration of cartilages and extension to lymph nodes, both of which are poor prognostic

indicators for laryngeal cancer. Five-year survival drops to less than 20% in almost all head and neck cancers if cervical lymph nodes are involved at the time of presentation. The role of tobacco smoking and alcohol consumption in the causation of laryngeal cancer show the potential for prevention. Early detection and adequate treatment will improve survival from this cancer in developing countries.

Lung

Survival from lung cancer was low in all registries. Though five-year survival increases if the disease is diagnosed in early stages, screening has not been effective in reducing mortality (Parkin & Pisani, 1996). Mass screening with chest X-ray and sputum cytology is not recommended to control lung cancer.

Squamous-cell carcinoma is the most common histological type of lung cancer, accounting for 36–59% of cases in different regions (Parkin & Sankaranarayanan, 1994; Parkin *et al.*, 1997). Small-cell lung cancer accounts for 10–25% of lung cancers in most regions; the proportion of small-cell lung cancer in developed countries is higher than that observed in developing countries.

Surgery remains the main modality of treatment, offering the best prospects of long-term survival in selected, small, localized non-small-cell lung cancers. Radiotherapy is useful for palliative treatment if the cancer is inoperable. The five-year relative survival for this type of cancer in the US SEER registries (for all races) was 13.8% in the period 1974–76 and 15.0% in the period 1983–89. Small-cell lung cancer has a very aggressive clinical course, with widespread metastases frequently present at the time of diagnosis. It is not amenable to surgical treatment. Though there have been advances in the treatment of small-cell lung cancer with combination chemotherapy and radiotherapy, the five-year survival from this cancer is still very low: it improved from 3.5% during the period 1974–76 to 4.9% in 1983–89 for all races in the US SEER registries (Miller *et al.*, 1993). It is unlikely that differences in the distribution of cell types can account for any of the observed differences in survival from lung cancer, as the prognosis from non-small-cell lung cancer is also poor.

Investment in early diagnosis and treatment is unlikely to reduce the high mortality from lung cancer. It would be prudent for developing countries to concentrate on the control of tobacco smoking to prevent lung cancer, thereby avoiding increased health care expenditure on costly treatment and palliative care in the future.

Melanoma of skin

Survival from skin melanoma was lower in the developing-country regions from which data were available than in the USA. Five-year survival has steadily improved in the USA since 1950, mainly owing to early detection activities (Miller *et al.*, 1993).

This is a relatively uncommon cancer in the populations studied, and its epidemiology in Asian populations, including subtypes of melanoma and its site distribution, differs from that of 'Western' populations. In white populations, melanomas occur principally on the trunk in males and the lower limbs in females. In black and Asian populations, the sole of the foot is the most frequent site. Several studies suggest that anatomical location and thickness of melanomas are important prognostic factors (Berwick *et al.*, 1994). The differences in survival among populations are probably due to differences in the above factors. Lesions in the extremities are associated with a good prognosis, while lesions on the trunk are associated with poor survival outcome. Patients with thick lesions experience poor survival compared with those with thin lesions.

Surgery is the mainstay of treatment for skin melanoma, and early detection is an important method by which survival could be improved in developing countries. In fair-skinned populations, the importance of prevention by controlling exposure to the sun needs to be emphasized.

Female breast

Five-year age-standardized relative survival in all registries in this study was considerably lower than the survival rates for the USA for periods 1974–86 and 1986–91. With the exception of Shanghai, the developing-country rates were also lower than in the USA in the period 1967–73. Survival in Shanghai (in 1988–91) was similar to Europe, while other developing-country regions had lower survival.

The proportion of localized breast cancers in the eight developing-country regions ranged from 3% in Khon Kaen to 38% in Cuba, as compared with 59% in the USA (Table 5).

For localized breast cancer, survival in Chiang Mai was only slightly lower than that in the USA (Table 6), although it is rather low in all the other registries. For disease with regional spread, survival is rather lower in developing countries than in the USA. These findings provide important indications for breast cancer control in developing countries.

The gain in long-term survival from breast cancer in developed countries over the last three decades is probably due both to early diagnosis and

to advances in treatment (Ewertz, 1993; Miller *et al.*, 1993; Nab *et al.*, 1994a, 1994b; Olivotto *et al.*, 1994; Garne *et al.*, 1997). Widespread use of mammography in screening for breast cancer has resulted in an increasing incidence of localized breast cancers. Clinical trials over the last three decades have also contributed considerably to the optimization and advancement of treatment in breast cancer (Bonnadonna *et al.*, 1976; Early Breast Cancer Trialists' Collaborative Group, 1992, 1995). During a period of increasing use of mammographic screening, conservative surgery (shift from radical mastectomy to simple mastectomy; increasing breast conservation surgery in localized breast cancer), redefined role of radiotherapy and increasing use of adjuvant therapy with antineoplastic drugs and/or tamoxifen in developed countries, survival from breast cancer has steadily improved. Adjuvant therapy is now routinely used in women with regional disease and in selected high-risk groups with node-negative breast cancer. Improvements in breast cancer survival coinciding with the introduction of adjuvant systemic therapy have been attributed to this aspect of treatment (Olivotto *et al.*, 1994).

The rather poorer survival from localized breast cancer in developing countries, compared with similar tumours in the USA, could be a reflection both of stage misclassification (due to limited investigative facilities) and the limited availability of adequate therapy. The poor survival in women with regional disease in developing countries could be due to inadequate treatment, particularly the difficulty of providing adjuvant treatment. However, stage misclassification due to limited investigative facilities could be another important factor.

The comparatively high survival from breast cancer in Shanghai (72.7% five-year survival) deserves further discussion. This registry covers a predominantly urban area with several outlets for cancer diagnosis and treatment, supported by early detection activities for cancer sites such as stomach, breast and cervix. Unfortunately no information on the stage distribution of breast and other cancers was available from Shanghai. Nevertheless, the results reported from a randomized trial of breast self-examination in Shanghai indicate that a high proportion of cases are diagnosed at an early stage (Thomas *et al.*, 1997). Thus, in women in the control group (who had not been trained in breast self-examination) 55% of new cancer cases were stage I, and 49% were 2 cm or less in diameter. This suggests a high level of awareness of breast cancer in the Shanghai population.

Table 6. Relative survival by clinical extent of disease for selected cancers

Registry	Years survived	Lip				Tongue				Oral cavity			
		L	R	D	U	L	R	D	U	L	R	D	U
Cuba	One					67.5	64.4	60.2	33.4	87.3	62.3	68.3	70.8
	Three					35.5	30.4	43.5	13.8	66.0	28.9	71.9	50.1
	Five					35.9	24.2	23.2	13.4	63.8	27.8	76.5	46.3
Madras	One	64.4	69.9	50.4	100.9	83.6	68.0	40.8	70.9	87.0	77.8	53.6	76.3
	Three	54.6	55.1	0.0	102.8	59.2	39.2	7.1	29.3	59.5	48.6	21.9	33.3
	Five	57.7	37.5	0.0	104.8	51.0	26.1	7.4	15.6	38.8	34.6	14.0	20.7
Chiang Mai	One	92.7	56.4	–	–	94.2	48.0	0.0	0.0	62.4	38.8	0.0	67.8
	Three	87.9	51.5	–	–	71.4	29.8	0.0	0.0	51.4	20.3	0.0	71.3
	Five	87.0	57.6	–	–	75.7	31.0	0.0	0.0	48.7	14.8	0.0	76.3
US SEER White, 86–91	Five									81.4	43.3	20.0	33.1

Registry	Years survived	Colon				Rectum				Colorectum			
		L	R	D	U	L	R	D	U	L	R	D	U
Cuba	One	77.7	63.3	27.3	26.1	84.7	66.2	31.9	40.4	81.0	64.4	28.8	30.9
	Three	68.7	47.6	11.8	20.4	65.1	40.5	15.3	26.3	67.1	44.8	13.0	22.4
	Five	65.5	40.8	11.7	16.7	58.5	36.1	12.5	26.6	62.3	38.9	12.1	19.9
Chiang Mai	One	91.4	83.4	17.5	71.8	81.0	69.0	25.0	80.8	86.3	75.7	20.1	78.2
	Three	90.1	61.8	7.0	59.8	75.4	34.9	6.3	44.2	82.9	47.4	6.8	47.9
	Five	91.1	57.3	4.8	64.1	80.7	27.7	2.2	22.9	86.5	41.2	3.8	31.4
US SEER White, 86–91	Five	93.3	66.4	7.8	32.9	88.2	55.1	4.9	37.2	91.6	63.3	7.1	34.7

Registry	Years survived	Larynx				Breast				Cervix			
		L	R	D	U	L	R	D	U	L	R	D	U
Cuba	One					94.5	86.1	46.0	71.7	89.8	70.7	32.7	65.2
	Three					85.3	64.8	24.7	59.1	77.1	42.3	30.3	48.1
	Five					78.7	51.7	23.7	50.9	74.2	37.1	29.1	44.6
Bangalore	One					91.6	85.1	50.6	77.3	86.0	78.5	48.5	72.0
	Three					72.0	55.2	23.1	55.4	63.8	52.1	30.8	51.5
	Five					61.3	40.7	14.3	40.4	53.2	39.2	21.2	38.3
Barshi	One									96.7	52.5	40.4	71.7
	Three									70.1	24.0	20.6	56.3
	Five									62.7	18.6	20.8	57.4
Bombay	One					96.8	87.9	47.7	87.9	90.8	84.0	43.2	75.9
	Three					86.1	60.6	19.0	71.3	83.1	50.1	9.0	53.8
	Five					79.9	46.1	10.4	65.8	81.2	37.3	6.0	45.2
Madras	One	88.5	75.3	23.7	50.1	88.8	88.5	54.3	82.0	98.1	89.0	50.1	88.2
	Three	66.9	48.9	16.7	34.6	79.9	64.1	32.4	57.2	86.1	69.2	26.0	74.3
	Five	59.5	37.4	17.7	18.3	58.2	54.4	22.9	47.0	74.1	59.5	14.1	62.7
Rizal	One					97.3	88.0	32.2	82.1	89.2	66.7	49.6	63.9
	Three					95.3	51.5	6.6	64.3	81.3	23.6	17.3	43.8
	Five					83.5	32.2	6.8	50.2	71.4	12.3	18.2	34.5
Chiang Mai	One	82.2	46.9	43.9	62.3	100.3	92.2	60.8	50.5	99.2	92.0	71.4	35.4
	Three	52.2	20.6	0.0	53.6	98.0	69.1	35.1	0.0	93.3	74.0	43.7	14.1
	Five	50.7	14.6	0.0	43.5	95.0	58.0	23.8	0.0	91.7	68.1	37.1	10.8
Khon Kaen	One					90.8	92.2	82.0	91.8	97.2	85.5	62.2	82.5
	Three					93.9	63.9	41.4	80.3	84.7	63.5	29.8	66.6
	Five					79.4	48.8	25.5	62.6	77.4	52.6	26.4	61.1
US SEER White, 86–91	Five	84.7	55.5	39.0	45.8	96.7	76.4	20.2	55.6	91.7	51.8	8.6	63.1

The generally high survival reported from Chiang Mai province in Thailand may be due to a special interest in the local health services in the early detection and treatment of breast cancer.

The results indicate that early detection linked with appropriate treatment can improve survival from breast cancer in developing countries. Mammography-based screening is not feasible in many developing countries, in view of the high technology and costs involved; there is a need to evaluate more affordable, low-cost, low-technology screening methods such as physical breast examination. There is currently insufficient evidence either for or against teaching breast self-examination as a control measure for breast cancer. Any benefit from teaching breast self-examination remains largely unproved (Semiglazov et al., 1992; UK Trial of Early Detection of Breast Cancer Group, 1993; Thomas et al., 1997). However, a small increment in survival from breast cancer was noted around 1955 in Denmark following several campaigns promoting breast self-examination by the Danish Cancer Society during 1951–55 (Ewertz, 1993). Formulation of treatment policies within the health services based on current evidence from clinical research is likely to improve treatment outcomes for breast cancer at various stages, and may help to ensure appropriate utilization of the health service resources devoted to therapy.

Uterine cervix

Age-standardized relative survival reported from developing-country regions, with the exception of Shanghai and Chiang Mai, was lower than in Europe in 1978–85 and in the USA in 1967–73 and later. The proportion of localized cervical cancer in the developing-country regions (with the exception of Cuba) was considerably lower than in the USA for the period 1986–91 (Table 5), indicating that the poor survival in developing-country regions was, in part, due to advanced disease at presentation.

For localized cervical cancer, survival was lower in all developing-country registries (except Chiang Mai) than in the USA. However, five-year survival was above 80% in Bombay, above 70% in Cuba, Madras, Rizal and Khon Kaen and above 60% in the rural region of Barshi in India (Table 6). The outcome from regional disease in Madras, Chiang Mai and Khon Kaen was similar to that in the USA. These results indicate that good survival can be achieved in developing-country regions if early detection and adequate treatment can be ensured.

Radiotherapy and surgery produce similar results for early invasive cervical cancer, and intracavitary radiotherapy, with or without external radiotherapy, is the treatment of choice in such lesions. More advanced lesions (stages II to IV) are treated with a combination of external radiotherapy and intracavitary radiation.

Intracavitary radiation therapy, using radium or caesium sources, provides a high dose near the tumour where radiation is desired, and the radiation dose rapidly diminishes in regions outside the tumour. Survival rates are the same with both manual and remote afterloading intracavitary methods, though the latter method minimizes the exposure to radiation of health personnel. Many different types of equipment are available for delivery of external-beam radiotherapy. The high-energy era began in 1956 with the development of cobalt 60 teletherapy machines. Today, linear accelerators provide a wide range of high-energy photons with a buildup of energies 3–4 cm beneath the skin, whereas the maximum buildup for cobalt 60 and 4 MeV beams is less than 1 cm below the skin. Though the skin-sparing effect is desirable, there is little evidence to suggest that survival within stage has been greatly improved by the increasing use of linear accelerators for external radiation, rather than cobalt machines (Pontén et al., 1995). Cobalt machines are much less costly, and easier to operate and maintain in developing countries, than linear accelerators.

The health services in the registry regions studied are mostly equipped with cobalt 60 teletherapy machines and use both manual and remote afterloading intracavitary therapy with either radium or caesium sources. Radiotherapy techniques and dosage for cervical cancer are highly standardized, which has probably contributed to the reasonable results obtained in most registry regions.

Cervical cancer is the most common cancer among women in developing countries (Parkin et al., 1993). Though incidence rates are either stable or slowly declining in many countries (Coleman et al., 1993), it is still a major cause of death in young women in developing countries (Pisani et al., 1993). Potential gains provided by early detection and treatment are thus important from the point of view of short-term control measures, but prevention should be the goal for long-term control.

Organized cervical cytology screening has been shown to be effective in reducing mortality from cervical cancer (Hakama et al., 1986) but such programmes are not possible in developing countries owing to technical and fiscal constraints (Sankaranarayanan & Pisani, 1997). The efficacy of alternative low-technology, early detection approaches for either prevention or early detection have yet to be demonstrated. Unaided visual inspection, widely recommended as an early detection screening procedure a few years ago (Stjernsward et al., 1987), performs poorly in detecting cervical lesions, and is unlikely to be cost-effective (Sankaranarayanan et al., 1997). Some recent studies indicate that visual inspection with acetic acid (VIA) is a promising test for early detection of cervix cancer and its precursors (Sankaranarayanan et al., 1998a; 1998b).

The investigators at the Barshi registry have demonstrated that health education to increase people's awareness of risk factors, symptoms, signs and treatment of cervical cancer, linked with case-finding and therapy, improves detection, compliance with therapy and survival from cervical cancer (Jayant et al., 1995; see Chapter 10). The improvement in outcome from cervical cancer in Sweden before the introduction of widespread cervical cancer screening in that country provides further observational evidence of the effectiveness of increased awareness linked with facilities for diagnosis and treatment in the control of cervical cancer (Pontén et al., 1995).

Corpus uteri

The incidence of this cancer in developing countries is low in comparison with the USA and Europe. The age-standardized relative survival from cancer of the corpus uteri in the developing-country registries was lower than that in the USA for the periods 1967–73, 1974–86 and 1986–91. The results from all registries, with the exception of Shanghai, were low compared with survival rates in Europe. This cancer, with its characteristic symptoms of menorrhagia or postmenopausal bleeding, particularly in obese women with diabetes or hypertension, arouses clinical suspicion and is thus more likely to be diagnosed early. Surgery is the mainstay of treatment: radiotherapy is useful for inoperable cases and for reducing local recurrences in patients with myometrial invasion, poorly differentiated tumours and capillary-lymphatic space invasion. The comparatively high survival in registries with data for this cancer indicate the potential benefits of early diagnosis and treatment by local health services.

Ovary

Age-standardized relative survival rates from Khon Kaen, Chiang Mai and Cuba were comparable with those in the USA for the period 1967–73, while the rate from Shanghai resembled that in the USA for the period 1974–86. Results from these developing-country registries compared favourably with survival

in Europe. Improvement in survival in the USA has been attributed both to early diagnosis and to increasing use of cytoreductive surgery and systemic chemotherapy combinations in treatment in moderately advanced lesions, particularly cisplatin/carboplatin based chemotherapy.

Ovarian cancer has the highest case-fatality rate of all the gynaecological cancers. Epithelial malignancies account for 85–90% of all ovarian cancers. More than three-quarters of ovarian cancers are advanced by the time they are diagnosed. The lack of specific symptoms and signs of early ovarian cancer precludes the possibility of early detection by clinical suspicion. The recent introduction of transvaginal ultrasonography and testing for CA 125 have opened up the possibility of diagnosing asymptomatic ovarian cancers. However, there is, as yet, no evidence that these techniques can be used effectively for screening to reduce mortality from ovarian cancer (NIH Consensus Development Panel on Ovarian Cancer, 1995). While surgery alone is adequate in very early ovarian cancers, treatment of moderately advanced and advanced lesions involves cytoreductive and debulking surgery and appropriate chemotherapy and, less frequently, radiotherapy.

Prostate

Age-standardized relative survival from prostate cancer in developing-country registries was low compared with that for the USA for the periods 1967–73, 1974–86 and 1986–91 (Table 4). The increments in survival in the US populations over time seems to be due to the increasing use of digital examination procedures, pathological examination of tissue removed during surgery for benign prostate hypertrophy, imaging methods and testing for prostate-specific antigen (PSA). These procedures lead to the detection of an increasing number of clinically insignificant lesions, many of which would have remained subclinical during the patient's lifetime if not actively sought. The result is a rapidly increasing 'incidence' of prostate cancer, with correspondingly large gains in survival, but with no accompanying change in mortality (Smart, 1997; Brawley, 1997).

Progress in the treatment of prostate cancer is limited to refinements in surgical and radiotherapy techniques for localized cancers and less toxic hormonal therapy with leuprolide or flutamide for advanced patients. In spite of the advances in the treatment of localized cancers, the 'wait and treat' policy still remains a valid option for localized prostate cancer patients. Very little difference in outcome is observed from the different types of hormonal therapy for advanced prostate cancer.

Survival in developing-country regions resembles the survival achieved in patients with nonlocalized cancer in the USA (Miller *et al.*, 1993). This is perhaps not surprising. Prostate cancer is an uncommon cancer in Asia, and medical personnel are less likely to look for it than those in developed countries. The patient is thus likely to present at a relatively late stage of the disease.

Testis

Age-standardized relative survival from the three developing-country registries providing data for this cancer was lower than those from the USA and Europe. Survival in Shanghai was similar to survival in the USA in 1967–73.

Approximately 95% of malignant tumours of the testis are germ-cell tumours. There has been a dramatic improvement in outcome from testicular germ-cell tumours over the last three decades, owing to substantial progress in management (cisplatin-containing chemotherapy regimens; improved surgical and radiotherapy techniques; better salvage of patients failing initial treatment and patients with advanced disease) and follow-up care (radioim-munoassay for testing human *B* fraction of chorionic gonadotrophin (HCG) and alpha-fetoprotein (AFP); salvage therapies for relapses) (Bosl & Mortzer, 1997). The improved survival has been followed by dramatic decreases in mortality. These advances in therapy have yet to become widespread in developing countries owing to technical and fiscal constraints: the survival differential seems to be predominantly due to this phenomenon.

Urinary bladder

The survival rates reported from the developing-country registries were lower than those from the USA. This poor survival seems to be due to advanced disease at presentation, as well as possible inadequacies of treatment. In particular, there may be difficulties in providing the optimum combination of surgery and radiotherapy in developing countries. The improvement in survival in the USA has been attributed to improvements in both detection and treatment (Miller *et al.*, 1993). Interpretation of survival data from bladder cancers should also take into account the pathological entities (carcinoma/papilloma) included in the analysis.

Hodgkin's disease

Age-standardized relative survival rates from developing-country registries were distinctly lower than those from the USA and Europe. The improvement in survival in the USA over the last three decades has been attributed to advances in treatment due to a better understanding of the natural history of the disease, particularly progress in radiotherapy for early disease, and the availability of effective combination chemotherapy to control advanced disease and salvage failures of initial treatment.

Among the histological subtypes, lymphocytic predominance and nodular sclerosis are associated with good prognosis, while mixed cellularity and lymphocyte depletion are associated with poor outcome. Mixed cellularity is the predominant histological type in Asian populations, as opposed to nodular sclerosis in the USA and Europe (Parkin *et al.*, 1997). Mixed cellularity and lymphocyte depletion subtypes often present with disease on both sides of diaphragm and B symptoms. Differences in the histological spectrum of disease should be taken into account when interpreting survival in different populations.

Non-Hodgkin lymphoma

Survival from non-Hodgkin lymphoma in the developing-country registries was considerably lower than in the USA, where an improvement in survival has been observed over the last three decades, particularly for the intermediate-grade and high-grade histological subtypes, owing to advances in diagnostic classification and treatment. Among the SEER white patients, 25.8%, 50.0% and 6.4%, respectively, were low-grade, intermediate-grade and high-grade histological subtypes; the rest were miscellaneous histological subtypes (Greiner *et al.*, 1995).

While radiotherapy is the treatment of choice for localized forms of low-grade lymphomas, single-agent or combination chemotherapy is the treatment of choice for advanced low-grade subtypes. Most intermediate-grade and almost all high-grade histological subtypes are treated with combination chemotherapy. There have been considerable advances in optimizing treatment regimens in terms of combinations of cytotoxic drugs, their dosage and duration of administration. These advances have generally resulted in the improvement of survival from intermediate-grade and high-grade disease, but not low-grade disease. It is essential to increase awareness of these advances by establishing special guidelines if equivalent improvements in survival are to be achieved in developing countries.

Leukaemia

Survival from leukaemias in the developing-country regions is poor and lower than that observed in the USA and Europe. The improvement

Table 7. Observed survival by clinical extent of disease for selected cancers

Registry	Years survived	Lip				Tongue				Oral cavity			
		L	R	D	U	L	R	D	U	L	R	D	U
Cuba	One					62.2	60.2	57.1	30.4	79.4	56.8	66.7	66.0
	Three					29.3	26.1	28.6	11.3	54.6	25.0	66.7	43.4
	Five					26.8	18.9	14.3	9.7	47.8	22.0	66.7	37.7
Madras	One	62.5	68.0	50.0	100.0	81.7	66.4	40.0	69.0	84.9	75.8	52.0	74.6
	Three	50.0	50.3	0.0	100.0	54.9	36.5	6.7	27.0	55.4	44.9	20.0	31.0
	Five	50.0	32.0	0.0	100.0	44.3	23.0	6.7	13.5	34.4	30.3	12.0	18.4
Chiang Mai	One	87.5	52.6	–	–	89.5	45.3	0.0	0.0	60.0	36.6	0.0	66.7
	Three	74.8	42.1	–	–	62.2	25.2	0.0	0.0	45.0	17.1	0.0	0.0
	Five	67.3	42.1	–	–	62.2	23.4	0.0	0.0	38.6	11.1	0.0	66.7

Registry	Years survived	Colon				Rectum				Colorectum			
		L	R	D	U	L	R	D	U	L	R	D	U
Cuba	One	72.4	60.5	23.9	23.3	79.8	62.2	28.0	35.5	75.8	61.2	25.2	27.4
	Three	59.4	42.0	9.5	16.5	56.4	34.6	12.7	20.7	58.0	39.0	10.6	17.9
	Five	52.4	33.0	8.4	12.1	46.2	28.7	9.6	18.4	49.6	31.3	8.8	14.2
Chiang Mai	One	89.2	81.5	16.9	66.7	78.9	67.3	24.1	79.7	84.2	74.0	19.4	75.8
	Three	83.4	57.7	6.3	50.0	68.4	32.4	5.6	42.3	76.0	44.1	6.1	44.2
	Five	74.3	51.2	4.1	50.0	68.4	24.4	1.9	21.1	72.2	36.6	3.2	27.6

Registry	Years survived	Larynx				Breast				Cervix			
		L	R	D	U	L	R	D	U	L	R	D	U
Cuba	One					92.5	83.7	43.6	68.2	88.8	69.6	31.1	63.8
	Three					80.3	60.6	22.3	53.9	75.0	40.5	27.6	45.5
	Five					70.9	46.4	20.4	44.1	70.9	34.2	24.2	41.0
Bangalore	One					90.3	83.7	49.7	76.2	84.8	77.4	47.6	70.8
	Three					68.9	52.6	21.9	53.1	61.1	49.9	28.2	49.0
	Five					56.9	37.6	13.0	37.6	49.5	36.5	19.3	35.2
Barshi	One									95.7	51.6	40.0	71.1
	Three									68.1	22.8	20.0	54.8
	Five									59.6	17.1	20.0	54.8
Bombay	One					95.5	86.7	46.8	86.3	90.0	83.0	42.6	74.9
	Three					82.5	58.2	18.0	67.3	80.8	48.2	8.6	51.5
	Five					74.4	43.0	9.5	59.5	77.4	35.0	5.6	41.8
Madras	One	86.0	73.4	23.1	48.8	87.3	87.1	53.5	81.0	97.1	87.9	49.2	87.3
	Three	61.2	45.1	15.4	32.0	75.9	61.2	30.9	55.1	83.6	66.6	24.6	72.0
	Five	51.2	32.6	15.4	16.0	53.5	50.3	21.2	44.1	70.4	55.8	12.8	59.4
Rizal	One					95.8	86.4	31.8	80.6	88.4	65.7	48.6	62.8
	Three					91.0	48.6	6.4	60.6	79.1	22.4	16.2	41.4
	Five					77.2	29.2	6.4	45.3	67.8	11.2	16.2	31.1
Chiang Mai	One	79.5	45.0	41.7	60.0	99.6	90.9	59.5	50.0	98.7	91.0	70.5	35.1
	Three	47.3	18.1	0.0	48.0	95.7	66.2	33.0	0.0	91.8	71.7	41.9	13.6
	Five	42.1	11.7	0.0	36.0	90.9	53.8	21.5	0.0	89.0	64.5	34.5	10.2
Khon Kaen	One					90.0	91.1	81.3	91.2	96.7	84.6	61.5	81.7
	Three					90.0	61.7	40.3	78.7	83.3	61.6	28.5	64.7
	Five					75.0	46.1	24.4	60.3	74.9	49.8	24.1	57.9

in survival from leukaemia in the USA is mostly a reflection of the dramatic increase in survival from acute lymphatic leukaemia, particularly in children, owing to advances in combination chemotherapy, prophylactic treatment of sanctuary sites and successful salvage of initial treatment failures and relapses. Survival from acute myeloid leukaemia remains poor, in spite of advances in combination chemotherapy and bone marrow transplantation. There has been no significant increase in survival from chronic leukaemias in the past three decades.

The comparative results given here include all leukaemias. There are proportionately more myeloid leukaemias in developing countries (Parkin et al., 1997) both in children and in adults, and this may, in part, explain the less satisfactory results in developing countries. The poorer survival in developing countries also stems from the inability to provide optimum treatment and supportive care to patients with acute lymphatic leukaemia, because of limited facilities and the high costs associated with such therapies. The general improvement in survival and mortality from paediatric neoplasms is the outcome of improved disease classifications, definition of risk groups and optimization and advances in therapy. The role of paediatric oncology as a speciality in implementing such advances in routine health services needs to be underlined if the improvements in survival from acute lymphatic leukaemia and other childhood neoplasms are to be translated to developing countries. Rational allocation of resources in health services towards treatment policies proven to be efficacious in improving survival and mortality is an important public health approach for improving outcomes from these neoplasms.

Conclusions

Fig. 1 summarizes the three broad categories of results obtained from the comparison of survival in developed and developing-country registries (Sankaranarayanan et al., 1996). The magnitude of differences in survival for patients with certain common cancers between the developing and developed countries are plotted against an axis representing the three major elements of cancer control, namely primary prevention, early detection and treatment. For tumours associated with poor prognosis, such as oesophagus, liver, lung and pancreas, the variation in survival rates and the differences observed between developed and developing-country regions were minimal. There are no effective screening tests or early detection

procedures for these cancers, and treatment is generally not effective, even when they are detected in early stages. Primary prevention is therefore the only available strategy to reduce mortality from these cancers.

The wide variation in survival observed in these registries cannot be entirely due to differences in the mechanisms and efficiency of data collection. Factors such as clinical extent of disease at presentation, efficiency and accessibility of the cancer-related health services available, treatment received, follow-up care and patient-related factors such as socioeconomic status, attitudes and compliance with treatment and aftercare are likely to be responsible for at least some of the observed differences. These factors may be particularly important for those cancer sites for which the outcome is influenced by treatment related to the clinical stage of the cancer at diagnosis.

There were greater differences in survival for cancer sites such as head and neck, large bowel, breast, melanoma, cervix, ovary and urinary bladder, which have a moderate-to-good prognosis if detected early and treated appropriately. The differences in survival are likely to be reduced by linking early detection with adequate treatment facilities. Some of these cancers are, of course, also amenable to primary prevention. Mortality from cervical cancer could be reduced by organized screening with cervical cytology.

The differences in survival between the developed and developing-country registries were even more striking for cancer sites such as testis, leukaemia and lymphoma, in which improved multimodality treatment has increased long-term survival. With appropriate logistics, the available resources can be used to deliver such treatment in developing countries, which is likely to reduce the differences observed in survival. The adoption of WHO recommendations on essential drugs for cancer chemotherapy should result in improved outcome from these cancers in low-resource settings (WHO, 1994).

The pattern emerging from comparison of survival rates in different countries calls for rational and balanced investment in a range of cancer control activities, covering the areas of primary prevention, screening, early detection, therapy, aftercare and palliative care.

The survival estimates reported from the 10 developing-country registries in this book probably include some of the best survival results currently possible in the third world, as the countries concerned are among those developing most rapidly, with better

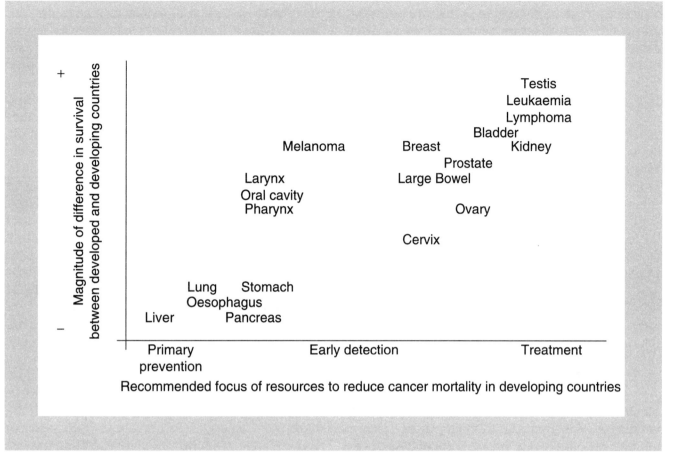

Figure 1. Relationship between differences in survival between developed and developing countries and prospects for reducing cancer mortality in developing countries

organized health care services and cancer control programmes than a number of other developing countries (in sub-Saharan Africa, for example). It is also true that cancer registries tend to be established in areas with at least basic cancer treatment facilities. It is quite likely that survival prospects from cancer are generally much lower than the estimates in this book in a number of developing countries from which data are not currently available.

Although the descriptive data available gives some indication of how cancer control measures should be developed, more information is required to identify the most suitable policies for particular local situations. From this angle, four types of approaches need to be emphasized.

(1) Population-based cancer registries covering sample populations are needed in many developing countries. These should operate within the framework of national cancer control programmes. The registries can provide the information base to target, monitor and evaluate the programme inputs. The emphasis here should be on getting good

information from selected populations within the country, rather than from the entire national population. A clear commitment from national governments and/or national medical research organizations to initiate and sustain population-based cancer registries is required. Guidelines for establishing and maintaining cancer registries have been well documented (Jensen *et al.*, 1991). The input by the cancer registries cited in this volume to their national cancer control programmes is commendable.

(2) 'High-resolution studies' of diagnosis, treatment and outcome for samples of patients from population-based cancer registries in developing countries are needed to identify the reasons for poor survival in some subgroups of developing-country populations. This will help to improve outcomes in such groups.

(3) Community-based intervention trials are required to identify effective low-technology, low-cost screening tests and prevention measures for

early diagnosis and prevention of invasive cancer in cancer sites such as breast, cervix, oral cavity, liver, oesophagus, and stomach, which are common in many developing-country regions. Fiscal and technical constraints and competing needs will not allow implementation of high-technology screening methods and interventions, as has been done in the developed countries. Operational research to implement proven interventions and treatments in local health services is also important, and should be promoted by the health services. A clear commitment from funding bodies and bilateral donor agencies to support research initiatives along the above lines will help to ensure the rational development of public health policies that will have a long-term beneficial impact on cancer control.

(4) Balanced investment in the development of adequate diagnostic and treatment facilities within the health services is important. Here the emphasis should be on developing all basic and essential services to diagnose and treat the common cancers seen in the region concerned. The improvement in survival due to treatment has been followed by impressive reductions in mortality from certain cancers. The improved therapies should be made available to the health services of developing countries by formulating guidelines for treatment, based on the results of clinical research and their applications elsewhere, if results comparable with those in the developed countries are to be achieved and the limited resources available for cancer care are to be judiciously used.

Common diagnostic methods involving plain and contrast X-rays, ultrasonography, biochemistry, endoscopy and cytology/pathology should be developed at the secondary care level. Investment in sophisticated diagnostic procedures (e.g. CT scanning, nuclear imaging, tumour markers) should be restricted to the tertiary care level.

A certain level of surgical services for common cancers needs to be developed at the secondary care level. However, facilities for specialized surgical care and more sophisticated procedures should be restricted to tertiary care services, in order to guarantee the standard and quality of care.

Services such as paediatric oncology, chemotherapy and radiotherapy should still be concentrated at the tertiary care level. The planning and delivery of radiotherapy is a complex procedure, which involves close cooperation among radiotherapists, physicists and technicians. Radiotherapy infrastructure is costly and requires a reasonably high level of technical sophistication. Hence this service should usually be available only in the tertiary medical care facilities, if health care resources are scarce. For most developing countries, cobalt 60 machines should be used rather than linear accelerators, in order to ensure maximum utility and cost-effectiveness. Similarly, brachytherapy services should use low dose-rate manual or remote afterloading for the cervix, and manual afterloading for head and neck sites. Very careful planning is required when setting up radiotherapy facilities in order to avoid an unnecessary drain on resources. Though WHO recommends one external radiotherapy machine per one million population, this could be easily stretched to one machine per 2–3 million population if prudent operational and fractionation practices are pursued for both radical and palliative therapies.

Though a number of chemotherapy drugs are currently available, WHO recommends 14 drugs as essential for treating the 10 most common cancers, and an additional nine agents for the satisfactory management of childhood cancers (WHO, 1994). Prudent chemotherapy policies are important if the maximum benefit is to be gained from systemic therapy approaches, while avoiding an unnecessary drain on scarce resources. Chemotherapy services should be developed and provided within tertiary care services. Limiting state subsidies for chemotherapy in sites where it is of unproved value, and devoting these resources instead to treatment in sites where it is of proven value, is a major policy change that health services should be encouraged to pursue.

A greater or lesser degree of supportive care, designed to alleviate both the psychological and the physical impact of cancer, should be developed at all levels of health care, including home-based care. Palliative care, aimed at the relief of the distressing symptoms of advanced incurable cancer, should also be available at all levels of health care. Guiding principles for the organization of palliative care have been well documented by WHO (WHO, 1996).

Consensus treatment protocols, appropriate for the technological and financial resources of the health service concerned, should be developed and implemented. Development of appropriate referral policies linking primary care (where clinical suspicion quite often initiates the referral process) with secondary and tertiary care facilities will help to ensure the optimum utilization of limited cancer care services within the health care system. Guiding principles have been drawn up for developing cancer health services as outlined above (WHO, 1995). The association between socioeconomic status and cancer survival has been well documented (Kogevinas *et al.*, 1991; Tomatis, 1995; Mackillop *et al.*, 1997). Health care systems designed, developed and motivated to provide equitable and ready access to equivalent standards of care in developing countries may be successful in narrowing the differences between developed and developing countries and between rich and poor communities within countries.

Acknowledgements

The authors gratefully acknowledge the support of the Finnish Cancer Society (for survival studies in India); the International Union Against Cancer (for training of participating registry staff in survival analysis through International Cancer Research Technology Transfer (ICRETT) fellowship awards); and the Association for International Cancer Research (AICR), St. Andrews, UK and the Gunnar Nielson Cancer Trust Fund, UK (for centralized analysis of data and the publication of this book).

References

Axtell, L.M., Asire, A.J., Myers, M.H. (1976) *Cancer Patient Survival; Report No. 5.* (DHEW Publication No. (NIH) 77-992). Bethesda, MD, National Cancer Institute

Berrino, F., Sant, M., Verdecchia, A., Capocaccia, R., Hakulinen, T. & Estève, J., eds. (1995) *Survival of Cancer Patients in Europe: the EUROCARE Study* (IARC Scientific Publications No. 132). Lyon, International Agency for Research on Cancer

Berwick, M., Dubin, N., Luo S.-T. & Flannery, J. (1994) No improvement in survival from malignant melanoma diagnosed from 1973 to 1984. *Int. J. Epidemiol.*, **23**, 673–681

Bonnadonna, G., Brusamolino, E., Valagussa, P., Rossi, A., Bruganatelli, L., Brambilla, C., De Lena, M., Tancini, G., Bajetta, E., Musumeci, R. & Veronesi, U. (1976) Combination chemotherapy as an adjuvant treatment in operable breast cancer. *N. Engl. J. Med.*, **294**, 405–410

Bosl, G.J. & Mortzer, R.J. (1997) Testicular germ cell tumour. *N. Engl. J. Med.*, **337**, 242–253

Brawley, O.W. (1997) Prostate carcinoma incidence and patient mortality. *Cancer*, **80**, 1857–1863

Chang, M.H., Chen, C.J., Lai, M.S., Hsu, H.M., Wu, T.C., Kong, M.S., Liang, D.C., Shau, W.Y. & Chen, D.S. (1997) Universal hepatitis B vaccination in Taiwan and the incidence of hepatocellular carcinoma in children. Taiwan Childhood Hepatoma Study Group. *N. Engl. J. Med.*, **336**, 1855–1859

Chu, K.C., Tarone, R.E., Chow, W-C., Hankey, B.F. & Ries, L.A.G. (1994) Temporal patterns in colorectal cancer incidence, survival, and mortality from 1950 through 1990. *J. Natl. Cancer Inst.*, **86**, 997–1006

Coleman, M.P., Estève, J., Damiecki, P., Arslan, A. & Renard, H. (1993) *Trends in Cancer Incidence and Mortality* (IARC Scientific Publications No. 121). Lyon, International Agency for Research on Cancer

Correa, P. & Chen, V.W. (1994) Gastric cancer. *Cancer Surveys*, **19/20**, 55–76

Early Breast Cancer Trialists' Collaborative Group (1992) Systemic treatment of early breast cancer by hormonal, cytotoxic, or immune therapy. *Lancet*, **339**, 1–15, 71–85

Early Breast Cancer Trialists' Collaborative Group (1995) Effects of radiotherapy and surgery in early breast cancer. An overview of the randomized trials. *N. Engl. J. Med.*, **333**, 1444–1455

Ewertz, M. (1993) Breast. *APMIS Suppl.*, **33**, 99–106

Fernandez Garrote, L., Sankaranarayanan, R., Lence Anta, J.J., Rodriguez Salva, A. & Parkin, D.M. (1995) An evaluation of the oral cancer control program in Cuba. *Epidemiology*, **6**, 428–431

Garne, J.P., Aspegren, K., Balldin, G. & Ranstam, J. (1997) Increasing incidence of and declining mortality from breast carcinoma. *Cancer*, **79**, 69–74

Greiner, T.C., Medeiros, L.J. & Jaffe, E.S. (1995) Non-Hodgkin's lymphoma. *Cancer*, **75** (Supplement 1), 370–380

Gupta, P.C., Mehta, F.S., Pindborg, J.J., Aghi, M.B., Bhonsle, R.B., Daftary, D.K., Murti, P.R. & Shah, H.T. (1986) Intervention study for primary prevention of oral cancer among 36 000 Indian tobacco users. *Lancet*, **1**, 1235–1239

Gupta, P.C., Mehta, F.S., Pindborg, J.J., Bhonsle, R.B., Murti, P.R., Daftary, D.K. & Aghi, M.B. (1992) Primary prevention trial of oral cancer in India: a 10 year follow-up study. *J. Oral Pathol. Med.*, **21**, 433–439

Hakama, M., Miller, A.B. & Day, N.E. (1986) *Screening for Cancer of the Uterine Cervix* (IARC Scientific Publications No. 76). Lyon, International Agency for Research on Cancer

IARC (1993) *IARC Monographs on the Evaluation of Carcinogenic Risks to Humans.* Vol. 56, *Some Naturally Occurring Substances: Food Items and Constituents, Heterocyclic Aromatic Amines and Mycotoxins.* Lyon, International Agency for Research on Cancer

IARC (1994a) *IARC Monographs on the Evaluation of Carcinogenic Risks to Humans,* Vol. 59, *Hepatitis Viruses.* Lyon, International Agency for Research on Cancer

IARC (1994b) *IARC Monographs on the Evaluation of Carcinogenic Risks to Humans,* Vol. 61, *Schistosomes, Liver Flukes and* Helicobacter pylori. Lyon, International Agency for Research on Cancer

Jayant, K., Rao, R.S., Nene, B.M. & Dale, P.S. (1995) Improved stage at diagnosis of cervical cancer with increased cancer awareness in a rural Indian population. *Int. J. Cancer*, **63**, 161–163

Jensen, O.M., Parkin, D.M., MacLennan, R., Muir, C.S. & Skeet, R.G. (1991) *Cancer Registration: Principles and Methods* (IARC Scientific Publications No. 95). Lyon, International Agency for Research on Cancer

Kogevinas, M., Marmot, M.G., Fox, A.J. & Goldblatt, P.O. (1991) Socio-economic differences in cancer survival. *J. Epidemiol. Community Health*, **45**, 216–219

Kosary, C.L., Ries, L.A.G., Miller, B.A., Hankey, B.F., Harras, A. & Edwards, B.K., eds. (1995) *SEER Cancer Statistics Review, 1973-1992: Tables and Graphs* (NIH Publication No. 96-2789). Bethesda, MD, National Cancer Institute

Krook, J.E., Moertel, C.G., Gunderson, L.L., Wieand, H.S., Collins, R.T., Beart, R.W., Kubista, T.P., Poon, M.A., Meyers, W.C., Mailliard, J.A., Twito, D.I., Morton, R.F., Veeder, M.H., Witzig, Cha, S. & Vidhyarthi, S.C. (1991) Effective surgical adjuvant therapy for high-risk rectal carcinoma. *N. Engl. J. Med.*, **324**, 709–715

Mackillop, W.J., Zhang-Solomons, J., Groome, P.A., Paszat, L. & Holowaty, E. (1997) Socioeconomic status and cancer survival in Ontario. *J. Clin. Oncology*, **15**, 1680–1689

Mathew, B., Sankaranarayanan, R., Sunilkumar, K., Kuruvila, B., Pisani, P. & Krishnan Nair, M. (1997) Reproducibility and validity of oral visual inspection by trained health workers in the detection of oral cancer and precancer. *Br. J. Cancer*, **76**, 390–394

Mathew, B., Sankaranarayanan, R., Binu, J., Gigi, T., Pisani, P., Thara, S., Pandey, M., Ramadas, K., Elizabeth, A., Iqbal, A., Najeeb, S., Parkin, D.M. & Krishnan Nair, M. (1999), Preliminary results from an oral cancer screening intervention trial in Kerala, India. In: Varma, A.K., (ed.), *Oral Oncology*, Vol. V, New Delhi, Macmillan India (in press)

Miller, B.A., Ries, L.A.G., Hankey, B.F., Kosary, C.L., Harras, A., Devesa, S.S. & Edwards, B.K., eds. (1993) *SEER Cancer Statistics Review: 1973-1990* (NIH Publication No. 93-2789), Bethesda, MD, National Cancer Institute

Moertel, C.G., Fleming, T.R., Macdonald, J.S., Haller, D.G., Laurie, J.A., Goodman, P.J., Ungerleider, J.S., Emerson, W.A., Tormey, D.C., Glick, J.H., Veeder, M.H. & Mailliard, J.A. (1990) Levamisole and fluorouracil for adjuvant therapy of resected colon carcinoma. *N. Engl. J. Med.*, **322**, 352–358

Nab, H.W., Hop, W.C.J., Crommelin, M.A., Kluck, H.M., van der Heijden, L.H. & Coebergh, J.W.W. (1994a) Changes in long term prognosis for breast cancer in a Dutch cancer registry. *Br. Med. J.*, **309**, 83–86

Nab, H.W., Hop, W.C.J., Crommelin, M.A., Kluck, H.M. & Coebergh, J.W.W. (1994b) Improved prognosis in breast cancer since 1970 in south-east Netherlands. *Br. J. Cancer*, **70**, 285–288

NIH Consensus Development Panel on Ovarian Cancer (1995) Ovarian cancer: screening, treatment and follow-up. *J. Am. Med. Ass.*, **273**, 491–497

Olivotto, I.A., Badjik, C.D., Plenderleith, I.H., Coppin, C., Gelmon, K.A., Jackson, S.M., Ragaz, J., Wilson, K.S. & Worth, A. (1994) Adjuvant systemic therapy and survival after breast cancer. *N. Engl. J. Med.*, **330**, 805–810

Parkin, D.M. & Pisani, P. (1996) Screening for lung cancer. In: Miller, A.B., ed., *Advances in Cancer Screening*. Boston, Kluwer Academic Publishers, pp. 121–128

Parkin, D.M. & Sankaranarayanan, R. (1994) Overview on small cell lung cancer in the third world: Industrialized countries, Third World, Eastern Europe. *Anticancer Res.*, **14**, 277–282

Parkin, D.M., Pisani, P. & Ferlay, J. (1993) Estimates of the world-wide incidence of eighteen major cancers in 1985. *Int. J. Cancer*, **54**, 594–606

Parkin, D.M., Whelan, S.L., Ferlay, J., Raymond L. & Young J., eds. (1997) *Cancer Incidence in Five Continents, Volume VII* (IARC Scientific Publications No. 143). Lyon, International Agency for Research on Cancer

Pisani, P. & Parkin, D.M. (1996) Screening for gastric cancer. In: Miller, A.B., ed., *Advances in Cancer Screening*. Boston, Kluwer Academic Publishers. pp. 113–120

Pisani, P., Parkin, D.M. & Ferlay, J. (1993) Estimates of the world-wide mortality from eighteen major cancers in 1985. Implications for prevention and projections of future burden. *Int. J. Cancer*, **55**, 891–903

Pontén, J., Adami, H.O., Bergström, R., Dillner, J., Friberg, J., Gustafsson, L., Miller, A.B., Parkin, D.M., Sparén, P. & Trichopoulos, D. (1995) Strategies for global control of cervical cancer. *Int. J. Cancer*, **60**, 1–26

Ries, L.A.G., Hankey, B.F., Edwards, B.K. (1990) *SEER Cancer Statistics Review, 1973-87* (NIH Publication No. 90-2789). Bethesda, MD, National Cancer Institute

Sankaranarayanan, R. (1997) Health care auxiliaries in the detection and prevention of oral cancer. *Oral Oncol. Eur. J. Cancer*, **33B**, 149–154

Sankaranarayanan, R. & Pisani, P. (1997) Prevention measures in the third world: are they practical? In: Franco, E. & Monsonego, J., eds., *New Developments in Cervical Cancer Screening and Prevention*. Oxford, Blackwell Science Publishers, pp. 70–83

Sankaranarayanan, R., Swaminathan, R. & Black, R.J. (for Study Group on Cancer Survival in Developing Countries) (1996) Global variations in cancer survival. *Cancer*, **78**, 2461–2464

Sankaranarayanan, R., Shyamalakumary, B., Wesley, R., Sreedevi Amma, N., Parkin, D.M. & Kristinan Nair M. (1998a) Visual inspection with acetic acid in the early detection of cervical cancers and precursors. *Int. J. Cancer*, (in press)

Sankaranarayanan, R., Wesley, R., Somanathan, T., Dhakad, N., Shyamalakumary, B., Sreedevi Amma, N., Parkin, D.M. & Krishnan Nair M. (1998b) Visual inspection of the uterine cervix after the application of acetic acid in the detection of cervical carcinoma and precursors. *Cancer,* **83**, 2150–2156

Sankaranarayanan, R., Syamalakumary, B., Wesley, R., Thara Somanathan, S., Chandralekha, B., Sreedevi Amma, N. & Parkin, D.M. (1997) Visual inspection as a screening test for cervical cancer control in developing countries. In: Franco, E. & Monsonego, J., eds., *New Developments in Cervical Cancer Screening and Prevention.* Oxford, Blackwell Science Publishers, pp. 411–421

Semiglazov, V.F., Moiseyenko, V.M., Bavli, J.L., Migmanova, N., Seleznyov, N.K., Popova, R.T., Ivanova, O.A., Orlov, A.A., Chagunava, O.A., Barash, N.J., Matitzin, A.N., Dyatchenko, O.T., Kozhevnikov, S.Y., Alexandrova, G.I., Sanchakova, A.V. & Musayev, B.T. (1992) The role of breast self-examination in early breast cancer detection: results of the 5-year USSR/WHO randomized study in Leningrad. *Eur. J. Epidemiol.,* **8**, 498–502

Smart, C.R. (1997) The results of prostate carcinoma screening in the U.S. as reflected in the Surveillance, Epidemiology, and End Results program. *Cancer,* **80**, 1835–1844

Stjernsward, J., Eddy, D., Luthra, U.K. & Stanley, K. (1987) Plotting a new course for cervical cancer screening in developing countries. *World Health Forum,* **8**, 42–45

Taira, K., Keiichi, M., Mitsuru, S., & Kazuo, O. (1993) Treatment results of gastric cancer patients: Japanese experience. In: Nishi, M., Ichikawa, H., Nakajima, T. & Tahara, E., eds., *Gastric Cancer.* Berlin, Springer-Verlag, pp. 319–330

Tanaka, H., Hiyama, T., Hanai, A. & Fujimoto, I. (1994) Interhospital differences in cancer survival: Magnitude and trend in 1975-1987 in Osaka, Japan. *Jpn. J. Cancer Res.,* **85**, 680–685

Thomas, D.B., Gao, D.L., Self, S.G., Allison, C.J., Tao, Y., Mahloch, J., Ray, R., Qin, Q., Presley, R. & Porter, P. (1997) Randomized trial for breast self-examination in Shanghai: methodology and preliminary results. *J. Natl. Cancer Inst.,* **89**, 355–365

Tomatis, L. (1995) Socioeconomic factors and human cancer. *Int. J. Cancer,* **62**, 121–125

UK Trial of Early Detection of Breast Cancer Group (1993) Breast cancer mortality after 10 years in the UK trial of early detection of breast cancer. *The Breast,* **2**, 13–20

WHO (1994) Essential drugs for cancer chemotherapy. *Bull. WHO,* **72**, 693–698

WHO (1995) *National Cancer Control Programmes: Policies and Managerial Guidelines.* Geneva, World Health Organization

WHO (1996) *Cancer Pain Relief: with a Guide to Opioid Availability,* second edition. Geneva, World Health Organization

Wiebelt, H. & Hakulinen, T. (1991) Do women survive cancer more frequently than men? *J. Natl. Cancer Inst.,* **83**, 579–580

Appendix

Relative survival from oral cavity cancer in developing countries

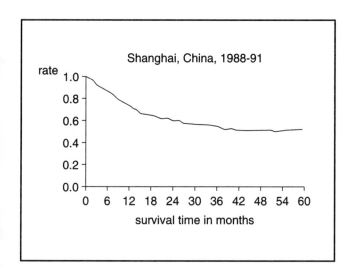

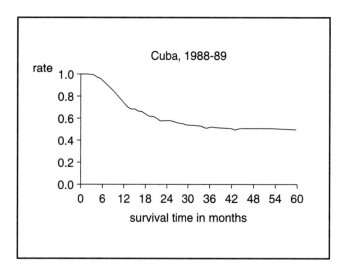

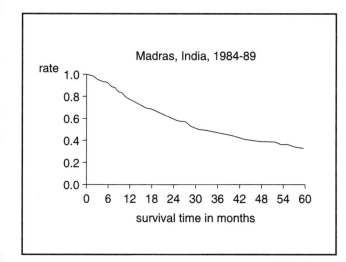

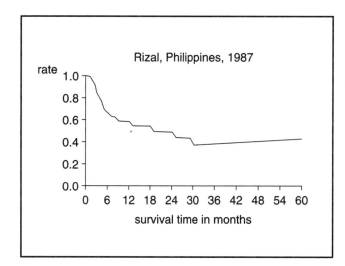

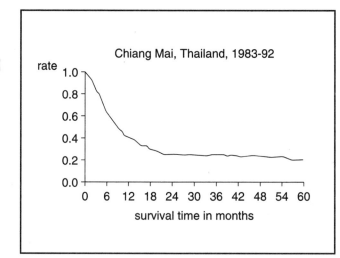

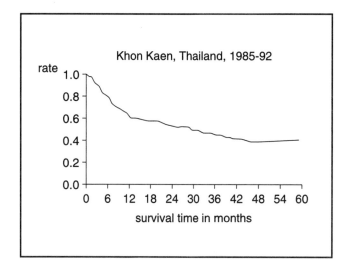

Relative survival from oesophageal cancer in developing countries

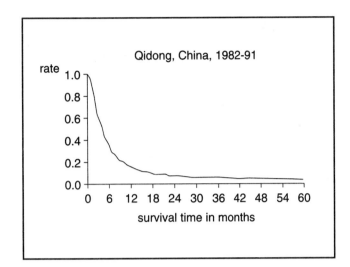

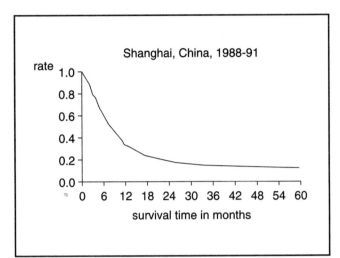

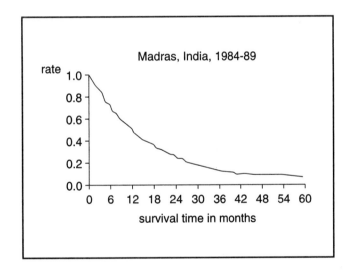

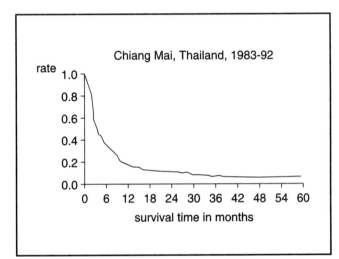

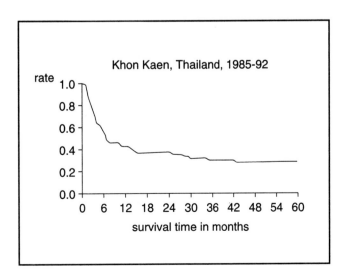

Relative survival from stomach cancer in developing countries

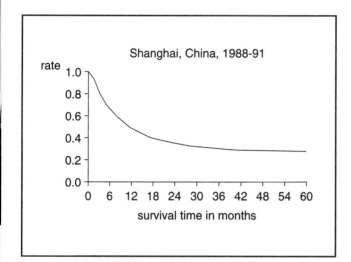

Shanghai, China, 1988-91

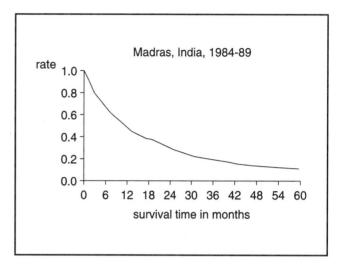

Madras, India, 1984-89

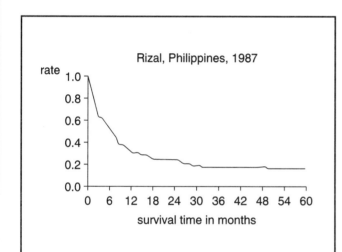

Rizal, Philippines, 1987

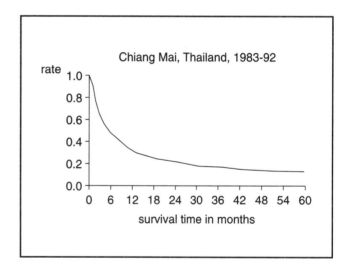

Chiang Mai, Thailand, 1983-92

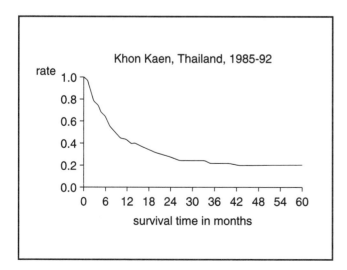

Khon Kaen, Thailand, 1985-92

Relative survival from colorectal cancer in developing countries

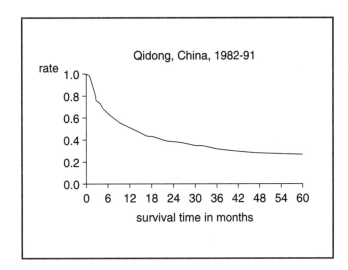

Qidong, China, 1982-91

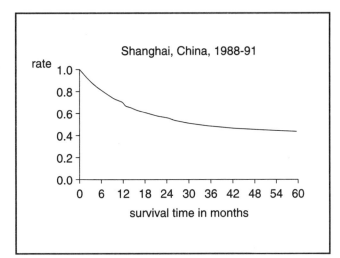

Shanghai, China, 1988-91

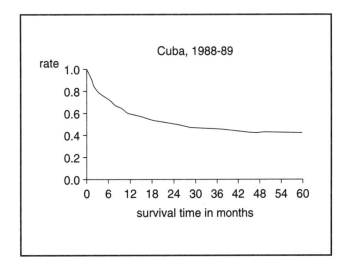

Cuba, 1988-89

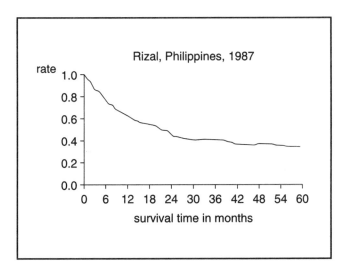

Rizal, Philippines, 1987

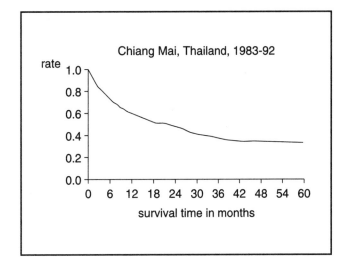

Chiang Mai, Thailand, 1983-92

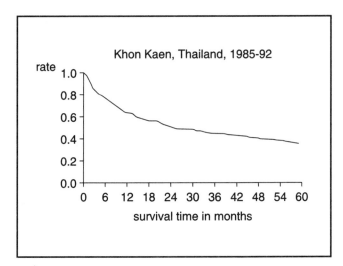

Khon Kaen, Thailand, 1985-92

Relative survival from liver cancer in developing countries

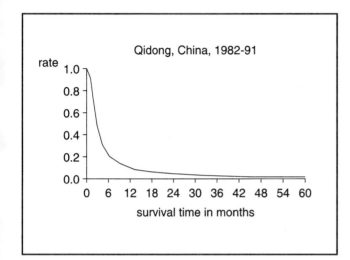

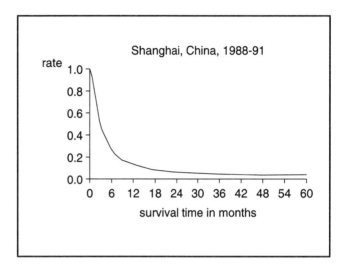

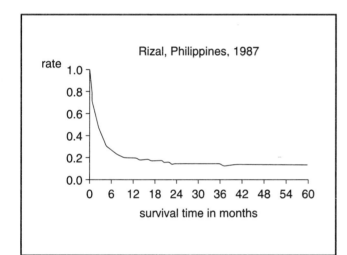

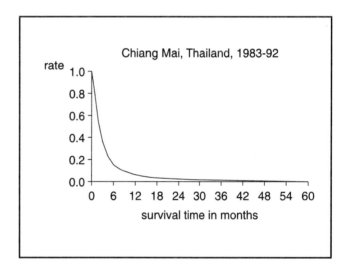

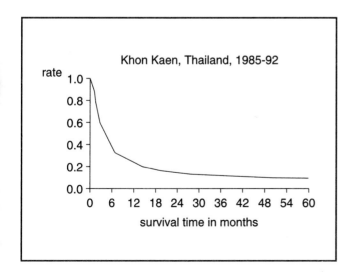

Relative survival from laryngeal cancer in developing countries

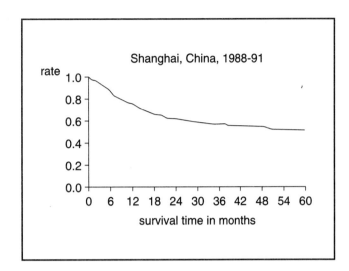

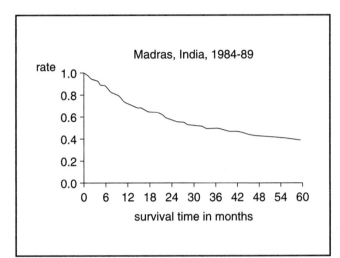

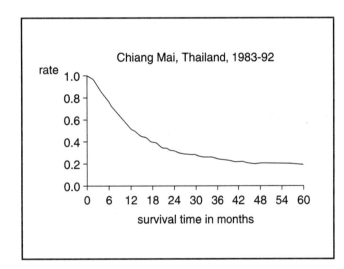

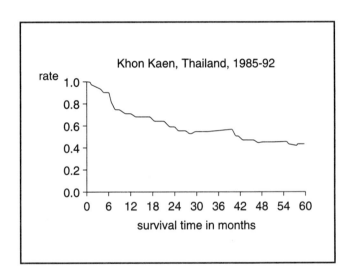

Relative survival from lung cancer in developing countries

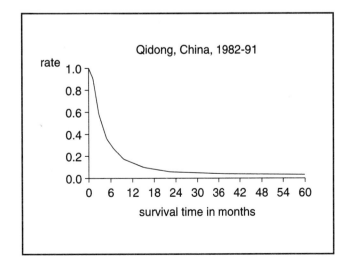

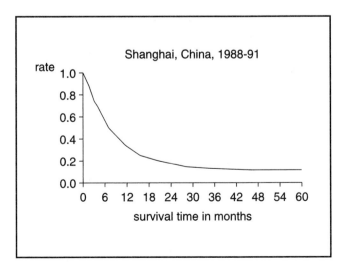

Relative survival from lung cancer in developing countries (Contd)

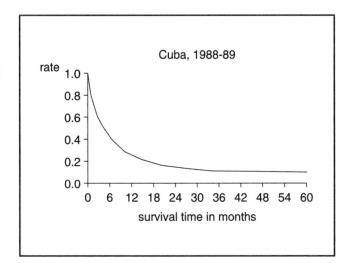

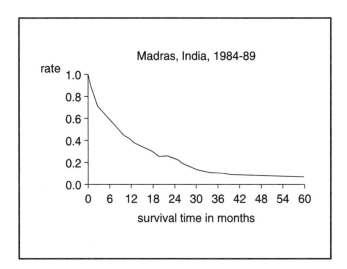

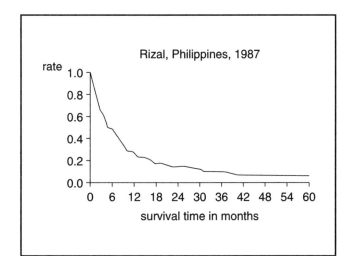

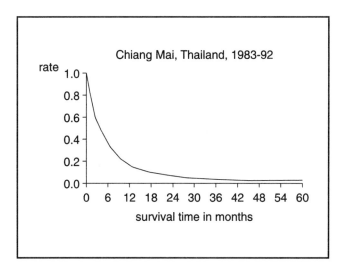

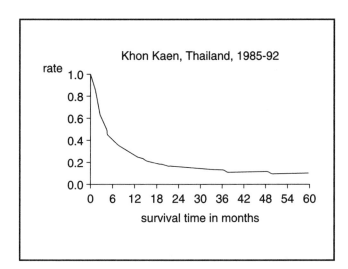

Relative survival from female breast cancer in developing countries

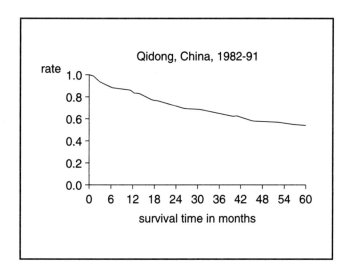

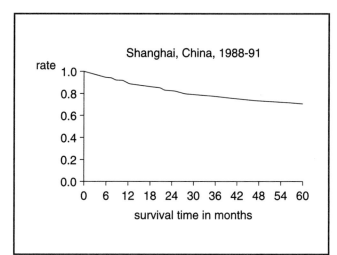

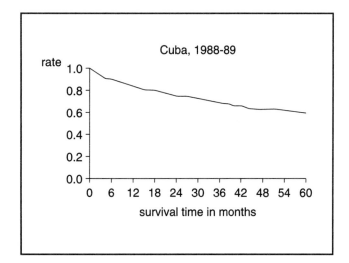

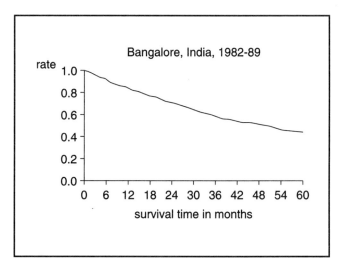

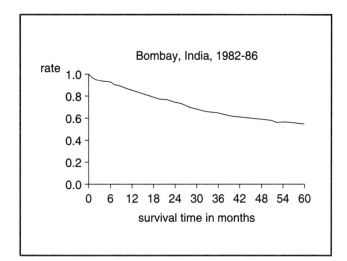

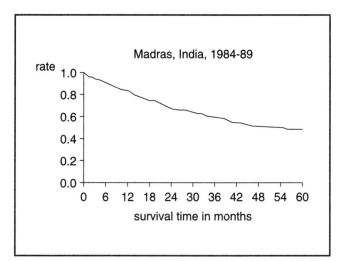

Relative survival from female breast cancer in developing countries (Contd)

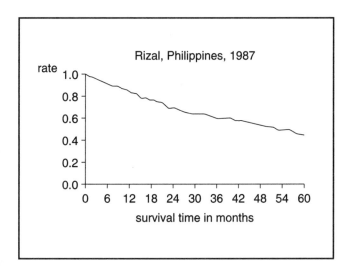

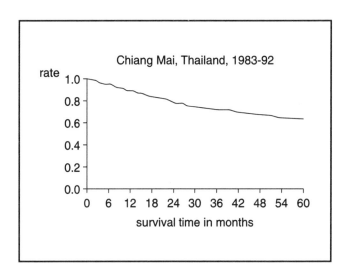

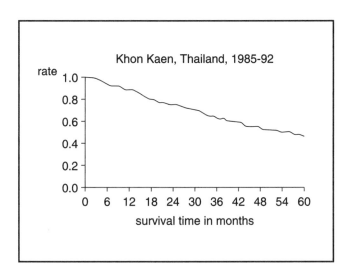

Relative survival from cervical cancer in developing countries

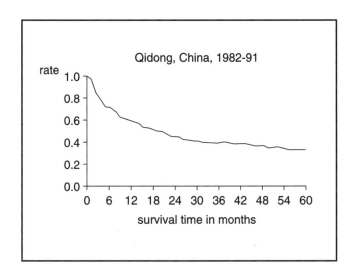

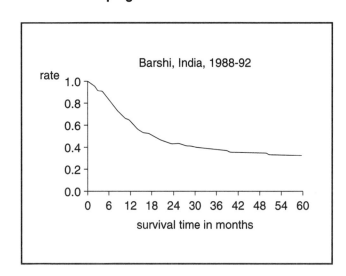

Relative survival from cervical cancer in developing countries (Contd)

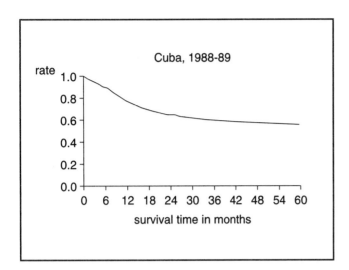

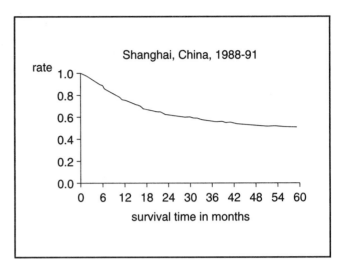

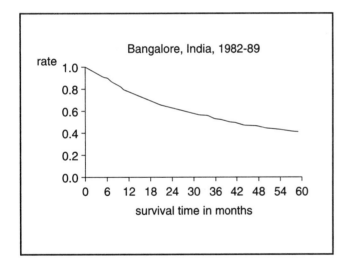

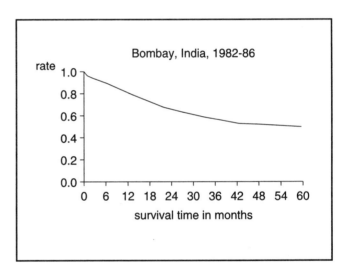

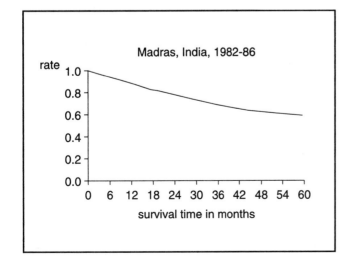

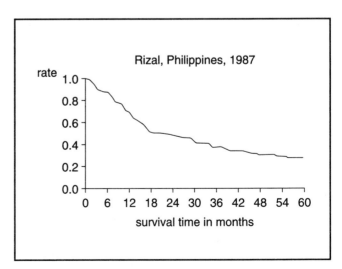

Relative survival from cervical cancer in developing countries (Contd)

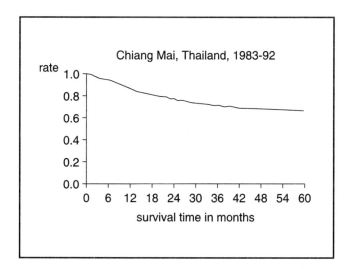

Chiang Mai, Thailand, 1983-92

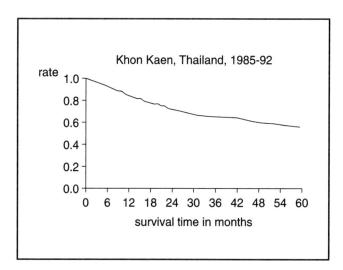

Khon Kaen, Thailand, 1985-92

Relative survival from ovarian cancer in developing countries

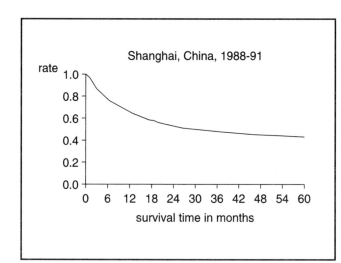

Shanghai, China, 1988-91

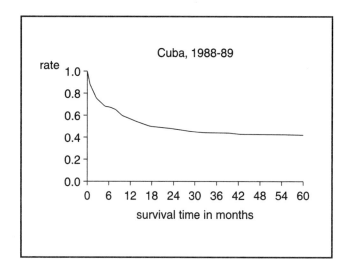

Cuba, 1988-89

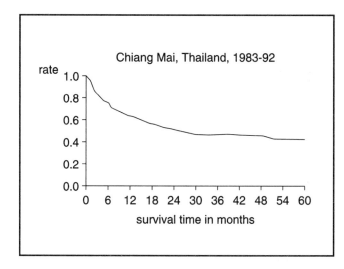

Chiang Mai, Thailand, 1983-92

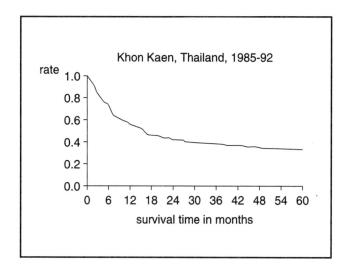

Khon Kaen, Thailand, 1985-92

Relative survival from Hodgkin's disease in developing countries

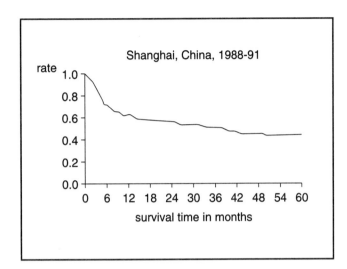

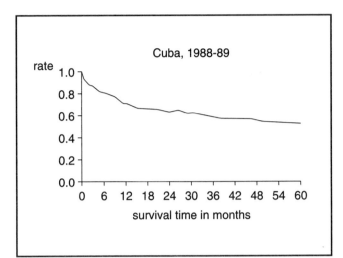

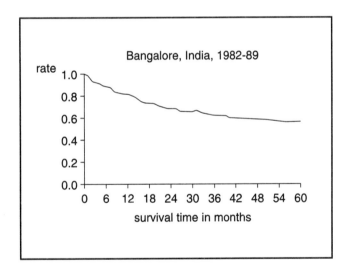

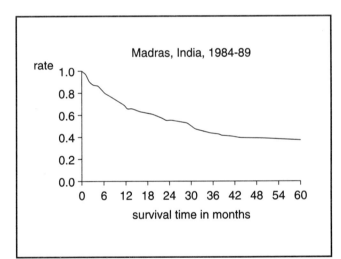

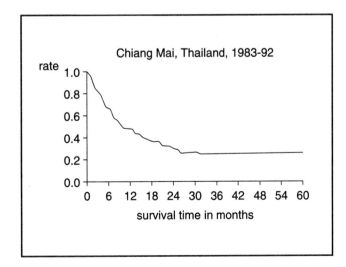

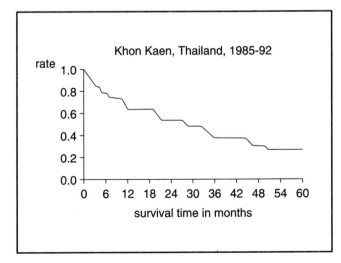

Relative survival from non-Hodgkin lymphoma in developing countries

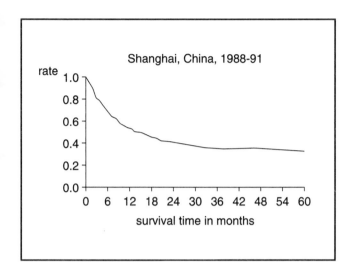

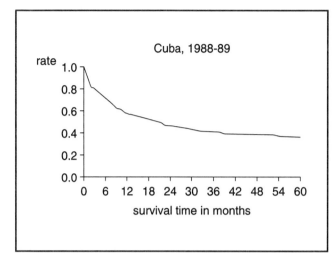

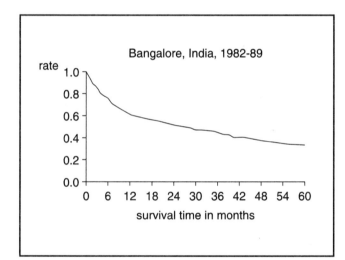

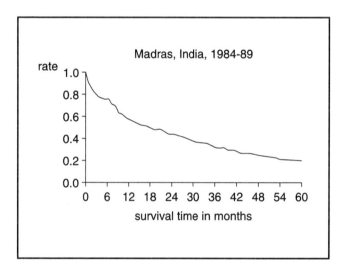

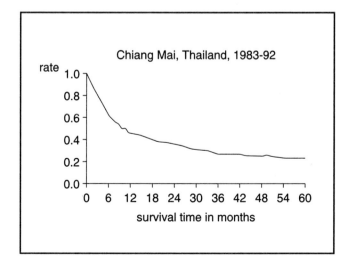

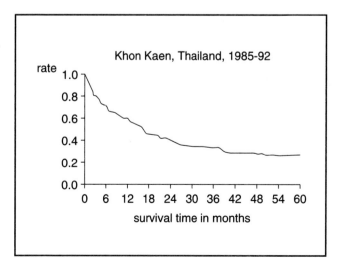

Relative survival from leukaemia in developing countries

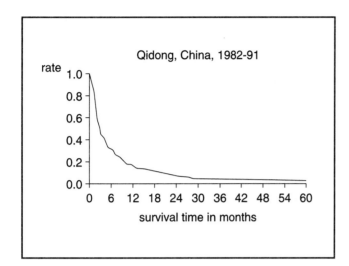

Qidong, China, 1982-91

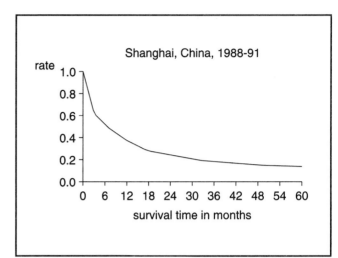

Shanghai, China, 1988-91

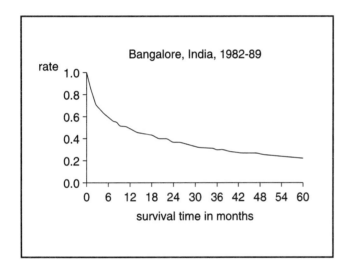

Bangalore, India, 1982-89

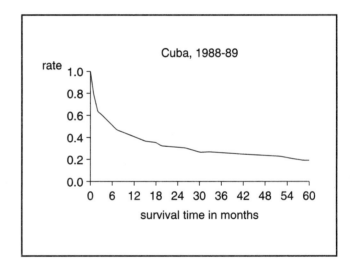

Cuba, 1988-89

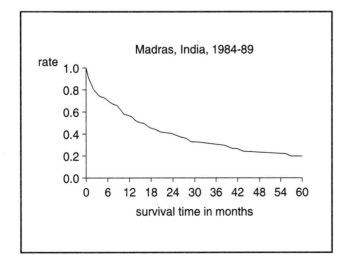

Madras, India, 1984-89

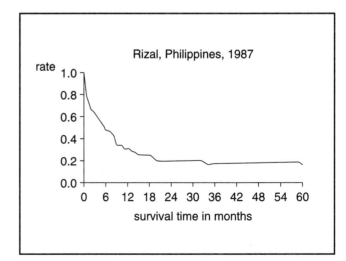

Rizal, Philippines, 1987

Relative survival from leukaemia in developing countries (Contd)

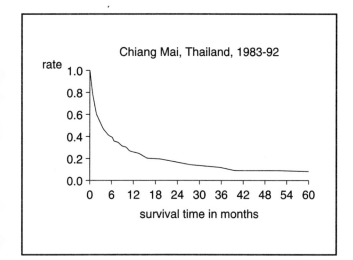

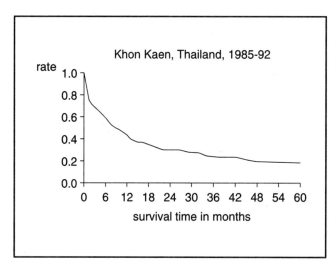

Achevé d'imprimer sur rotative
par l'imprimerie Darantiere à Dijon-Quetigny
en janvier 1999

Dépôt légal : 1er trimestre 1999
N° d'impression : 98-1058